Thieme

Radiology of Chest Diseases

Sebastian Lange, MD

Professor and Chairman
Department of Radiology
Knappschaftshospital
Recklinghausen
Germany

Geraldine Walsh, MRCP, FRCR, FRANZCR

Consultant Radiologist
Department of Radiology
Royal Berkshire Hospital
Reading
United Kingdom

With a contribution by Michael Montag

Third edition, fully revised and updated

1118 illustrations
35 tables

Thieme
Stuttgart · New York

Library of Congress Cataloging-in-Publication Data
is available from the publisher.

This book is a fully revised and expanded authorized translation of the 3rd German edition published and copyrighted 2005 by Georg Thieme Verlag, Stuttgart, Germany. Title of the German edition: Radiologische Diagnostik der Thoraxerkrankungen.

1st English edition 1990
1st Spanish edition 1990
1st Italian edition 1991
1st French edition 1991
1st Japanese edition 1993
1st Chinese edition 1994
2nd English edition 1998
2nd Chinese edition 2000
1st Brazilian edition (Portuguese) 2002

Translator: Terry Telger, Fort Worth, Texas, USA

Important note: Medicine is an ever-changing science undergoing continual development. Research and clinical experience are continually expanding our knowledge, in particular our knowledge of proper treatment and drug therapy. Insofar as this book mentions any dosage or application, readers may rest assured that the authors, editors, and publishers have made every effort to ensure that such references are in accordance with **the state of knowledge at the time of production of the book.**

Nevertheless, this does not involve, imply, or express any guarantee or responsibility on the part of the publishers in respect to any dosage instructions and forms of applications stated in the book. **Every user is requested to examine carefully** the manufacturers' leaflets accompanying each drug and to check, if necessary in consultation with a physician or specialist, whether the dosage schedules mentioned therein or the contraindications stated by the manufacturers differ from the statements made in the present book. Such examination is particularly important with drugs that are either rarely used or have been newly released on the market. Every dosage schedule or every form of application used is entirely at the user's own risk and responsibility. The authors and publishers request every user to report to the publishers any discrepancies or inaccuracies noticed. If errors in this work are found after publication, errata will be posted at www.thieme.com on the product description page.

© 2007 Georg Thieme Verlag,
Rüdigerstrasse 14, 70469 Stuttgart, Germany
http://www.thieme.de
Thieme New York, 333 Seventh Avenue,
New York, NY 10001, USA
http://www.thieme.com

Typesetting by primustype Hurler GmbH, Notzingen
Printed in Germany by Grammlich, Pliezhausen

ISBN-10: 3-13-740703-6 (GTV)
ISBN-13: 978-3-13-740703-4 (GTV)
ISBN-10: 1-58890-447-4 (TNY)
ISBN-13: 978-1-58890-447-8 (TNY)   1 2 3 4 5 6

To Maritta, Constantin,
Caroline, Christian, and Clemens

Sebastian Lange

To Colin

Geraldine Walsh

Preface

Almost a decade has passed since the publication of the second edition of *Radiology of Chest Diseases* in 1997. This period has seen tremendous advances in imaging technology.

Single-slice helical CT has given way to multi-detector row CT (MDCT), and with increasing numbers of detectors we move toward the concept of "isotropic" spatial resolution. This has been combined with decreased scan times and improved temporal resolution. The rapid evolution of CT technology has led to marked improvements in the quality of thoracic CT studies and has allowed us to contemplate and perform with some success cardiac evaluation and CT coronary angiography.

Positron emission tomography (PET)/PET-CT has been incorporated into everyday clinical practice in the past decade and today plays a significant role in imaging evaluation of thoracic disease, particularly in oncologic staging and assessment.

Advances in magnetic resonance imaging (MRI) today allow improved cardiac evaluation and particularly myocardial first-pass perfusion and viability assessment.

In this text, we have tried to convey how these exciting advances in technology fit into the clinical setting of cardiothoracic imaging evaluation.

We also recognize the ever-increasing availability and use of CT as an "early" second-line imaging tool in assessment of the patient with suspected pulmonary disease and have placed a greater emphasis on the role of high-resolution/thin-section CT in evaluation of parenchymal lung disease.

A new chapter on interventional procedures in the thorax describes a spectrum of procedures from the standard image-guided biopsy and drainage through to the more specialized interventions of pulmonary AVM and pulmonary false aneurysm embolization.

Once again, we hope that this text conveys the fascinating diversity of cardiothoracic radiology and that it will prove a useful guide to the practitioner in the everyday clinical setting.

Sebastian Lange, MD
Geraldine Walsh, MRCP, FRCR, FRANZCR

Table of Contents

1 Examination Technique and Normal Findings

2 Malformations

3 Infection and Inflammatory Disorders

4 Chronic Obstructive Pulmonary Disease and Diseases of the Airways

5 Inhalational Lung Diseases and Pneumoconioses

6 Tumors and Tumor-Like Lesions of the Lung

7 Pulmonary Hypertension and Edema

1 Examination Technique and Normal Findings

Indication and radiation exposure: All radiographic examinations should be medically indicated, and stricter criteria should be applied in selecting patients for thoracic CT—which gives a radiation dose in the range of 6–10 mSv—than for standard chest radiographs where the dosage is much lower at 0.02–0.05 mSv. In addition, the risk of side effects from contrast agents used in CT, angiography, radionuclide imaging, and magnetic resonance imaging (MRI) should always be weighed against the expected gain in diagnostic information.

Use of imaging studies: The frontal posteroanterior (PA) and lateral chest radiographs constitute the basic radiologic examination of the thorax. Radiographs should be acquired at full inspiration in the upright position, although in sick or debilitated patients supine or semi-supine anteroposterior (AP) views at functional residual capacity may be the only option.

Plain radiographic findings together with the presumptive clinical diagnosis will determine the need for further imaging studies. In current clinical practice, the most commonly requested second-line imaging investigations are CT, ventilation-perfusion scintigraphy (VQS), and ultrasound. Magnetic resonance imaging increasingly is being used in cardiac/myocardial assessment, and angiography continues to play a role in diagnosis as well as intervention.

Reading: Meticulous image interpretation is important. The "five D's" provide an effective strategy for reading all thoracic imaging procedures: **d**etect, **d**escribe, **d**iscuss, **d**ifferential diagnosis, and **d**ecide.

Detect: A methodical approach is important in image interpretation. In evaluation of the chest radiograph, the heart size, shape and contour, mediastinal/hilar contour and widening/size, the lungs, pleura, bony and soft tissue structures of the chest wall should be systematically assessed. Review areas include the apices, costophrenic angles, retrocardiac lung, and posterior mediastinum.

Describe and Discuss: If a pulmonary abnormality is detected, it may be assigned to one of the radiographic patterns in Chapter 13.

Differential diagnosis: Good results have been achieved with the "gamut approach" (Reeder and Felson 2003). Just as a musician deliberately strikes each note while practicing scales on a piano, every possible interpretation of a pattern should be considered when reading an image. At the very least, the reader should consider the various main disease categories. These include congenital malformations, inflammatory disorders, chronic obstructive pulmonary disease (COPD), inhalational diseases and pneumoconioses, neoplasia, vascular disorders, and trauma.

Decide: The ultimate goal of imaging is to make a definitive diagnosis. The clinical data frequently are important in making a definitive diagnosis. Sometimes, however, this is not possible and the radiologist can do no more than offer a differential diagnosis in which diagnoses are listed in order of probability. In this case cytology/histology may be required to make a definitive diagnosis.

The five D's for reading thoracic images
Detect
Describe
Discuss
Differential diagnosis
Decide

Disease categories that should be considered in making a differential diagnosis (acronym: Victim)
Vascular disease
Inflammation
Cancer and other tumors
Trauma
Inhalational disease
Malformation

Radiographic Examination

Frontal Chest Radiograph

The upright patient positions his anterior chest against the film cassette (Fig. 1.1 a, b). The dorsal aspects of the hands are placed on the hips, and the shoulders are rolled forward to project the scapulae outside the lungs. For better support, weak patients may place their arms around the cassette stand.

The patient wears a short lead apron. The upper border of the cassette is at the level of C7, and 35 × 35 to 40 × 40 cm size film is used, depending on patient size. The roentgen beam is collimated laterally on the skin surface over the lower ribs and is centered on the fourth thoracic vertebra (T4).

The radiograph is taken at full inspiration using, for example, a film-focus distance (FFD) of 185 cm and exposure parameters of approximately 125 kV, 5 mA, or automatic exposure control.

The AP projection is useful for imaging sick patients (Fig. 1.1 c, d). Bedridden patients are filmed in the supine position, and internal rotation of the shoulders aids in separating the scapulae (Fig. 1.1 e).

> **Characteristics of a technically acceptable frontal chest radiograph:**
> The spinous process of T3 is projected midway between the sternoclavicular joints, indicating the absence of chest rotation.
>
> The medial borders of the scapulae project outside the rib cage or touch the lateral aspects of the ribs.
>
> The thorax is completely imaged if the larynx and both costophrenic angles are visible.
>
> The degree of inspiration is adequate if the dome of the diaphragm projects caudal to the posterior part of the 9th rib.
>
> Exposure time is appropriate if the heart, diaphragm, and large pulmonary vessels are sharply defined. Overexposure is excluded if vascular shadows can be seen in the lung periphery.
>
> Underexposure is excluded if the larger lower lobe vessels and the thoracic vertebrae still are visible through the cardiac silhouette.

The technical parameters recommended for chest radiographs are listed in Table 1.1.

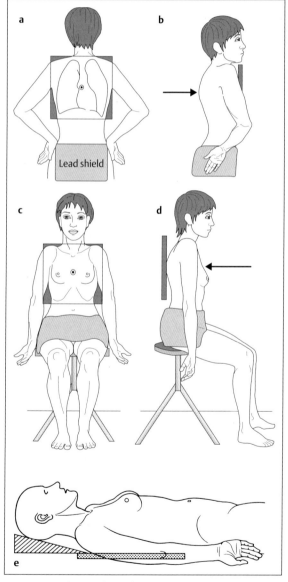

Fig. 1.1 a–e   Chest radiographs in PA and AP projections. **a, b** Standing PA radiograph. **c, d** Sitting AP radiograph. **e** Supine AP radiograph.

Table 1.1   Technical parameters for chest radiographs (Zimmer and Zimmer-Brossy 1992)

Technical specifications	Grid technique, wall cassette holder
Automatic exposure control:	
• PA	Side chamber
• Lateral	Central chamber
Film format	40 x 40 (30 x 40, 35 x 35)
Film-screen system	Film speed 400 (200)
Focus-film distance	150–200 cm
Kilovoltage	110–150 kV
Exposure:	
• PA	<20 ms
• Lateral	<40 ms
Scatter reduction grid	r/2(8)

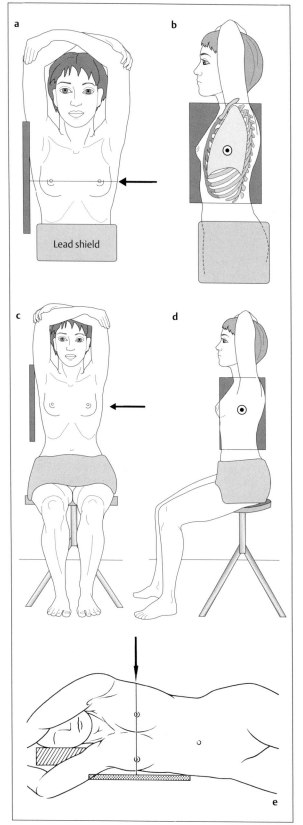

Lateral Chest Radiograph

The patient, wearing a lead apron, stands sideways against the cassette with arms raised. The roentgen beam is centered approximately 10 cm caudal to the axilla (Fig. 1.2 a, b).

The radiograph is taken at full inspiration using film size 30 × 40 or 35 × 35 cm. A FFD of 185 cm and settings of 125 kV, approximately 8 mA, or automatic exposure control are appropriate.

Debilitated patients are radiographed in the sitting position (Fig. 1.2 c, d) or, if necessary, in the lateral decubitus position with the head supported, the arms drawn forward and upward, and the legs slightly flexed to improve stability (Fig. 1.2 e).

> **Criteria for a technically acceptable lateral chest radiograph:**
> The entire lung is visible.
>
> The view is not rotated if the right and left posterior rib margins are superimposed.
>
> The arms are not superimposed on pulmonary structures.
>
> The image is not overexposed if the pulmonary vessels in the retrocardiac space are well defined.

The image is not underexposed if the large pulmonary vessels are visible through the cardiac silhouette.

Oblique Views

The patient is rotated in the frontal plane to approximately 45° with either the right (right anterior oblique or "fencer" position; Fig. 1.3 a) or left anterior chest wall (left anterior oblique or "boxer" position; Fig. 1.3 b) in

Fig. 1.2 a–e Lateral chest radiographs. **a, b** Standing lateral radiograph. **c, d** Sitting lateral radiograph. **e** Supine lateral radiograph.

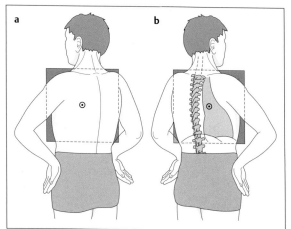

Fig. 1.3 a, b Oblique chest radiographs. **a** Right anterior oblique (*fencer*) position, **b** left anterior oblique (*boxer*) position.

contact with the cassette. The depth of inspiration, film size, FFD, and exposure parameters are the same as for the PA view.

Apical Lordotic View

The patient stands about 4 cm from the chest stand and arches the upper body backward until the shoulders touch the cassette. A FFD of 100 cm and 35–45° of cephalad tube angulation are appropriate. The beam is centered on the manubrium sterni (Fig. 1.**4**).

A technically acceptable image shows the lung apices projected clear of the scapulae.

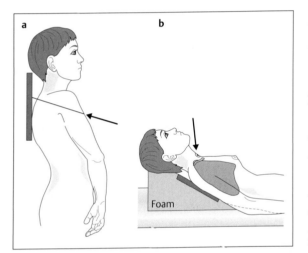

Fig. 1.**4 a, b**   Apical lordotic views. **a** Standing, **b** supine.

Fluoroscopy

Fluoroscopy is used occasionally today and is a valuable adjunct to the chest radiograph. It analyzes dynamic processes and facilitates localization of pathologic changes but it has a much lower spatial resolution than the chest radiograph.

Fluoroscopy is performed using an AP or PA beam at maximum shutter aperture. This permits comparison of the respiratory movements of the diaphragm and chest wall on both sides. The patient should breathe deeply, cough, blow his nose, and expire against a closed glottis to raise intrathoracic pressure (Valsalva maneuver). Finally, the patient attempts to inhale with the nostrils pinched shut; this lowers intrathoracic pressure (Müller maneuver). Sniffing is important since it elicits pure diaphragmatic motion and can thus magnify any asymmetric or paradoxical motion.

The above-described supplementary chest views together with fluoroscopy are used less frequently as CT becomes the mainstream second line imaging investigation in the assessment of thoracic disease.

Scatter-Reduction Grids

Grids are used to reduce scatter radiation, which degrades contrast in radiographic images.

Two main types are available:

Focused moving grids, which are used on a Bucky table. The strips in the grid are aligned to match the divergence of the primary beam (Fig. 1.**5 a**). Because the grid moves during the exposure, grid lines do not appear in the final image. There are two main sources of exposure errors with this type of grid system:

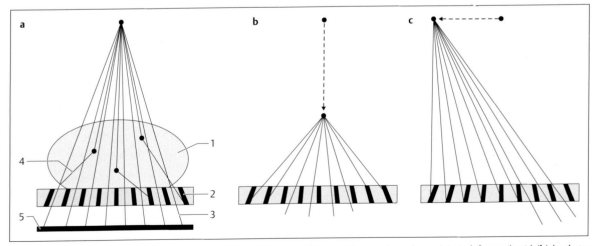

Fig. 1.**5 a–c**   Scatter-reduction grids. The strips of the grid converge toward the roentgen focus (**a**). A defocused grid (**b**) leads to underexposure of the lateral areas. An off-center grid (**c**) leads to asymmetrical exposure (modified from Laubenberger 1980).

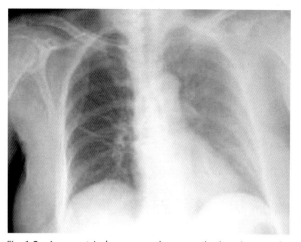

Fig. 1.**6** Asymmetrical exposure due to a tilted grid. Note the decreased lucency of the lung and "haziness" of the bones and soft tissues on the left side.

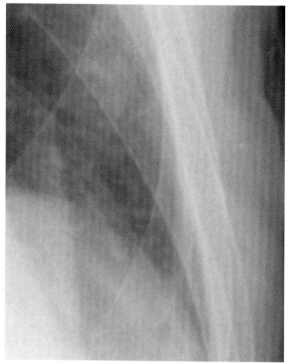

Fig. 1.**7** Stationary grid for bedside radiography. Vertical grid lines are visible on the image.

- *Defocused grid.* If the necessary focusing distance is not maintained between the grid and X-ray tube, the lateral portions of the image will be underexposed (Fig. 1.**5b**).
- *Off-center grid.* If the central ray is not aimed at the center of the grid (due to a poorly adjusted collimator, for example), the film will be asymmetrically exposed (Figs. 1.**5c**, 1.**6**).

Stationary grids with parallel strips are used for bedside radiography. Often it is difficult to position the patient as desired, and it is not unusual to work with a tilted grid. This also causes asymmetrical film exposure because the strips at one edge are aligned with the beam divergence while the strips at the other edge are not (Fig. 1.**7**). When an image made with a stationary grid is examined closely (e. g., with a magnifying lens), grid lines always can be seen.

The Normal Chest Radiograph

The chest radiograph requires a systematic evaluation (Figs. 1.**8** and 1.**9**) in which the
- chest wall,
- diaphragm,
- pleura,
- lungs, and
- mediastinum

are identified, analyzed, and described. To reinforce this approach, these regions will be considered in the above order.

Structures of the Chest Wall

■ Thoracic Skeleton

The thoracic skeleton comprises the ribs, vertebral column, scapulae, clavicles, and sternum.

Ribs

The posterior aspects of the ribs have an almost horizontal orientation, and they then extend obliquely forward from superolateral to inferomedial to the costochondral junction. Rib cartilages are not visible on chest radiographs except in the elderly when cartilage calcification

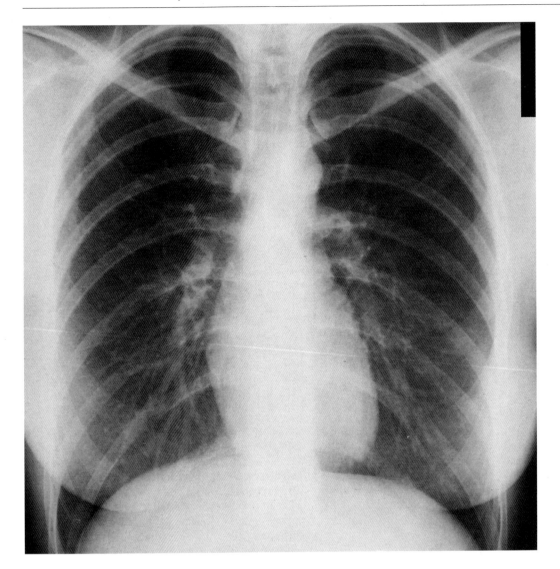

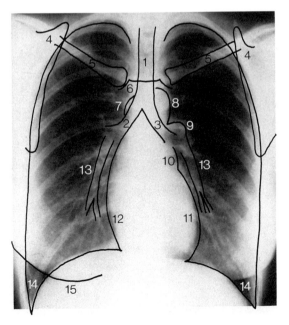

Fig. 1.8   PA chest radiograph.
1   Trachea
2   Right main bronchus
3   Left main bronchus
4   Scapula
5   Clavicle
6   Manubrium sternum
7   Azygos vein
8   Aortic arch
9   Left pulmonary artery
10 Upper left cardiac border, left atrial appendage
11 Lower left cardiac border, left ventricle
12 Right atrium
13 Lower lobe arteries
14 Lateral costophrenic angle
15 Breast shadow

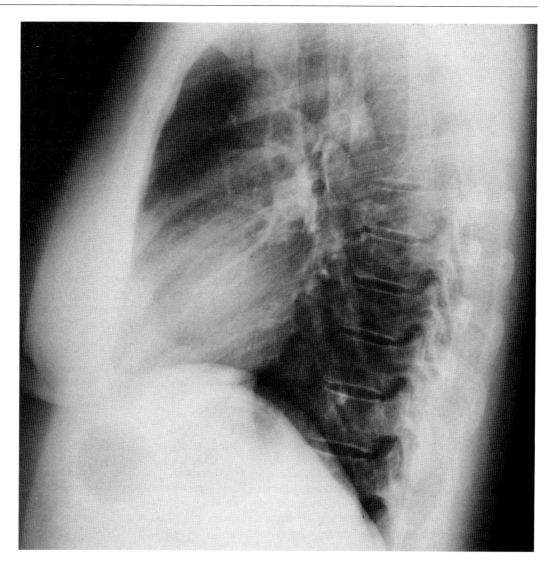

Fig. 1.**9** Lateral chest radiograph.
 1 Trachea
 2 Pretracheal vascular bundle
 3 Aortic arch
 4 Right upper lobe bronchus
 5 Left upper lobe bronchus
 6 Left pulmonary artery
 7 Right pulmonary artery in pretracheal vascular oval
 8 Axillary fold
 9 Scapula
10 Right posterior costophrenic angle (right hemidiaphragm visible as far as the sternum)
11 Left posterior costophrenic angle (left hemidiaphragm visible as far as the cardiac silhouette)
12 Gastric bubble
13 Transverse colon
14 Inferior vena cava

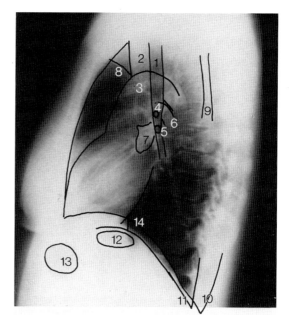

may be present. The dorsal aspects of the ribs appear denser because they have an almost circular anatomic cross section, while the ventral aspects are flatter and therefore more radiolucent. The ribs may have a slightly ill-defined inferior border due to thinning of the bone at the subcostal sulcus.

On the lateral view, the posterior rib segments project behind the vertebral bodies while the lateral portions appear as faint bands running obliquely forward and downward.

Vertebral Column

The vertebral column should be visible through the cardiac silhouette on a well-exposed frontal radiograph. The vertebral bodies, pedicles, spinous and transverse processes may be identified. On the lateral view, the superior and inferior articular processes may be identified.

Scapula

The medial and lateral borders, the inferior angle, the spine, and the coracoid process of the scapula may be identified on the frontal chest radiograph. On the lateral view, the scapulae project onto the vertebral column as dense vertical bands; their connection with the raised upper arms usually can be appreciated.

Clavicles

The clavicles extend horizontally from the acromioclavicular joints laterally to the sternoclavicular joints medially. They are projected over the lung apices on the frontal radiograph. A notch formed by the insertion of the costoclavicular ligament often is seen inferiorly at the sternal end of the clavicle (rhomboid fossa).

Sternum

On the frontal radiograph, only the manubrium, part of the body of the sternum, and the sternoclavicular articulations are delineated. The lateral view defines the cortical outlines and the synchondrosis between the manubrium and body (Louis' angle). The normal sternum shows a slight degree of anterior convexity. In the "funnel chest" deformity (pectus excavatum), the sternum is convex posteriorly and projects behind the anterior rib margins. In "pigeon chest" (pectus carinatum), the sternum is bowed forward, showing an exaggerated anterior convexity.

■ Soft Tissues of the Chest Wall

The soft tissues form the contour of the chest wall. They also may project over the intrathoracic organs as opacities and interface lines (Figs. 1.**10** and 1.**11**).

Skin Folds

Skin folds are especially prominent on supine radiographs of cachectic patients. They may form linear opacities and should not be mistaken for a pneumothorax.

Breast Shadow

The breast shadows decrease the lucency of the lower lung zones. Nipple shadows may mimic small pulmonary nodules and may be quite asymmetrical in appearance.

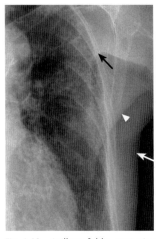

Fig. 1.**10** Axillary folds: posterior axillary fold (white arrow), anterior axillary fold (arrowhead), apex of axilla (black arrow).

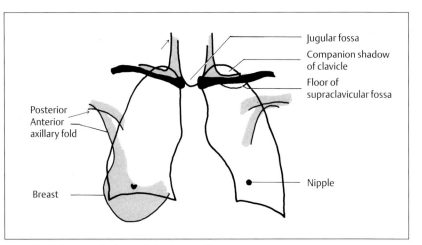

Fig. 1.**11** Soft-tissue shadows of the chest wall.

Axillary Folds

The anterior and posterior axillary folds have caudally concave contours, and their interface may project over the lung, occasionally mimicking a pneumothorax. A third caudally concave shadow representing the apex of the axilla sometimes may be seen in thin patients.

Clavicular Companion Shadows

This narrow soft-tissue stripe along the upper border of the clavicle represents soft tissue that is tangential to the x-ray beam (Fig. 1.**12**).

Sternocleidomastoid Muscle

The sternocleidomastoid muscle appears as an almost vertical soft-tissue opacity in the neck. It has a well-defined lateral border, and it merges inferiorly with the companion shadow of the clavicle.

Supraclavicular Fossa

Visible only in thin patients, the supraclavicular fossa appears as a thin horizontal line projected above or below the clavicle. It extends laterally beyond the lung, thus distinguishing it from an apical pneumothorax (see Fig. 1.**11**).

Jugular Fossa

In thin patients, both sternocleidomastoid muscles have sharp medial borders and their contours unite inferiorly in a U-shaped configuration. This may sometimes mimic widening of the trachea.

Upper Arms

The lateral radiograph projects the soft tissues of the upper arm over the anteroapical lung. Usually the left and right upper arms can both be seen and their contours are continuous with the posterior axillary fold.

Diaphragm

The diaphragm forms the inferior boundary of the thorax. It is slightly curved towards the lung. In normal individuals, the angle between the chest wall and diaphragm is acute in inspiration. These angles border on the lung, so they are clearly visible laterally in the PA view and posteriorly in the lateral view (lateral and posterior costophrenic angles). The angle between the diaphragm and heart (cardiophrenic angle) is usually acute. In deep inspiration, the diaphragm moves sufficiently caudad to allow visibility of the 10th rib in the right cardiophrenic angle. During expiration, the dome of the diaphragm moves upward by approximately 3–7 cm.

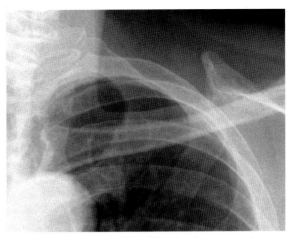

Fig. 1.**12** Companion shadow of the clavicle (tangential projection of the skin over the clavicle) and the vertical shadow of the sternocleidomastoid muscle.

The right hemidiaphragm may lie up to 4 cm cranial to the left hemidiaphragm. The caudal surface of the diaphragm is not visible unless it is outlined on the left by the gastric bubble or on the right by air between the liver and diaphragm, as can occur in both pneumoperitoneum and colonic interposition (Chilaiditi syndrome).

Individual muscle slips may give the smooth contour of the diaphragm a scalloped or serrated appearance in the lateral costophrenic angle. This normal variant may be especially pronounced in emphysema.

If the distance between the lower border of the lung and the gastric air bubble is more than 1 cm, a pathologic process such as a subpulmonic effusion should be suspected. This sign is especially valuable in the lateral projection.

Several features can be used to differentiate the left and right hemidiaphragms. On the lateral chest radiograph, the left hemidiaphragm is usually lower anteriorly and higher posteriorly with the gastric bubble lying inferiorly. Its contour extends anteriorly only to the posterior border of the cardiac silhouette. The right hemidiaphragm is usually higher anteriorly and lower posteriorly. Its contour may be traced throughout its posteroanterior course from the posterior costophrenic angle forward to the sternum (Fig. 1.**13**).

Pleura

■ Anatomy and Physiology

The pleura consist of two layers. The parietal pleura lines the chest cavity and is fused with the chest wall, diaphragm, and mediastinum. The visceral pleura invests the surface of the lung and merges with the parietal pleura at the hilum. A capillary space containing a film of fluid permits relative motion between the two layers.

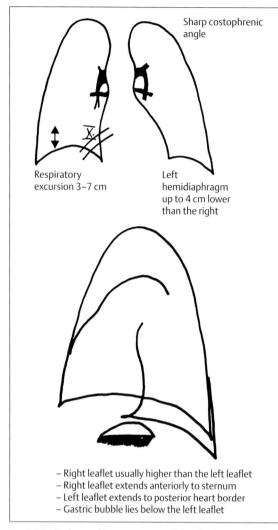

Fig. 1.**13**   Radiographic appearance of the diaphragm.

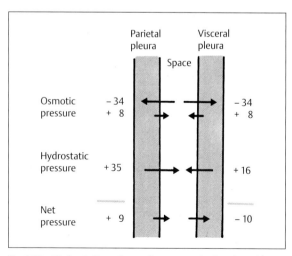

Fig. 1.**14**   Hydrostatic and oncotic pressure in the pleural layers (from Müller and Fraser 2001).

Apposition of the pleural leaves is made possible by a negative pressure within the pleural cavity (approximately –5 cm H_2O); this counteracts the elastic recoil of the pulmonary interstitium. Because of the intrinsic weight of the lung, this partial vacuum is greater in the apical region than at the base (Paré and Fraser 1983).

Negative pressure is important in keeping the lungs inflated. Serum inflow would tend to equalize this pressure were it not for the low protein content of the pleural fluid and the oncotic "suction" of the adjacent capillary blood, which tends to draw fluid from the pleural space. Negative pressure is maintained even though approximately 100 mL of fluid flows from the parietal pleura to the visceral pleura each day. This is possible because of the unequal hydrostatic pressures in the chest wall and pulmonary capillaries (Fig. 1.**14**).

■ Radiographic Anatomy

The peripulmonary pleura invests the surface of the lung, and the interlobar pleura lines the fissures between the lobes. Radiographically, the peripulmonary pleura appears only as an interface between the lung and soft tissues. The interlobar pleura which comprises the fissures, on the other hand, often is directly visible as a hairline shadow.

Peripulmonary Pleura

A dense stripe 0.5 mm in width may occasionally be seen in the area where the lung abuts the chest wall, diaphragm, and mediastinum. This stripe does not represent the pleura; it is a visual artifact caused by the collateral inhibition or stimulation of retinal receptors (Mach effect; Fig. 1.**15**). This is easily confirmed by covering the lung with a piece of paper next to the stripe and noting that the stripe is gone (Fig. 1.**16**).

The peripulmonary pleura has several radiographically distinct components (Coussement and Butori 1978; Fig. 1.**17**).

Companion Shadow of the Second Rib

The apical pleura appears in profile as a stripe, 2 mm in width, at the inferior border of the posterior aspect of the second rib (Fig. 1.**18**).

Companion Shadow of the Lateral Chest Wall

The pleural line, if seen tangentially, usually is smooth but occasionally bulges into the intercostal spaces, creating a scalloped contour. In obese patients an extrapleural fat stripe, several millimeters in width, may be visible between the inner surface of the ribs and the lung edge; this should not be confused with pleural thickening or a small pleural effusion. Occasionally the sub-

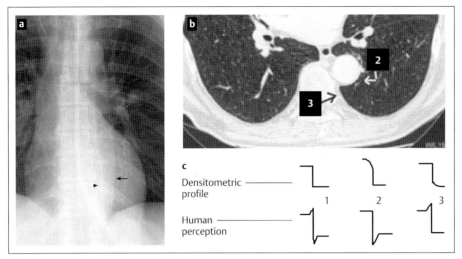

Fig. 1.**15 a–c**   The Mach effect. The contour of the aorta on a chest radiograph (**a**) appears to be accompanied by a dark stripe (arrow), and the paravertebral space appears to be bounded by a bright stripe (arrowhead). These are optical illusions due to accentuation of contrast in the human retina. When two homogeneous areas of different brightness are apposed (1 in **c**), the actual densitometric profile (top row in **c**) is not perceived. Instead, the bright area appears even brighter while the dark area appears somewhat darker (bottom row in **c**). If the bright area darkens toward the boundary, the contrast appears to be accentuated only in the dark area (2 in **b** and **c**). If the dark area gradually lightens toward the boundary, a bright edge will be perceived (3 in **b** and **c**).

costal muscle fibers elevate the pleura, producing a wavy contour (see Fig. 1.**16**).

Basal Pleural Reflection

A line may be seen passing medially and horizontally from the deepest point of the lateral costophrenic angle. This is seen particularly well on overexposed radiographs. It corresponds to the pleural reflection at the posterior costophrenic angle.

Apical Pleural Cap

Anteriorly the lung extends to the level of the clavicle, but posteriorly it projects more superiorly. On the lateral view, the soft-tissue shadow of the upper arm usually is superimposed usually on the lung apex. However, if the shoulders are lowered, the lung apex with its accompanying pleural shadow may be seen.

Posterior Pleural Stripe

On the lateral view, the posterior pleural stripe is visible in profile along the posterior ribs. The pleural stripe extends inferiorly to the posterior costophrenic angle and the diaphragmatic reflection. On the lateral view, the pleural line can help in identifying right and left diaphragmatic leaflets (see Fig. 1.**13**).

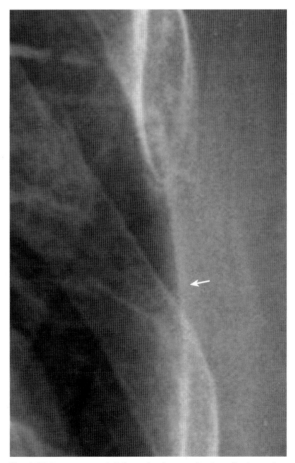

Fig. 1.**16** An apparent bright stripe is perceived at the boundary between the lung and soft tissue as a result of the Mach effect (see Fig. 1.**15**).

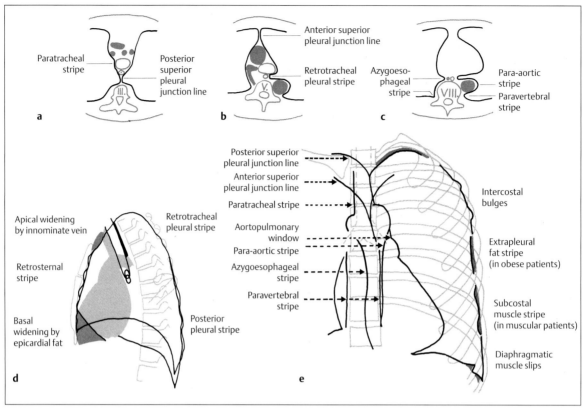

Fig. 1.**17 a–e**   Pleural reflections (from Heitzman 1993, Meschan 1981).

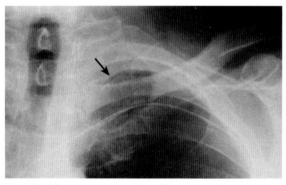

Fig. 1.**18**   The companion shadow of the second rib corresponds to the lung apex or the boundary between air and soft tissue. The catheter position defines the course of the subclavian vein.

pleural border is smoother because of the interposed heart. In the basal part of the retrosternal stripe, epicardial fat frequently displaces the left anterior lung border from the chest wall, producing a triangular retrosternal opacity (cardiac incisure).

Posterior Superior Pleural Junction Line

The pleura sweeps medially from both sides as a continuation of the companion shadow of the 2nd rib, unites at the level of the T3/4 intervertebral space, then passes as a vertical stripe to the aortic arch. This creates a Y-shaped shadow that corresponds to the posterior pleural reflection (see Figs. 1.**17 d**, 1.**19**). It is composed of four layers of pleura and corresponds to the course of the superior intercostal veins.

Retrosternal Stripe

On the lateral view, the retrosternal stripe is relatively wide superiorly behind the manubrium. Here, the brachiocephalic vein is interposed between the lung and sternum. The stripe is narrower in its midportion, where the right and left anterior lung borders may be differentiated. The right pleura protrudes into the intercostal spaces and thus has a wavy contour; it is frequently projected over the body of the sternum. The left anterior

Anterior Superior Pleural Junction Line

This pleural reflection corresponds to the course of the innominate and subclavian veins. It forms a Y-shaped configuration, the limbs of which originate from the inferior margins of the sternoclavicular joints. They course caudally, medially, and, on uniting, slant to the left. The anterior junction line complex extends inferiorly to the heart and encompasses the potential space of the anterior mediastinum (see Figs. 1.**17 e**, 1.**19**).

Azygoesophageal Stripe

The right lung extends in front of the vertebral column and forms the azygoesophageal recess. It borders the azygos vein and the esophagus and forms a mediastinal pleural stripe in a paramedian location, paralleling the course of the esophagus (see Figs. 1.17 e, 1.20).

Paravertebral Stripe

The posterior parts of the lungs are contiguous to the lateral aspects of the vertebral bodies. Pleura seen in tangent to the roentgen beam in this region forms a visible stripe on the left side. On the right side, the stripe is seen only if it is widened by aging or pathologic processes such as degenerative osteophyte formation, hematoma, or tumor (see Figs. 1.15 a, 1.17 e). On the left side, the paravertebral stripe can reach a width equal to half the diameter of the descending aorta.

Para-aortic Stripe

This accompanies the descending aorta on the left side. Comparison of the paravertebral and para-aortic stripes reveals an interesting visual phenomenon: The aortic border to the lung is a convex arch; this produces a negative Mach effect, resulting in an apparently darker stripe paralleling the descending aorta. The paravertebral soft tissues have a concave boundary with the lung; this results in a positive Mach effect creating the impression of a white border stripe (Figs. 1.15 a, 1.17 e, 1.20).

Right Paratracheal Stripe

This corresponds to the mediastinal pleural reflection on the tracheal wall. The inferior widening of the stripe is due to the horizontally orientated arch of the azygos vein. The width of the paratracheal stripe should not exceed 4 mm. It frequently is superimposed on the superior vena cava. A well-exposed view, conventional or computed tomography (CT) will demonstrate the paratracheal stripe, azygos vein, and superior vena cava and will determine the true width of this stripe (see Fig. 1.17 e).

Retrotracheal Stripe

On the lateral radiograph, this stripe blends with the posterior border of the trachea and should not exceed 3 mm in width (see Fig. 1.17 d).

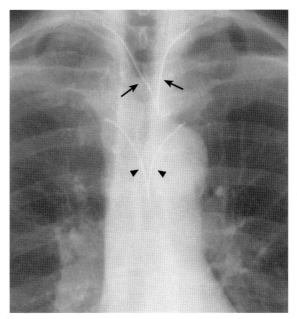

Fig. 1.**19** The posterior pleural reflection (= posterior superior pleural junction line, arrows) and anterior pleural reflection (= anterior superior pleural junction line, arrowheads).

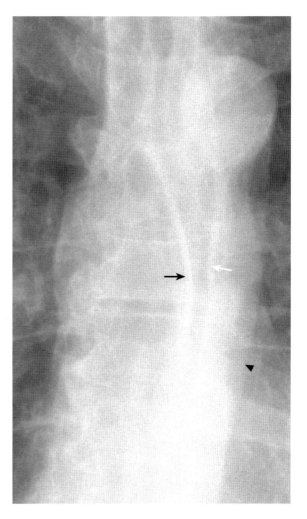

Fig. 1.**20** The azygoesophageal stripe (black arrow), the left lateral esophageal wall with air in the esophagus (white arrow), and the para-aortic stripe (arrowhead).

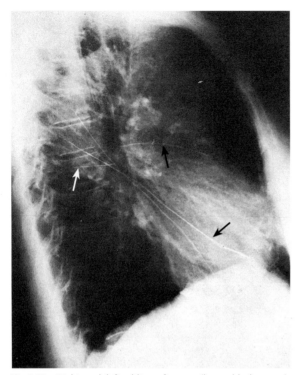

Fig. 1.**21**   Right and left oblique fissures (lower black arrow), horizontal fissure (upper black arrow), and left accessory fissure (white arrow).

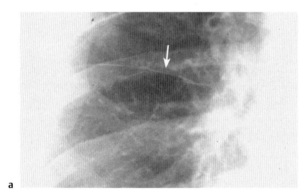

a

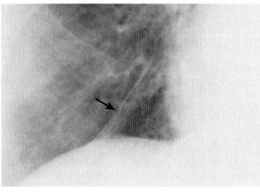

b

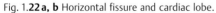

Fig. 1.**22 a, b** Horizontal fissure and cardiac lobe.

Interlobar Fissures

Two layers of visceral pleura separate the pulmonary lobes and, occasionally, the segments. These duplications are visible when a significant segment is imaged in profile. The following are frequently seen on the chest radiograph:

Major (Oblique) Fissures

Very occasionally, a tenting of the diaphragmatic pleura is seen on the PA chest radiograph; this corresponds to the caudal end of the major fissure. On the lateral view, the major fissures are seen as fine linear shadows that course obliquely in an anteroinferior direction (Fig. 1.**21**).

The union of the right horizontal fissure with the oblique fissure may help to distinguish between the right and left oblique fissures. In addition, the left oblique fissure usually runs more vertically than the right. The major fissures merge with the ipsilateral diaphragmatic leaflets allowing further distinction between right and left sides (see Fig. 1.**13**).

Minor (Horizontal) Fissure

In the right midzone, there is a fissure between the upper and middle lobes extending to, but not crossing the hilar shadow (Fig. 1.**22**). Occasionally this line is accompanied by a second, parallel stripe representing a second section of the horizontal fissure seen in tangent to the x-ray beam. On the lateral view, the minor fissure appears as a horizontal line extending anteriorly from the major fissure to the sternum (see Fig. 1.**21**).

Azygos Lobe Fissure

The azygos vein normally runs medial to the right lung. In 0.5 % of the population, it has a more lateral course and descends along a fissure in the upper lobe. This forms a curvilinear shadow in the right upper zone which has the shape of an inverted comma (Figs. 1.**23**, 1.**24**). The azygos fissure contains four layers of pleura.

Cardiac Lobe

In 10 % of the population, the mediobasal segment of the right lower lobe is separated from the other basal segments. On the PA view, this inferior accessory fissure is seen as a line lateral to the cardiophrenic sulcus (see Fig. 1.**22**).

Other Accessory Fissures

In 6 % of the population, the apical segment of the lower lobe is separated from the basal segments by an accessory fissure. On the lateral view, this is seen as a horizontal line extending from the oblique fissure to the posterior chest wall. Other unusual accessory lobes and fissures are illustrated in Figures 1.**25** and 1.**26**.

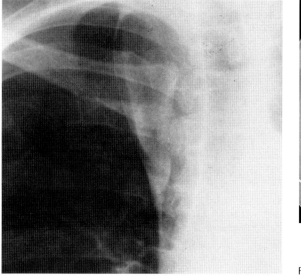

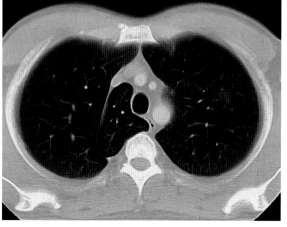

Fig. 1.**23 a, b**   Azygos lobe.

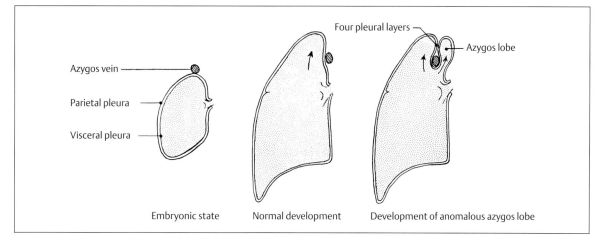

Azygos vein
Parietal pleura
Visceral pleura

Four pleural layers
Azygos lobe

Embryonic state   Normal development   Development of anomalous azygos lobe

Fig. 1.**24**   Development of an azygos lobe (from Meschan 1981).

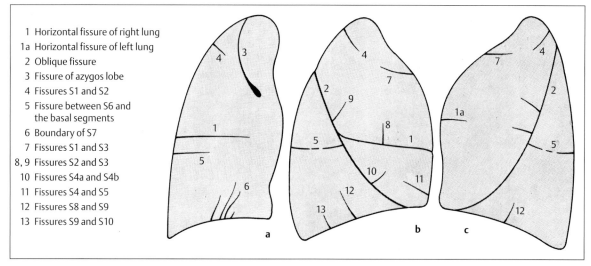

 1 Horizontal fissure of right lung
1a Horizontal fissure of left lung
 2 Oblique fissure
 3 Fissure of azygos lobe
 4 Fissures S1 and S2
 5 Fissure between S6 and
    the basal segments
 6 Boundary of S7
 7 Fissures S1 and S3
8, 9 Fissures S2 and S3
 10 Fissures S4a and S4b
 11 Fissures S4 and S5
 12 Fissures S8 and S9
 13 Fissures S9 and S10

Fig. 1.**25 a–c**   Interlobar and accessory fissures. **a** PA view of right lung. **b** Lateral view of right lung. **c** Lateral view of left lung (from W. Teschendorf 1975).

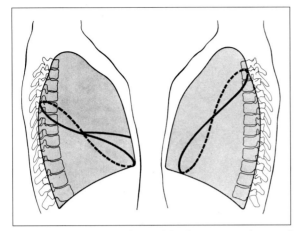

Fig. 1.**26** Lateral views of the interlobar fissures. Note the typical propeller shape of the oblique fissure, formed by the costal margin (solid line) and the mediastinal margin (broken line) (from H. Uthgenannt, Linear opacities. In: W. Teschendorf 1975).

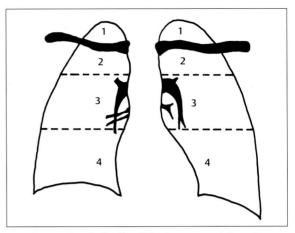

Fig. 1.**27** Landmarks for identifying lung zones. 1 Apex, 2 upper zone, 3 midzone, 4 lower zone.

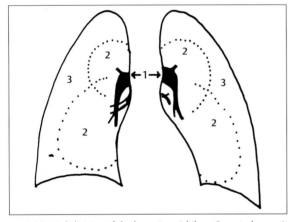

Fig. 1.**28** Subdivision of the lungs into 1 hilum, 2 central or perihilar region, and 3 peripheral region.

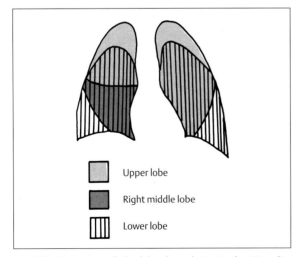

Upper lobe

Right middle lobe

Lower lobe

Fig. 1.**29** Projection of the lobar boundaries in the PA radiograph (from Bohlig 1975).

Lung Parenchyma

The frontal chest radiograph displays the lungs as they lie to either side of the mediastinum. For orientation purposes, the lungs may be divided into upper, middle, and lower zones by two horizontal lines drawn through the upper and lower borders of the hilum (Fig. 1.**27**). The apical subdivision of the upper zone (lung apex) lies superior to the clavicle.

The lungs may also be divided into central (perihilar) and peripheral (subpleural) regions. The latter is the 4-cm wide parenchymal zone at the periphery of the lobes that is devoid of radiologically visible vessels (Fig. 1.**28**).

Subdivision of the lungs into upper, middle, and lower zones is possible when the topography is known (Fig. 1.**29**). However, accurate subdivision and lesion localization are possible only when all of the interlobar fissures are visible.

The basic unit of gas exchange, the alveolus, is radiologically invisible because of its minute size. The human lung contains approximately 300 million alveoli arranged like clusters of grapes around the dichotomously branching bronchial tree. The diameter of the alveolar wall capillaries is just sufficient to allow passage of erythrocytes. The alveolar wall consists of flattened epithelial cells (type I pneumocytes) and granular type II pneumocytes. Type I pneumocytes line the alveolus and are apposed to the endothelial cells of the alveolar wall capillaries. Granular pneumocytes, usually five to eight in number, lie between epithelial cells and produce surfactant. This phospholipid reduces surface tension within the alveolus and allows expansion (Müller and Fraser 2001).

The alveoli together with the bronchioles, nerves, and blood vessels are the functional units of the lung (Fig. 1.**30**):

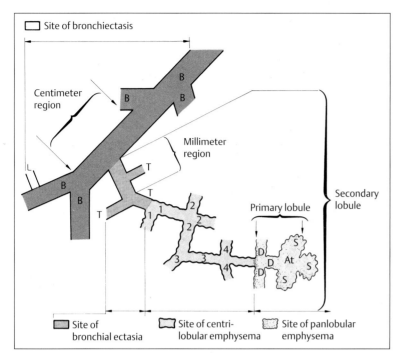

Site of bronchiectasis

Centimeter region

Millimeter region

Primary lobule

Secondary lobule

Site of bronchial ectasia

Site of centri-lobular emphysema

Site of panlobular emphysema

Fig. 1.**30** Branching pattern of the bronchial tree (Meschan).
B   Bronchi
L   Lobular bronchioles
T   Terminal bronchioles
1–4 Respiratory bronchioles
D   Alveolar ducts
At   Atrium
S   Alveolar sac

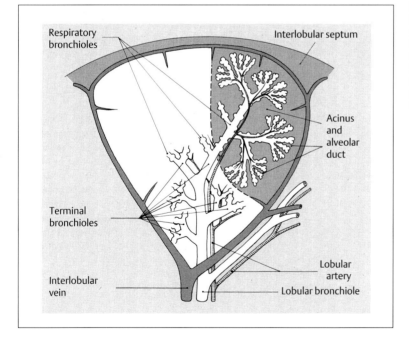

Respiratory bronchioles

Interlobular septum

Acinus and alveolar duct

Terminal bronchioles

Lobular artery

Lobular bronchiole

Interlobular vein

Fig. 1.**31** The secondary pulmonary lobule. The lobular bronchiole and artery enter the lobule centrally, and peripherally the interlobular veins course within the interlobular septa. The lobular bronchiole branches into terminal bronchioles, which aerate the acini. The terminal bronchioles give rise to respiratory bronchioles which supply the primary lobules (Schinz 1983).

Primary Lobule

A primary lobule is the smallest functional unit of the lung. It comprises all the structures distal to a respiratory bronchiole including the 16 to 40 alveoli. The normal adult has approximately 23 million primary lobules. Because of their small size, primary lobules are not visible on chest radiographs (Fig. 1.**31**).

Acinus

An acinus consists of all structures distal to the terminal bronchiole, including vessels, nerves, and connective tissue. It has a diameter of 4 to 8 mm and contains approximately 10 to 20 primary lobules. Müller and Fraser (2001) describe the acinus as the functional unit in which perfusion and ventilation are coordinated. When

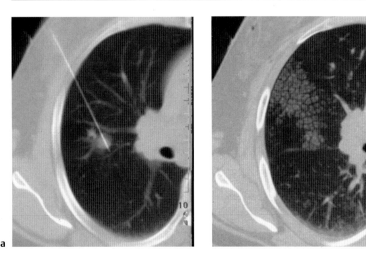

a   b

Fig. 1.**32a, b** Pulmonary hemor-rhage during percutaneous fine needle aspiration (FNA) of a pulmo-nary mass (**a**). The resulting pulmo-nary opacification has an "acinar" pattern (**b**).

infiltrated, the acinus appears radiologically as an ill-defined opacity approximately 0.5 cm in diameter (acinar shadows). Peribronchiolar infiltration or consolidation may have a similar radiographic appearance and thus may mimic acinar shadowing (Rau 1980; see Figs. 1.**31**, 1.**32**).

Secondary Lobule

The secondary lobule is the smallest structural unit of lung parenchyma that is surrounded by a connective tissue septum. Heitzman (1993) describes it as the principal physiologic functional unit of the lung. It contains 3–12 acini and measures 1.0–2.5 cm in diameter. When the connective tissue septa between secondary lobules (i. e. interlobular septa) become abnormally thickened, they are visible on both the chest radiograph (Kerley lines) and on high-resolution CT (HRCT) images (see Fig 1.**48**). Normal interlobular septa occasionally may be seen on HRCT images in the peripheral subpleural lung.

Lung Segments

These are 10 functionally autonomous bronchovascular and bronchopulmonary units on each side. They are wedge shaped with their apices directed toward the hila. When they are infiltrated or atelectatic, they produce characteristic appearances (Fig. 1.**33**). Occasionally, some of these segments may be separated from the rest of the lung by accessory fissures (see Fig. 1.**25**).

Lobes

The right lung is divided into three lobes, the left lung into two lobes, and all are separated from one another by interlobar fissures lined by two layers of visceral pleura. In 50 to 70% of cases, the interlobar fissures are incomplete. Lobar consolidation and atelectasis can be identified by their characteristic radiographic appearances (see Figs. 1.**26**, 1.**33**).

Tracheobronchial System

The bronchi form a system of dichotomous branching channels that conduct air to the alveoli and gas-exchange surfaces. Inhaled gases must pass through an average of 14 bronchial divisions (8–25) before reaching the alveoli.

The walls of the trachea and main bronchi are reinforced by incomplete cartilage rings which prevent luminal collapse. In the segmental bronchi, this reinforcement dwindles to irregular cartilage plates that become smaller and less numerous in the subsegmental and smaller bronchi. The bronchiolar walls are devoid of cartilage.

The tracheobronchial system has a mucosal lining that secretes approximately 10 to 100 mL of mucus daily. Covering the mucosa are myriad ciliated cells that beat rhythmically in the direction of the oropharynx and mouth (mucociliary escalator), helping to remove inhaled foreign bodies and irritants from the lung.

Only the trachea, main and lobar bronchi can be identified on the chest radiograph. Their lumina appear as radiolucent bands or, when seen end-on, as elliptical and circular lucencies outlined by the faint linear density of the bronchial wall.

Trachea

On the frontal chest radiograph, the trachea appears as a broad, lucent band traversing the medial part of the superior mediastinum. Its walls are parallel, and the cartilage rings produce a slight scalloping of its contour. The left lower tracheal wall is usually indented by the aortic arch, and rarely the right border is indented by the azy-

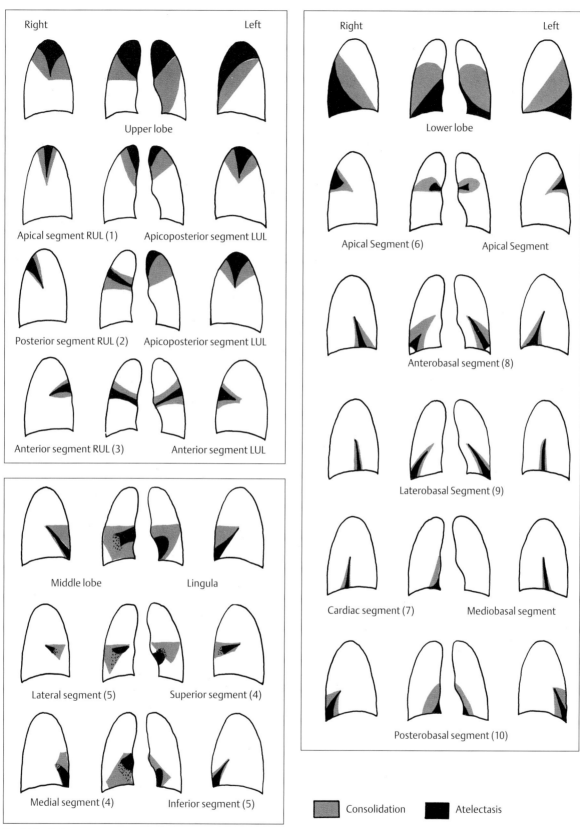

Fig. 1.**33**   Pulmonary segments.

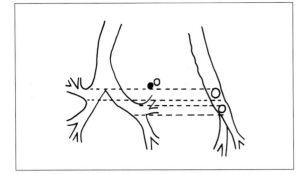

Fig. 1.**34** Radiographically visible bronchi. The lateral projection gives an en-face view of the right and left upper lobe bronchi. In the PA projection, the anterior segmental bronchus of the upper lobe is occasionally seen end-on, adjacent to the segmental artery.

gos vein. On the lateral projection, the trachea appears as a lucent band in the upper mediastinum that passes caudally and posteriorly at a slightly oblique angle.

Tracheal Bifurcation

At the bifurcation, the trachea divides dichotomously into the main bronchi which extend obliquely inferolaterally. This division is symmetrical up to the age of about 15 years, when the right main bronchus gains a more vertical orientation. This explains why aspiration occurs more frequently on the right side. The angle of bifurcation is 55 to 70° in adults; an angle greater than 90° is considered pathologic.

Upper Lobe Bronchi

On the frontal projection, they arise from the main bronchi in an almost horizontal plane; the origin of the right upper lobe bronchus is slightly superior to that of the left upper lobe bronchus. On the lateral view, the upper lobe bronchi may be seen end-on as elliptical lucencies below the tracheal band. The more superiorly lying right upper lobe bronchus is seen inconsistently; the more inferior left upper lobe bronchus is clearly demarcated by the lower lobe artery arching over it (see Figs. 1.**9**, 1.**34**).

Bronchus Intermedius and Lower Lobe Bronchi

On the right side, the main bronchus continues distally as the bronchus intermedius and then as the right lower lobe bronchus after giving branches to the right upper and middle lobes, respectively. The left main bronchus divides into the upper and lower lobe bronchi, and the left lower lobe bronchus descends caudally and rather more steeply than on the right side. On the frontal chest radiograph, these bronchi are usually but not invariably visible as radiolucent bands. On the right side, the lower lobe artery lies lateral to the bronchus.

Vascular System

■ Anatomy and Physiology

The lung has a dual blood supply with partial communication between the two systems: the pulmonary and the bronchial arterial systems.

The pulmonary system includes the pulmonary arteries, the perialveolar capillaries, and the pulmonary veins. All blood pumped from the right heart enters this system, is arterialized in the pulmonary capillaries, and then is pumped through the left heart into the systemic circulation.

The bronchial system has a predominantly nutritive function. The paired bronchial arteries arise from the descending aorta and accompany the bronchi along their course. In the perihilar regions, the blood drains via bronchial veins into the azygos-hemiazygos system. In the peripheral lung, the bronchial arteries open into the perialveolar capillary network creating an anastomosis between the two vascular networks.

Functionally, the pulmonary vascular system resembles the systemic venous system with pressures of 5 to 20 mmHg. This is significantly lower than in the systemic arteries, in part because the pulmonary vessels are highly compliant (Fig. 1.**35**).

In a normal resting adult, blood flows through the lungs at a rate of approximately 5 L/min. Only about 25 % of the lung capillaries are perfused in this resting state. When cardiac output increases during exercise, additional capillaries are recruited and the major vessels dilate. There is only a slight concomitant increase in pulmonary artery pressures (see Fig. 1.**35**).

The compliance of the pulmonary vessels is also responsible for the normal orthostatic perfusion gradient (orthostatic caudalization) that exists in the lungs. In the upright position and on deep inspiration, there is an increasing perfusion gradient from lung apex to base. This is manifest radiographically as more dilated vascular shadows in the basal zones. Since the hydrostatic pressure is somewhat higher at the base than at the apex, it causes greater dilatation of the basal vessels. On expiration, the basal vessels are compressed by the intrinsic weight of the lung, and the hydrostatic pressure effect is eliminated (Figs. 1.**36**–1.**39**).

In pathologic conditions which give rise to pulmonary venous hypertension, the normal orthostatic perfusion gradient is lost, and perfusion may be directed preferentially to the upper zones.

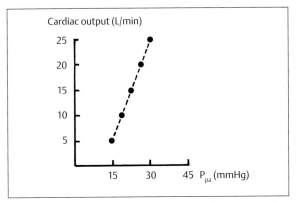

Fig. 1.**35**   Compliance of the pulmonary vascular system. A five-fold increase in the cardiac output from 5 to 24 L/min causes only a two-fold increase in the mean pulmonary artery pressure (P_{pa}).

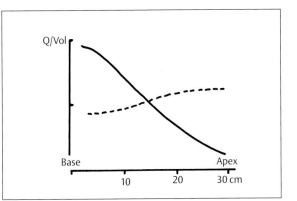

Fig. 1.**38**   Effect of degree of lung expansion on the distribution of pulmonary blood flow. In the upright position and in inspiration, blood flow increases from apex to base. In the supine position and in expiration, the apical and basal flows equalize. Blood flow per unit lung volume (Q/Vol) is shown on the ordinate (Fuchs and Voegeli 1973). Upright inspiration (solid line), upright expiration or supine position (broken line).

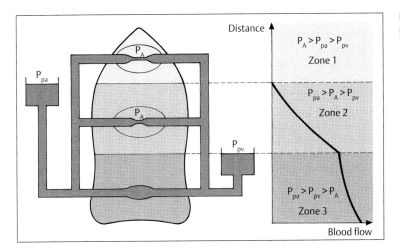

Fig. 1.**36**   The "waterfall" model of the pulmonary circulation. In the erect position and in deep inspiration, the apical vessels are collapsed while the basal vessels are dilated. The basal blood supply depends on the arteriovenous pressure difference. Blood flow in the midzone is determined by the arterial-alveolar pressure gradient. Hence the flow at that level is not regulated by the a-v pressure difference, just as the flow across the rim of a waterfall is independent of the height of the waterfall. P_{pa} pulmonary arterial pressure, P_A alveolar pressure, P_{pv} pulmonary venous pressure (Fuchs and Voegeli 1973).

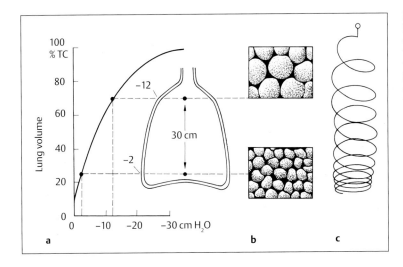

Fig. 1.**37a–c**   Gravitational effects on the lung. **a** Pulmonary pressure–volume curve. Due to the weight of the lung, intrapleural pressure has a higher negative value at the lung apex than at the lung base. This results in greater lung expansion and larger volume of the alveoli in the apical and upper zones. **b** Nonlinearity of the pressure–volume curve means that greater pressure is needed to inflate the apical alveoli since they already are greatly expanded. Because of this, inspired air is distributed predominantly to the basal segments. **c** A suspended coil spring is somewhat analogous to the lung: pulling on the bottom of the spring will cause relatively greater expansion of the lower segments than the upper segments. TC = total capacity (Fuchs and Voegeli 1973).

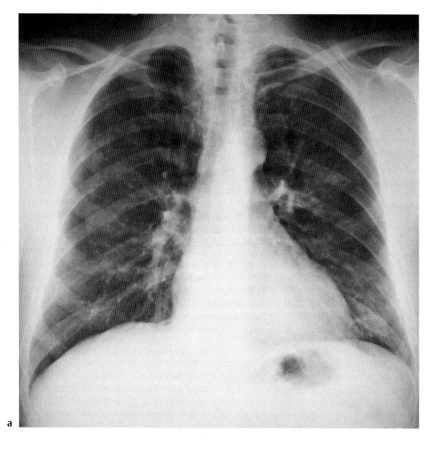

a

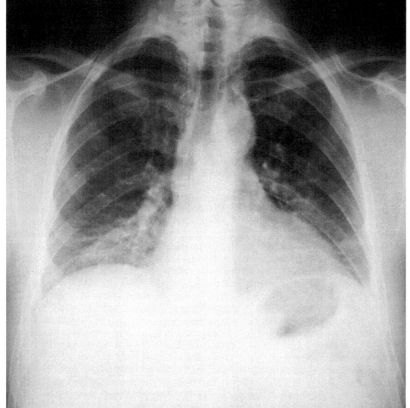

b

Fig. 1.**39 a, b**   Inspiratory and expiratory radiographs. Note the decrease in thoracic size on expiration, the apparent widening of the cardiac silhouette, the apparent mediastinal widening, and the compression of the basal pulmonary vessels.

■ Radiographic Anatomy of the Vascular System

The pulmonary vasculature is responsible for the branching linear markings seen on chest radiographs. Other structures such as the bronchial walls, bronchial vessels, lymphatic vessels, and interstitium are too small or too faint to be visible. Small vessel shadows appear as an overlapping network of branches in which arteries are indistinguishable from veins. However, several features allow differentiation between larger arteries and veins (Figs. 1.**40**, 1.**41**).

Arteries and Veins

The pulmonary arteries accompany the bronchi; the veins do not. Thus, a vascular shadow accompanying a lobar bronchus represents an artery. This relationship is best appreciated on conventional and computed tomographic images. When seen end on, a bronchus and its accompanying artery resemble a pair of spectacles with one opaque lens (see Fig. 1.**41**). Felson (1973) called this the "seminoma" pattern in reference to the orchidectomy necessitated by that disease. Since the bronchial tree is visible only to the level of the segmental bronchi on chest radiographs, the presence of an adjacent bronchus is useful only for identifying larger arteries.

Origin of the Pulmonary Arteries

The pulmonary arterial bifurcation occurs at a more cranial level than the entry of the pulmonary veins into the left atrium. This accounts for the steep descending course of the lower lobe arteries and the almost horizontal course of the lower lobe veins. The veins may be recognized by the fact that their shadows cross the lower lobe artery, which in turn is identified by its typical course and peribronchial position. Conversely, in the upper zones, the veins lie lateral to the arteries and have a more vertical orientation.

Pulmonary Veins

The lower lobe veins enter the left atrium anterior to the bronchi, while the lower lobe arteries lie posteriorly. The retrocardiac vascular bundle is always clearly visible on the lateral projection; its anterior components are veins, its posterior components are arteries.

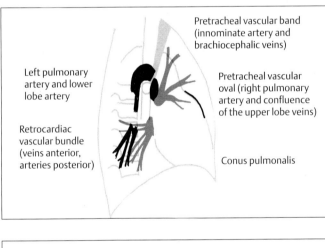

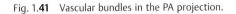

Fig. 1.**40**   Vascular bundles in the lateral projection.

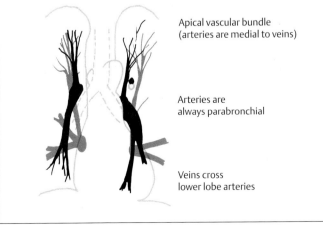

Fig. 1.**41**   Vascular bundles in the PA projection.

Main Pulmonary Artery

On the lateral view, the main pulmonary artery lies superior to the upper cardiac shadow and extends to the trachea in an anteriorly convex arch. On the PA view, the main pulmonary artery is visible only when it forms a border along the upper left cardiac outline. This may be due to slight right anterior rotation of the chest (cardiac waist) or may occur as a normal variant in young females.

Right Pulmonary Artery

From its origin, the right pulmonary artery runs horizontally to the right side, passing anterior to the airway. On the lateral view, it appears as a pretracheal elliptical shadow. Pulmonary arterial and venous branches frequently are superimposed on one another, giving the appearance of radiating branches. The horizontal limb cannot be seen on the PA view, but its branches form most of the right hilar shadow: the upper pole by the upper lobe segmental arteries, and the mid and lower hilum by the interlobar and lower lobe arteries.

Left Pulmonary Artery

Shortly after its origin at the bifurcation, the left pulmonary artery divides anterior to the left main bronchus into the upper lobe artery, which passes superiorly, and the lower lobe artery, which initially accompanies the left main bronchus and then courses inferiorly with the lower lobe bronchus. Thus, the upper pole of the hilum is formed by the left pulmonary and left upper lobe arteries while the mid and lower hilum are formed mainly by the lower lobe artery. Overall, the hilar point lies more superiorly on the left side than on the right side. The more distal lower lobe artery may lie adjacent to or be superimposed on the cardiac silhouette. On the lateral view, the left main bronchus appears as a lucent circle or ring shadow, and as the lower lobe artery arches over it, a characteristic shadow is formed.

Lower Lobe Veins

These vessels drain the lower lobes and pass to the left atrium as horizontal vascular shadows. Easily recognized on PA tomograms, they appear on the chest radiograph as linear shadows which cross the steeply descending arteries. On the lateral view, the veins form the anterior portion of the retrocardiac vascular bundle. Occasionally, individual pulmonary veins may be identified as they run medially to enter the left atrium.

Upper Lobe Veins

These veins drain the upper lobes and lingula and pass inferomedially to enter the left atrium. In the upper zones, they comprise the lateral vascular shadows of the apical vascular bundle. On the right, they frequently cross the lower lobe artery at the level of the horizontal fissure. On the lateral view, the upper lobe veins follow an anteroposterior course, are projected onto the cardiac silhouette, and converge toward the left atrium. Together with the right pulmonary artery, they may form a large pretracheal oval shadow.

The Mediastinum

The mediastinum lies between the lungs and is bounded superiorly by the thoracic inlet, posteriorly by the vertebral column, anteriorly by the sternum, and inferiorly by the diaphragm. It is customary to subdivide the mediastinum into anterior, middle, and posterior compartments (Fig. 1.**42**). This subdivision is useful, since certain disease processes predominate in specific compartments.

On the frontal view, the mediastinum appears as a central shadow in which the air-filled lumina of the trachea and main bronchi may be identified. The esophageal lumen may occasionally be visible because of swallowed air or contrast medium. A calcified aortic wall may be visible in older patients. Other mediastinal structures can be identified only at sites where they border the adjacent lung.

On the frontal view, the right mediastinal border is formed by the brachiocephalic (innominate) vessels and more inferiorly by the superior vena cava, the horizontal limb of the azygos vein, and the right atrium. The left mediastinal border is formed from above downward by the brachiocephalic vessels, left subclavian artery, the aortic knuckle, the pulmonary artery, the left atrial appendage, and the left ventricle. On both sides, epicardial fat pads may occupy and obliterate the cardiophrenic angles.

A well-exposed radiograph also demonstrates the characteristic pleural stripes (see Fig. 1.**20**), including the para-aortic and paraspinal lines and the azygoesophageal stripe.

On the lateral radiograph, the air-filled trachea may be seen descending within the mediastinal shadow. The anterior contour of the mediastinum is formed inferiorly by the right ventricle where it lies adjacent to the lower sternum. More superiorly, the right ventricular outflow tract, the anterior border of the ascending aorta, and the pretracheal band of brachiocephalic vessels form the anterior mediastinal contour. The retrosternal space is the triangular lucent area separating the vascular shadows and the sternum.

The posterior cardiac border is formed by the left atrium as it merges imperceptibly with the left ventricle. The triangular density occupying the angle between the posterior cardiac border and the diaphragm corresponds to the inferior vena cava.

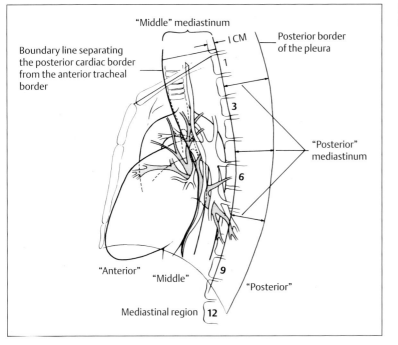

Fig. 1.**42** Mediastinal compartments (Meschan 1981).

Conventional Tomography

▦ Technique

Conventional tomography is used much less frequently today due to increasing availability and use of cross-sectional imaging and particularly of computed tomography.

The purpose of tomography is to demonstrate specific body planes free of superimposed shadows. This is accomplished by simultaneous motion of the X-ray tube and cassette around a fulcrum which lies in the plane of interest (Figs. 1.**43** and 1.**44**). Only objects in the plane of interest appear in focus; the motion blurs out tissues which lie outside this focal plane.

The sitting position is most appropriate for conventional tomography, but supine and lateral positions also may be used. When possible, tomograms should be obtained in two projections using a sufficiently large film size (24 × 30 or even 35 × 35 cm). Unnecessary exposures can be avoided by determining the plane of interest from plain radiographs. For thoracic studies, linear tomography with craniocaudal motion is recommended. A tomographic angle of 30 to 40° with exposure parameters of 0.6 s, 110 kV, and 8–20 mAs is appropriate. A compensating filter should be mounted near the tube for the simultaneous imaging of hilar and pulmonary structures.

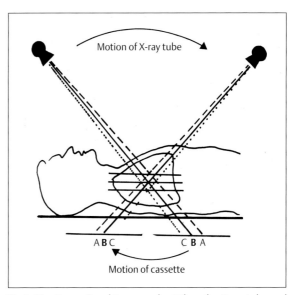

Fig. 1.**43** Conventional tomography. When the X-ray tube and cassette are moved simultaneously in opposite directions, only the structures in the plane of interest are in focus. Detail of objects outside the focal plane are blurred.

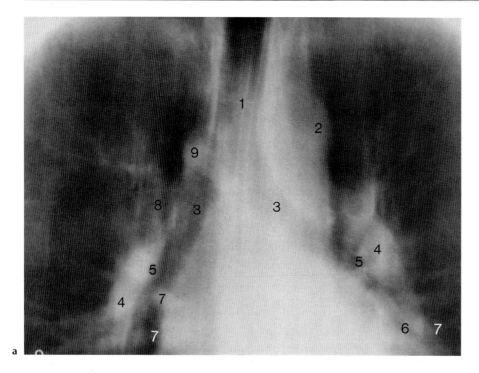

a

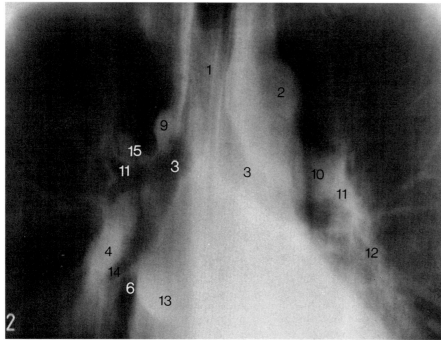

b

Fig. 1.**44a–e** Chest tomograms.
a AP tomogram 10 cm
b AP tomogram 12 cm
c AP tomogram 14 cm
d Lateral tomogram 5 cm left of midline
e Lateral tomogram 7 cm left of medial plane

 1 Trachea
 2 Aortic arch
 3 Main bronchus
 4 Lower lobe artery
 5 Apical lower lobe segmental bronchus
 6 Lower lobe bronchus
 7 Laterobasal veins
 8 Upper lobe vein
 9 Azygos vein
10 Pulmonary artery

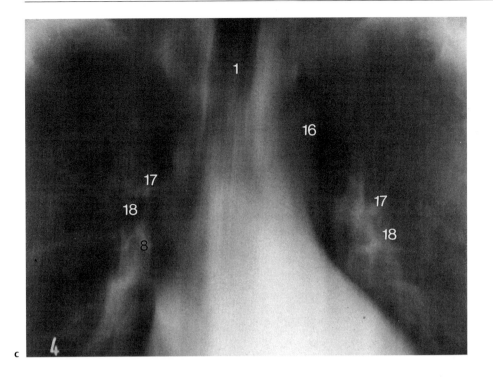

c

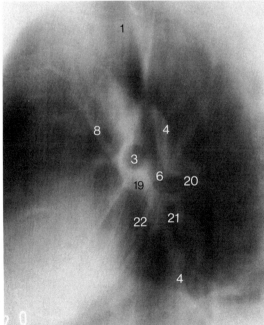

d

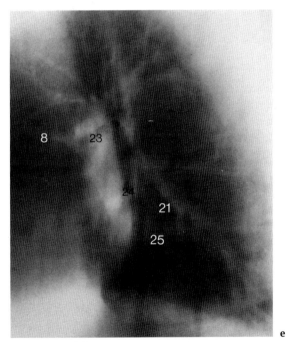

e

11 Upper lobe bronchus
12 Lingular bronchus
13 Systemic venous confluence at right atrium
14 Right middle lobe bronchus
15 Upper lobe artery
16 Aorta
17 Anterior upper lobe segmental artery
18 Anterior upper lobe segmental bronchus

19 Venous confluence
20 Apical lower lobe segmental bronchus and artery
21 Posterobasal lower lobe segmental bronchus and artery
22 Anterobasal lower lobe segmental bronchus and artery
23 Anterior upper lobe segmental bronchus and artery
24 Laterobasal lower lobe segmental bronchus and artery
25 Lower lobe vein

Computed Tomography

■ Technique

CT data are acquired by passing a collimated beam through a transverse section of the patient's body. The emergent beam then is measured by a semicircular array of detectors. During data acquisition, both the X-ray tube and detector array rotate around the patient so that the plane of interest is scanned from all directions. This gives a large number of attenuation values (e. g., 400 000), which then are recorded and processed by a computer to produce a digital image of the relevant plane (Fig. 1.**45**).

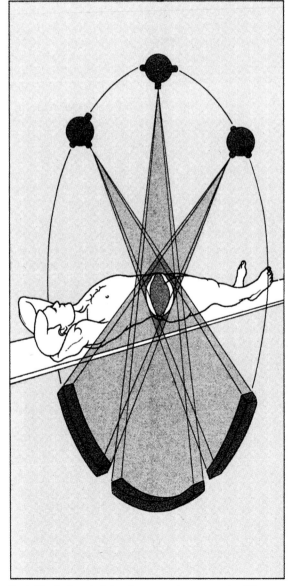

Fig. 1.**45** Basic principle of computed tomography (Wegener 1992).

All CT examinations initially require acquisition of a preliminary AP scout view from which the cranial and caudal limits of the study are determined. The standard CT examination is acquired at full inspiration though supplementary data acquired in expiration may be useful, particularly in the investigation of small airway disease. Contrast medium is infused preferably into an antecubital vein during the examination (e. g., 100–140 mL of approximately 300 mg iodine/mL, 3–4.5 mL/sec, 15–25 s delay). Reconstructed images usually are displayed at standard mediastinal (window width/center = 350/40) and lung (window width/center = 1500/–700) window settings.

Incremental CT

Early generation CT scanners used an incremental or single-slice technique in which one axial image was acquired during a breath-hold. The CT table then advanced up to 10 millimeters and a second image was acquired.

Helical and Multidetector CT

Helical CT involves acquisition of a volumetric data set through the anatomic region of interest during a single breath-hold. There is continuous patient movement with simultaneous scanning by a constantly rotating gantry and detector system. Initial helical CT systems employed a single detector but technology has advanced rapidly and today, 4, 16, and 64 multi-detector row CT systems (MDCT) are in clinical use.

MDCT systems allow increasingly faster image acquisition over any given craniocaudal distance (z axis) in a single breath-hold. Hence, with increasing numbers of detectors, collimation is decreased leading to improved spatial resolution. Coronal and sagittal reformatted images and three-dimensional (3D) reconstructions may be acquired from this volumetric data set and evaluation of the former in particular is becoming routine in interpretation of CT studies (Fig. 1.**46 a–c**).

High-Resolution CT

HRCT acquiring 1–2 mm collimation images at 10–15 mm intervals and employing a high frequency reconstruction algorithm was the standard CT technique for evaluation of diffuse parenchymal lung disease for many years. The advent of MDCT allows reconstruction of these "high-resolution" images from the volumetric data set and this now is an option if a "global" examination of the thorax is required. However, when lung parenchymal evaluation only is required, the traditional HRCT technique still is appropriate and this noncontiguous image acquisition gives a considerably lower radiation dose (1.5–2 mSv) than standard helical/MDCT where the dose is in the order of 6–10 mSv.

■ Computed Tomography in Cardiology

Conventional coronary angiography remains essential in planning and guiding catheter-based intervention and surgery in patients with significant coronary artery disease. However, CT shows considerable promise in the assessment of asymptomatic and early-stage disease (Schoenhagen et al. 2004).

The complex cyclical motion of the heart requires an imaging modality with high temporal resolution and images need to be referenced to the cardiac cycle. The temporal resolution of conventional angiography is 10 msec, that of electron-beam CT (EBCT) is 50–100 msec and that of MDCT is 50–300 msec. Therefore, CT image acquisition should be during the phase of minimal cardiac motion, i.e., late diastole. MDCT has the advantages over EBCT of a higher signal-to-noise ratio and higher spatial resolution.

Noncontrast CT is used for coronary artery calcium quantification. Coronary artery calcium scores at EBCT have been shown to correlate with total atherosclerotic plaque (both calcified and noncalcified) and also have been shown to have a predictive value for future coronary events (Secci et al. 1997). MDCT recently has emerged as an alternative to EBCT for coronary artery calcium assessment (Becker et al. 2001). The traditional scoring method has been the Agatston scoring system, which gives a calcium score based on maximum CT number and area of calcium (Agatston et al. 1990). Alternatives include volume and mass scoring (Callister et al. 1998, Detrano et al. 1995).

MDCT coronary angiography allows three-dimensional/volumetric scanning of the entire heart in a single breath-hold. Typical imaging parameters for 16 MDCT are 16 × 0.75 mm collimation, 0.42-sec rotation time, 140 kVp, and 400–500 mAs and for 64 MDCT are 64 × 0.6 mm collimation, 0.33-sec rotation time, 120 kVp, 850 mAs.

Data are gated retrospectively to reconstruct images during the diastolic phase of the cycle. Curved multiplanar reformats along the axes of the coronary arteries are possible as are maximum intensity projection (MIP) and volume-rendered reconstructions.

While the temporal resolution of MDCT is less than that of conventional angiography, it has the advantage of vessel-wall and plaque depiction in addition to its ability to assess luminal dimensions. Therefore, MDCT allows assessment of calcified and noncalcified plaque together with changes in vessel architecture including arterial remodeling. This is significant as noncalcified plaque may be more unstable and prone to rupture giving rise to acute coronary events. Positive remodeling also is associated with acute coronary syndromes (Schoenhagen et al. 2000, Yamagishi et al. 2000).

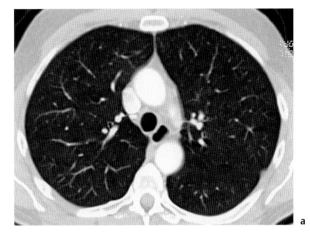

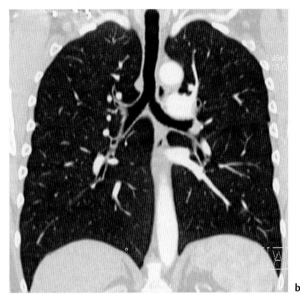

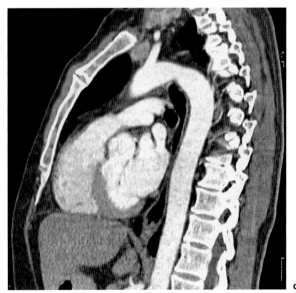

Fig. 1.**46** Axial image (**a**) from a volumetric MDCT study with coronal (**b**) and sagittal(**c**) reformats.

■ CT of the Normal Lung

Volumetric CT in the thorax performed on MDCT gives collimation of 1.5–3 mm and allows for much better resolution of pulmonary parenchymal structures than was possible when incremental CT with 8–10 mm collimation images were acquired as standard practice. When 1–1.5 mm collimation noncontiguous HRCT images are acquired, excellent visualization of lung parenchymal detail is also possible.

The visibility of a structure depends, in part, on attenuation differences between it and adjacent structures. For example, an interlobular septum with an anatomical thickness of only 0.1 mm will be imaged only if it intersects the plane of section at right angles; it will not be detected if it is parallel to the section. This is because the perpendicular septum will occupy a much greater proportion of the voxel, increasing its average radiographic density.

The following structures are visible in healthy subjects (Naidich 1991):

- The *bronchovascular bundle* is composed of bronchi, arteries, and their associated connective tissue. An artery and bronchus always follow a parallel course and have equal outer diameters, which taper towards the lung periphery as the airways and vessels ramify into progressively smaller channels. A bundle running perpendicular to the CT section will appear as a round soft-tissue density adjacent to an air-containing ring. A bundle in the plane of the CT section will appear as branching arterial streaks accompanied by the tubular lines of the bronchial wall. A bundle

crossing the section obliquely will produce oval or elliptical rings and shadows. Since the thickness of the bronchial wall is only about 1/6 to 1/10 of its luminal diameter, bronchi are visible only to about their 8th division, or to the junction of the central and peripheral halves of the lung. Vessels, on the other hand, may be traced as far as their 16th division, or to about 1 cm from the pleural surface (Fig. 1.**47**).

- *The pulmonary veins* appear as branched structures unattended by an airway. Since arteries in the outer half of the pulmonary lobe can no longer be identified by their accompanying bronchi, veins are indistinguishable from arteries in the lung periphery.

- *Interlobular septa*: The secondary lobule is surrounded by interlobular connective tissue septa which form a polyhedral network completely permeating the lung parenchyma. These septa are well developed in the peripheral portions of the lung, and they are best appreciated in the anterolateral and diaphragmatic regions. Septa in the perihilar lung are invisible unless they are pathologically thickened due to edema, infiltration, or fibrosis. Portions of the septa may show small nodular densities which represent veins coursing through the periphery of the lobule.

- *The secondary pulmonary lobule* usually can be identified in the peripheral lung only by its surrounding connective tissue septum. The lobular artery at the center of the lobule appears as a punctate or comma-shaped structure on thin section CT (Fig. 1.**48**).

- *The fissures* are less than 0.4 mm thick and frequently are visible on today's thin collimation CT studies. They are visible in thicker sections only if they

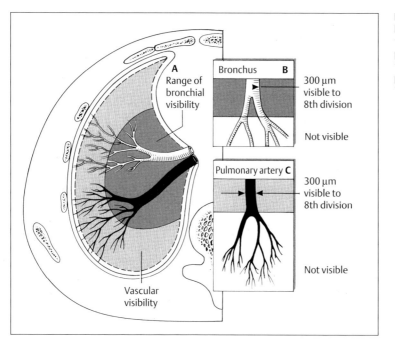

Fig. 1.**47** Limits of thin section CT for delineation of normal bronchovascular structures. Normal bronchi are not visible in the peripheral lung due to their narrow walls, whereas arteries and veins can be traced peripherally to the subpleural lung (Engler 1982).

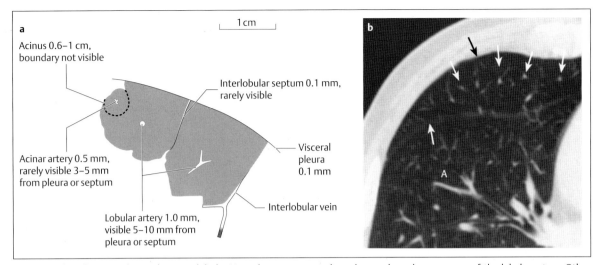

a

1 cm

Acinus 0.6–1 cm,
boundary not visible

Interlobular septum 0.1 mm,
rarely visible

Acinar artery 0.5 mm,
rarely visible 3–5 mm
from pleura or septum

Visceral
pleura
0.1 mm

Lobular artery 1.0 mm,
visible 5–10 mm from
pleura or septum

Interlobular vein

b

A

Fig. 1.**48 a, b**   The secondary pulmonary lobule. Note the punctate, y-shaped, or v-shaped appearance of the lobular artery. Other structures are occasionally visible (Naidich 1999).

traverse the section at almost a right angle, but the position of the major fissures can be indirectly determined by noting the adjacent relative avascularity of the lung (Fig. 1.**49**). The major fissures appear as sharp lines of soft-tissue density on high-resolution CT. The minor fissure runs parallel to the plane of section, so even on high-resolution CT its position usually must be inferred from the relative avascularity in the adjacent lung. However, on these thin sections (1 to 2 mm) the minor fissure, which usually has a somewhat superiorly convex shape, may pass through the section two or more times, appearing as a sharp, wavy line. The fissures may be readily appreciated on reformatted images particularly in the sagittal plane.

• *Pleura*: Unlike the fissures, the pleura borders on soft tissue structures at the lung-chest wall interface and, given its width (0.2 to 0.4 mm), is not demonstrated easily by CT. The chest wall comprises the visceral pleura, the parietal pleura, the very thin extrapleural fat stripe, the endothoracic fascia, the internal intercostal muscle, the intercostal fat, and the ribs (Fig. 1.**50**). Given the obliquity of the ribs in the lateral portion of the chest, axial CT scanning can demonstrate the boundary between the lung and intercostal space. This boundary is marked by the narrow intercostal stripe, which consists of pleura, fascia, and the internal intercostal muscle and contrasts sharply with the intercostal fat. Posteriorly, the pleura and endothoracic fascia lie on the paravertebral fat and appear as a very fine stripe called the paravertebral line. Pleura in close proximity to a rib can be identified only if it is pathologically thickened.

■ Normal Findings—CT Thorax

(See Figs. 1.**49**, 1.**51**–1.**55**).

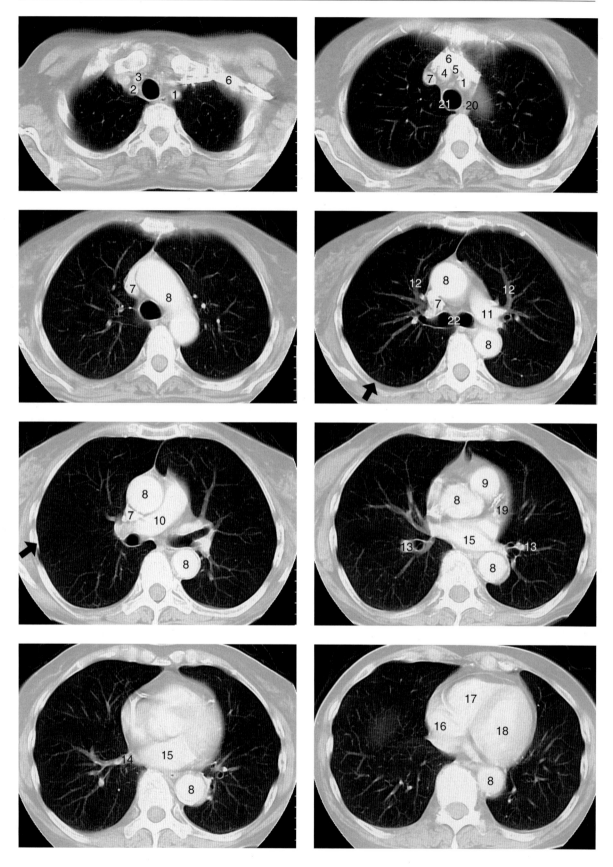

◁ Fig. 1.**49**   Computed tomography (CT)
1   Left subclavian artery
2   Right subclavian artery
3   Right carotid artery
4   Innominate Artery
5   Left carotid artery
6   Subclavian vein
7   Superior vena cava
8   Thoracic aorta
9   Main pulmonary artery
10   Right pulmonary artery
11   Left pulmonary artery
12   Upper lobe artery
13   Lower lobe artery
14   Pulmonary veins
15   Left atrium
16   Right atrium
17   Right ventricle
18   Left ventricle
19   Left anterior descending coronary artery
    (with atherosclerotic calcification)
20   Esophagus
21   Trachea
22   Tracheal bifurcation

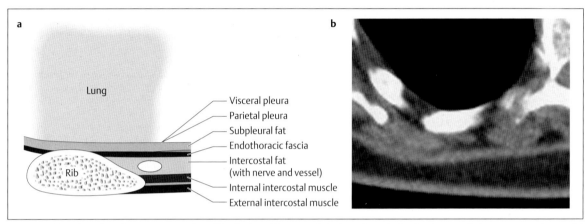

Fig. 1.**50 a, b**   The "pleural stripe," consisting of both pleural layers and the intrathoracic fascia, shows soft-tissue attenuation on CT. Note also the intercostal fat stripe with its vessels and the intercostal muscles (Naidich 1999).

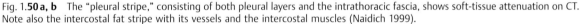

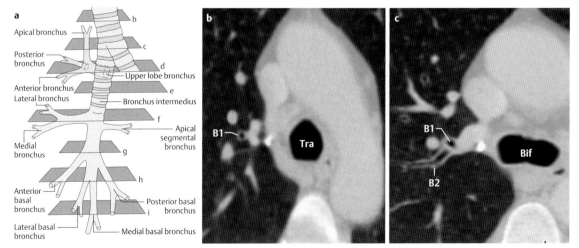

Fig. 1.**51 a–c**   Branching pattern of the right main bronchus.
Tra   Trachea
Bif   Bifurcation

B1   Apical segmental bronchus RUL
B2   Posterior segmental bronchus RUL

Fig. 1.**51 d–i**   ▷

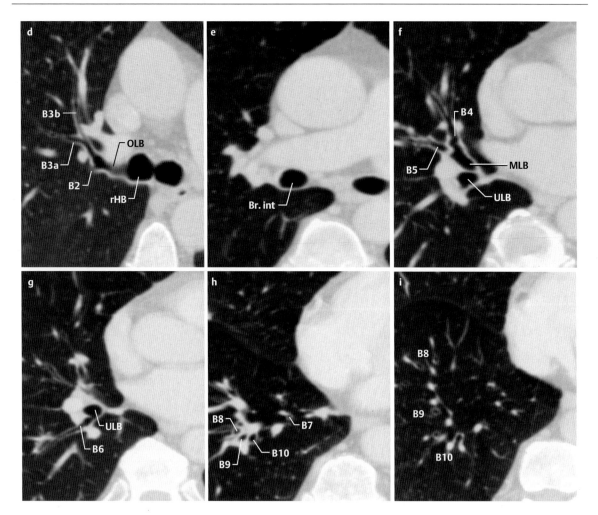

Fig. 1.**51 d–i** Branching pattern of the right main bronchus.

Tra	Trachea	B4	Segmental bronchus to medial segment RML
Bif	Bifurcation	B5	Segmental bronchus to lateral segment RML
RMB	Right main bronchus	B6	Apical segmental bronchus to RLL
ULB	Upper lobe bronchus	B7	Medial basal (cardiac) segmental bronchus RLL
MLB	Middle lobe bronchus	B8	Anterior basal segmental bronchus RLL
LLB	Lower lobe bronchus	B9	Lateral basal segmental bronchus RLL
B1	Apical segmental bronchus RUL	B10	Posterior basal segmental bronchus RLL
B2	Posterior segmental bronchus RUL	RUL	Right upper lobe
B3	Anterior segmental bronchus RUL	RML	Right middle lobe
		RLL	Right lower lobe

▷

Fig. 1.**52** Branching pattern of the left main bronchus.

ULB	Upper lobe bronchus
LLB	Lower lobe bronchus
Eso	Esophagus
LIN	Lingular bronchus
B1/B2	Apicoposterior bronchus
B3	Anterior bronchus
B4	Superior lingular bronchus
B5	Inferior lingular bronchus
B6	Apical segmental bronchus
B7	Medial basal bronchus
B8	Anterior basal bronchus
B9	Lateral basal bronchus
B10	Posterior basal bronchus

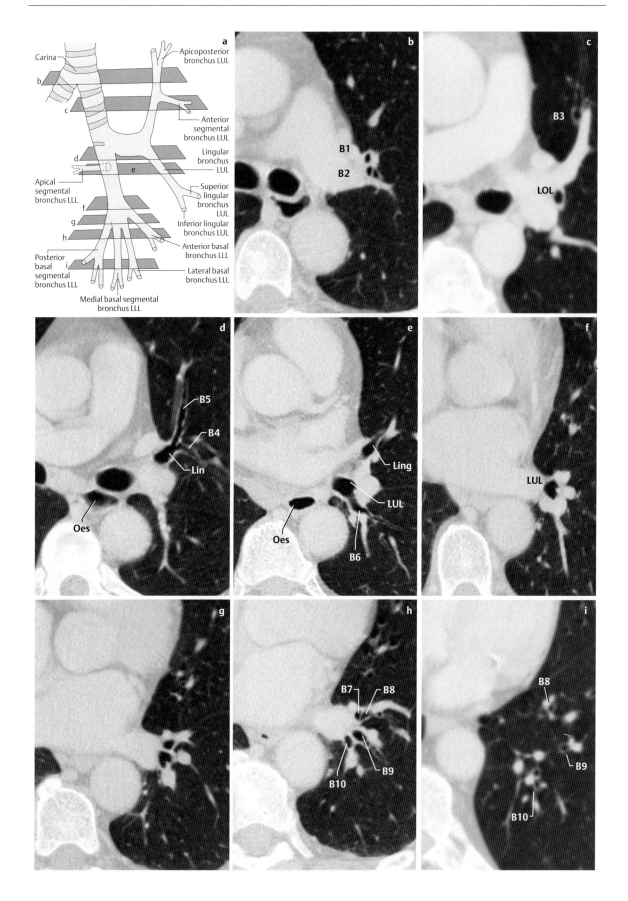

a Carina, Apicoposterior bronchus LUL, Anterior segmental bronchus LUL, Lingular bronchus LUL, Apical segmental bronchus LLL, Superior lingular bronchus LUL, Inferior lingular bronchus LUL, Anterior basal bronchus LLL, Posterior basal segmental bronchus LLL, Lateral basal bronchus LLL, Medial basal segmental bronchus LLL

b B1, B2

c B3, LOL

d B5, B4, Lin, Oes

e Ling, LUL, Oes, B6

f LUL

g

h B7, B8, B10, B9

i B8, B9, B10

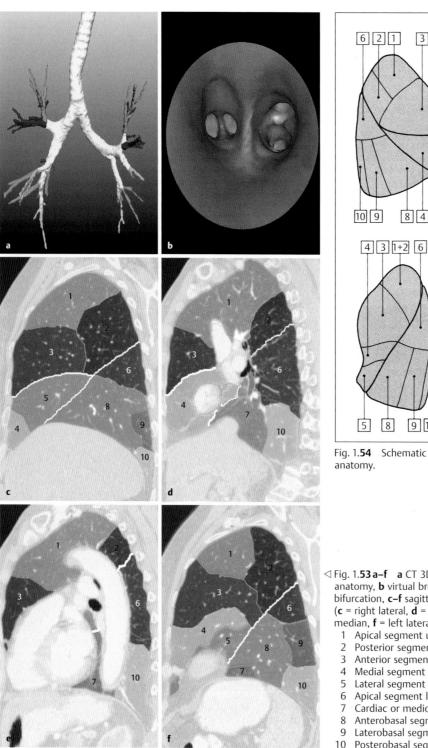

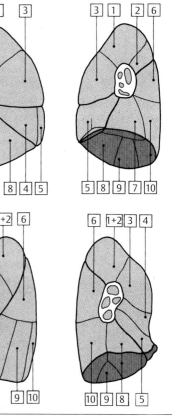

Fig. 1.**54**   Schematic representation of segmental lung anatomy.

◁ Fig. 1.**53 a–f**   **a** CT 3D reconstruction of bronchial anatomy, **b** virtual bronchoscopy at the level of the bifurcation, **c–f** sagittal sections through the lung (**c** = right lateral, **d** = right paramedian, **e** = left paramedian, **f** = left lateral).
  1 Apical segment upper lobe
  2 Posterior segment upper lobe
  3 Anterior segment upper lobe
  4 Medial segment RML or superior segment lingula
  5 Lateral segment RML or inferior segment lingula
  6 Apical segment lower lobe
  7 Cardiac or mediobasal segment
  8 Anterobasal segment
  9 Laterobasal segment
 10 Posterobasal segment

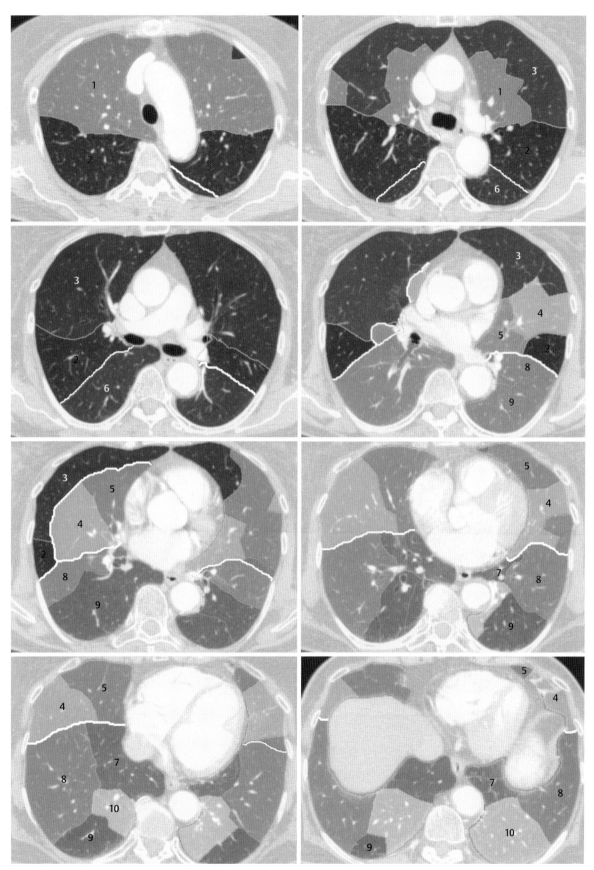

Fig. 1.**55** Axial CT images through the thorax showing lobar and segmental lung anatomy.

Radionuclide Imaging

Radionuclide imaging documents the distribution of a radionuclide-labeled pharmaceutical within the body with emitted radioactivity recorded by a gamma camera.

Lung Scintigraphy

Radionuclide lung imaging documents the regional distribution of pulmonary blood flow (perfusion scanning) and of alveolar ventilation (ventilation scanning). Ventilation-perfusion scintigraphy still plays a significant role in investigation of pulmonary embolism particularly in young adults with a normal chest radiograph. Ventilation scintigraphy may also be helpful in evaluating the activity and coordination of the ciliary apparatus of the bronchial mucosa (mucociliary escalator; Fig 1.56).

Perfusion Scintigraphy

The supine patient performs a series of deep inspirations, then technetium (Tc 99 m)-labeled albumin microspheres or macroaggregates are injected into the antecubital vein (Fig. 1.57). These albumin particles with a diameter of 10 to 40 μm, lodge in the pulmonary vascular bed, embolizing about 1 of every 10 000 capillaries.

Ventilation Scintigraphy

Gases or aerosols may be used to evaluate lung ventilation. Gases used include xenon (^{133}Xe and ^{127}Xe) and krypton (Kr 81 m). Shortcomings associated with these agents include expense, low gamma ray energy, and inability to allow six-view ventilation and consequently, aerosols are widely used in clinical practice. Tc 99 m-diethylenetriaminepentaacetic acid (DTPA) is the most widely used aerosol. The patient breathes through a face mask until the count is sufficiently high for imaging. When aerosols are used, Tc 99 m is the radionuclide for both ventilation and perfusion studies and simultaneous image acquisition is not feasible. The ventilation study usually is performed first, as aerosol particles are cleaned through the alveolar membrane relatively quickly.

When assessing ventilation only, delayed images may provide information on radionuclide clearance from the lungs and thus on the regional activity of the mucociliary system (see Fig. 1.56).

Ventilation-Perfusion Scintigraphy

Comparison of ventilation and perfusion images allows identification of unmatched perfusion defects (Fig. 1.58). A probability score for pulmonary embolism then is possible based on VQS and chest radiographic findings.

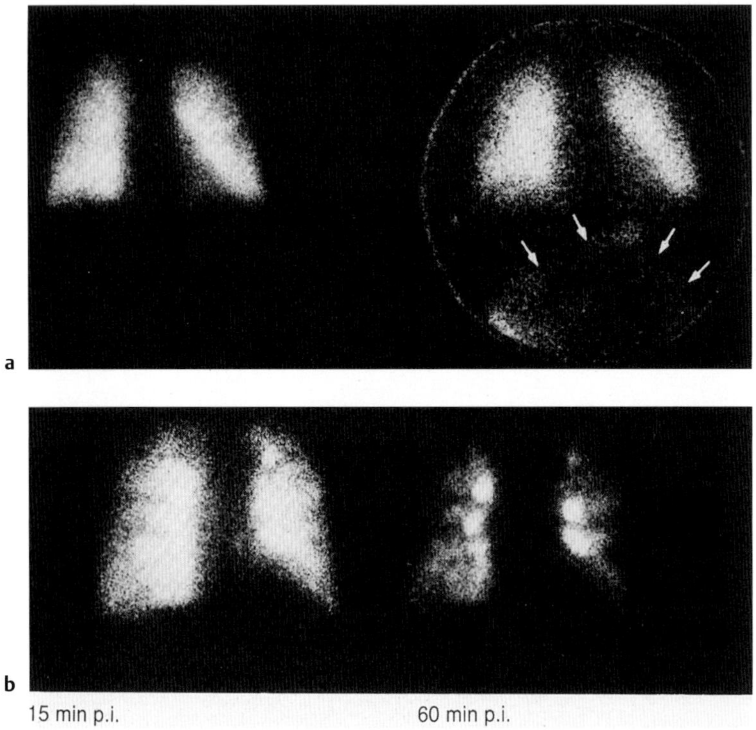

a

b

15 min p.i.   60 min p.i.

Fig. 1.56 a, b   Scintigraphic evaluation of mucociliary transport. a Normal study.
b Chronic obstructive pulmonary disease (COPD) with patchy central deposition of tracer.
(→ swallowed radionuclide appearing in the bowel).

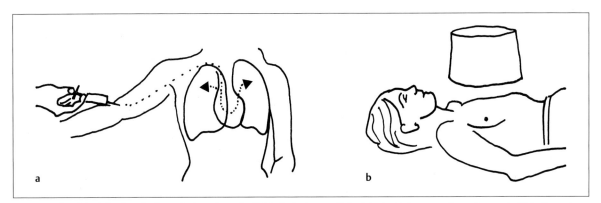

Fig. 1.**57 a, b**   Principle of perfusion scintigraphy. **a** Radiolabeled microparticles injected intravenously are trapped within the pulmonary capillaries. **b** Gamma camera imaging of distribution of radioactivity.

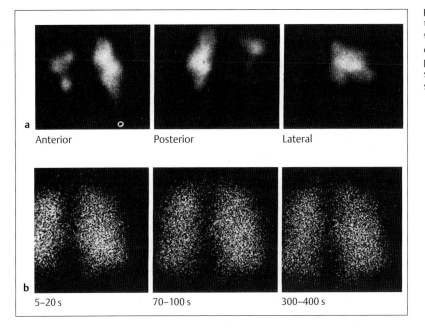

Fig. 1.**58 a,b   a** Ventilation (10 mCi ^{133}Xe) and **b** perfusion scans (4 mCi ^{99m}Tc-MAP) in patient with pulmonary embolism. Images show characteristic pattern of multiple unmatched perfusion defects with normal ventilation study.

Myocardial Perfusion Scintigraphy

Radionuclide imaging of the myocardium (Fig. 1.**59**) documents the extent and distribution of both ischemic and infarcted myocardium. Both thallium-201 and technetium-99 may be used for myocardial scintigraphy.

Both agents are administered by intravenous injection.

When Thallium-201 is used, it activates the sodium-potassium ATPase enzyme system at the cell membrane level and this transports the isotope into the myocardial cell. Following initial uptake of 201-Tl in myocardial cells, redistribution occurs with thallium being washed out of cells into the vascular compartment from which it then is available for re-extraction. 201-Tl has the disadvantage of low gamma radiation and high radiation dose to the kidneys.

Isonitrile compounds such as hexakis-2-methoxyisobutylisonitrile (HMIBI) bound to Tc 99 m may also be used. These have the advantage of higher gamma energy. However, there is no redistribution and rest imaging requires a second injection.

Normal scintigraphic studies show a relatively homogeneous distribution of radionuclide throughout the myocardium. Regions of decreased activity signify areas of diminished blood flow.

Radionuclide uptake by myocardial cells is determined during exercise or pharmacological stress and then at rest. Approximately 100 MBq of thallium-201 chloride or 240 MBq of Tc 99 m-HMIBI are injected intravenously during exercise, and image acquisition begins immediately. Gamma camera equipment with SPECT capability is routinely used. The distribution of tracer uptake by the myocardium is documented. Rest images are acquired approximately 30 minutes later.

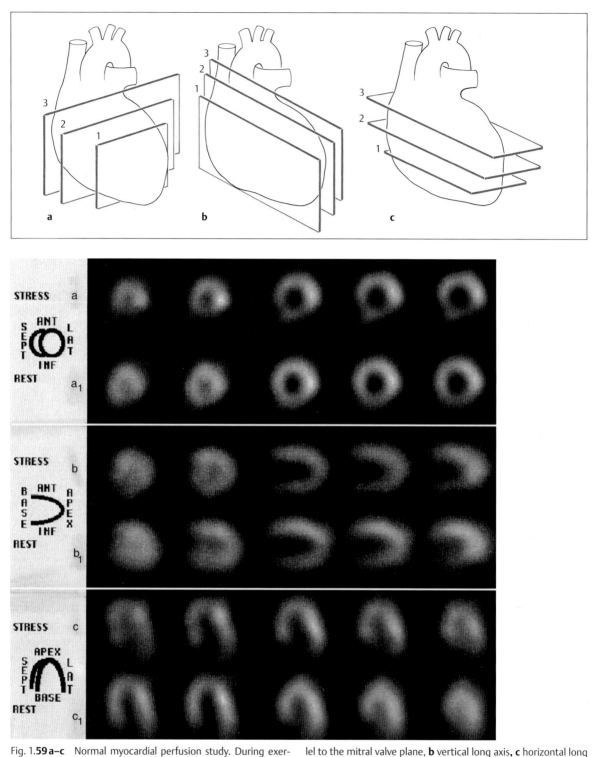

Fig. 1.**59a–c** Normal myocardial perfusion study. During exercise or pharmacologic stress, thallium-201 is distributed homogeneously throughout the left ventricular myocardium with subsequent imaging in three perpendicular planes: **a** Short axis parallel to the mitral valve plane, **b** vertical long axis, **c** horizontal long axis. The examination subsequently is repeated at rest (**a₁, b₁, c₁**). Both exercise/stress and resting thallium studies show homogeneous uptake with no areas of decreased perfusion.

Image analysis allows differentiation of infarcted myocardium from regions of reversible ischemia. An area of decreased tracer activity which is present on both stress and resting images usually indicates irreversible ischemia/infarction. Reversible ischemia shows decreased tracer activity during stress but reverts to normal on the rest images. This occurs because a stenosed coronary artery may allow normal perfusion at rest, but perfusion

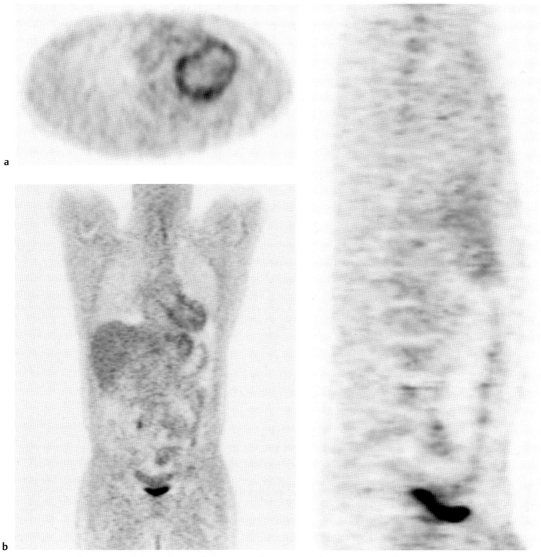

a

b

c

Fig. 1.**60**   Axial (**a**), coronal (**b**) and sagittal (**c**) images from a normal 18FDG-PET study

diminishes relative to normal myocardium during stress as the stenosed vessel cannot allow the physiologic increase in blood flow which normally is seen during stress and exercise.

"Hibernating" myocardium retains its cellular integrity but blood flow is reduced so significantly that it cannot sustain the high energy requirement of contraction. Rest-redistribution-reinjection protocols with 201-Tl attempt to distinguish hibernating from infarcted myocardium (Hossein et al. 1999).

Positron Emission Tomography (PET) and PET-CT

PET is a molecular imaging technique which allows visualization of both physiologic and pathologic processes (Fig. 1.**60 a–c**). 18F fluorodeoxyglucose (FDG) is the most frequently used radiopharmaceutical in clinical PET imaging. This glucose analogue is transported across cell membranes by glucose transporter proteins, is phosphorylated and with the exception of the liver, becomes trapped metabolically. Malignant cells are associated with an increased glycolytic rate. PET has become increasingly important in oncologic imaging and relies on imaging the distribution of FDG which shows increased accumulation in neoplastic lesions relative to normal tissue.

18F degrades to $18O_2$, a positron, and a neutron. The neutron travels a short distance in the human body typically less than 1 mm for 18F. Once most of its energy is lost, the neutron annihilates with a nearby electron and two photons, each having energy of 511 keV, are produced. These photons leave the site of annihilation in opposite directions and travel at 180° to each other. They subsequently reach the detector ring surrounding the body.

Simultaneous detection of two 511-keV photons in two detectors in the ring indicates that an annihilation has occurred somewhere along the column connecting the two detectors, and this event is recorded as a coincidence.

PET-CT is a unique combination of cross-sectional anatomy provided by CT and metabolic information provided by PET. Both are acquired during a single examination and are fused. This combined modality study allows accurate localization of increased FDG activity to specific anatomical locations.

Patients having PET/PET-CT studies are required to fast for 4–6 hours and are asked to avoid caffeinated and alcoholic beverages. Blood glucose is measured prior to injection and a normal blood glucose level is preferable. Administration of insulin to diabetic patients for glucose control is controversial as it may exaggerate physiologic uptake in muscles. Strenuous activity should be avoided before and after injection as it too may lead to increased muscle uptake of FDG (Kapoor et al. 2004).

Ultrasound

The role of ultrasound in the thorax is limited to evaluation of the soft tissues of the chest wall and the pathologically distended pleural space. The large impedance difference between the soft tissues and the aerated lung prevents sonographic visualization of the pulmonary parenchyma. Pleural effusions are visualized easily with sonography. It also is possible to determine if chest-wall and circumscribed pleural lesions are solid or fluid and if subacute/chronic effusions have become loculated.

While ultrasound plays a limited role in chest imaging, echocardiography plays a very major role in evaluation of the heart, but a discussion of this modality is beyond the scope of this text.

Pulmonary Angiography

Advances in CT technology and particularly the development of CT pulmonary angiography have led to a marked decrease in the use of conventional pulmonary angiography. Traditionally, it was regarded as the "gold standard" for investigation of pulmonary embolism. It involved a transfemoral approach using the Seldinger technique (Fig. 1.**61**) with an initial test injection excluding the presence of thrombus in the right heart and main pulmonary artery and allowing progression to selective pulmonary artery injections (see Fig. 1.**62**).

Today its use is largely confined to specialist centers where it continues to be used in the assessment of some patients with pulmonary hypertension and in the evaluation of pulmonary stenoses and malformations.

Accurate mortality and morbidity figures for pulmonary angiography were difficult to determine, with some series reporting mortality rates of 0.5 to 1.0% (Mills 1980, PIOPED Study 1990), while in others there were no deaths (Cheely 1981).

■ Normal Findings

See Figures 1.**62** and 1.**63**.

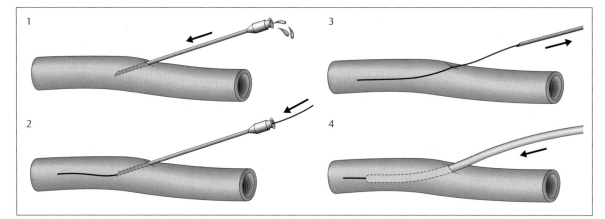

Fig. 1.**61**   Percutaneous arterial catheterization using the Seldinger technique.

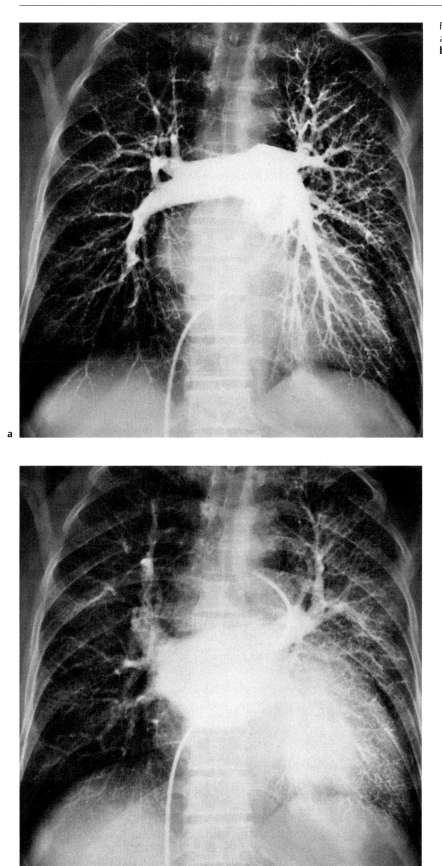

Fig. 1.**62 a, b** Normal pulmonary angiogram. **a** Arterial phase, **b** Venous phase.

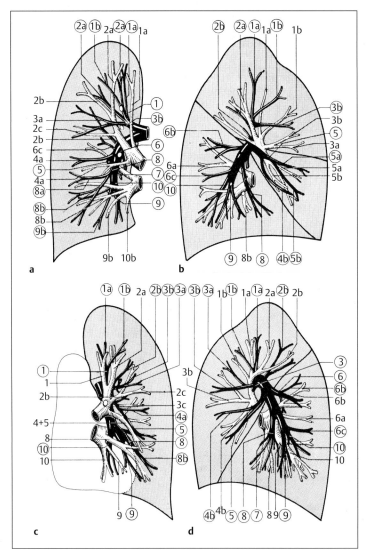

Fig. 1.**63 a–d**   Pulmonary vessels (from Uthgenannt: Linear densities. In: W. Teschendorf: *Röntgenologische Differentialdiagnostik*. Vol. I/1, 5th ed. Stuttgart: Thieme 1975).

Arteries (circled numbers):

1   Apical segmental artery, 1 a apical branch, 1 b anterior branch
2   Posterior segmental artery; 2 a apical branch, 2 b lateral branch
3   Anterior segmental artery; 3 a lateral branch, 3 b anterior branch
4   Lateral artery of right middle lobe and superior lingular artery of left upper lobe; 4 a posterior branch, 4 b anterior branch
5   Medial artery of right middle lobe and inferior lingular artery of left upper lobe; 5 a superior branch, 5 b inferior branch
6   Apical or superior artery of lower lobe; 6 a medial branch, 6 b superior branch, 6 c lateral branch
7   Mediobasal lower lobe artery with anterior and posterior branches
8   Anterobasal lower lobe artery; 8 a lateral branch, 8 b basal branch
9   Laterobasal lower lobe artery; 9 a lateral branch, 9 b basal branch
10 Posterobasal lower lobe artery; 10 a laterobasal branch, 10 b mediobasal branch, 10 c posterior branch

Veins (noncircled numbers)

1   Apical vein of upper lobe; 1 a apical branch (between S 1 a and S 1 b), 1 b anterior branch (between S 1 b and S 3 b)
2   Posterior vein of upper lobe; 2 a apical branch (between S 1 a and S 2 a), 2 b posterior branch (between S 2 a and S 2 b), 2 c intermediate branch (between S 2 b and S 3 a), lateral branch (between S 3 a and S 3 b), interlobar branch (interlobar subpleural S 2 a)
3   Anterior vein of upper lobe; 3 a superior branch (between S 3 b1 and S 3 b2), 3 b inferior branch (between S 3 b2 and S 4 b), 3 c (left side only) lateral branch (between S 3 a and S 4 a)

4   Lateral vein of right middle lobe; 4 a posterior branch (between S 4 a and S 4 b), 4 b anterior branch (between S 4 b and S 5 a) and superior lingular vein of left upper lobe; 4 a posterior branch (between S 4 a and S 5 b), 4 b anterior branch (between S 4 b and S 5)
5   Medial vein of right middle lobe; 5 a superior branch (between S 5 a and S 5 b), 5 b inferior branch (interlobar subpleural branch in S 5 b) and inferior lingular vein of left upper lobe; 5 a superior branch (between S 5 a and S 5 b), 5 b inferior branch (between S 5 b and S 5 b2)
6   Apical or superior vein of lower lobe; 6 a medial branch (between S 6 a and S 10), 6 b superior branch (between S 6 b and S 6 c, and between S 6 b1 and S 6 b2), 6 c lateral branch (between S 6 c and S 8 a)
7   Mediobasal vein of lower lobe; 7 a anterior branch (between S 7 a and S 7 b), 7 b posterior branch (between S 7 b and S 10 b)
8   Anterobasal vein of lower lobe; 8 a lateral branch (between S 8 a and S 8 b), 8 b basal branch (between S 8 b, S 7 a and S 9 b)
9   Laterobasal vein of lower lobe; 9 a lateral branch (between S 9 a and S 9 b), 9 b basal branch (between S 9 b and S 10 a)
10 Posterobasal vein of lower lobe; 10 a lateral branch (between S 10 a and S 10 b), 10 b medial branch (between S 10 c and S 10 b)

Bronchography

Bronchography traditionally has been used in evaluation of the airways. CT ± flexible bronchography has largely replaced this procedure which is no longer available at most institutions.

■ Normal Findings

See Figures 1.**64** and 1.**65**.

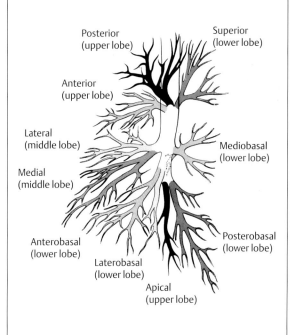

a

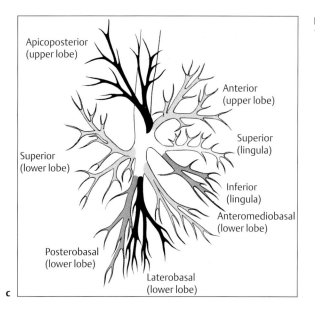

c

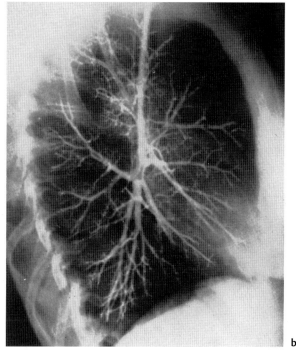

b

Fig. 1.**64 a–c** Normal lateral bronchogram (from Meschan 1981).

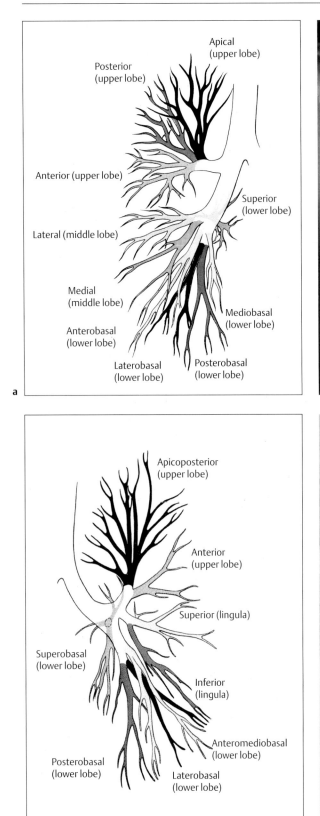

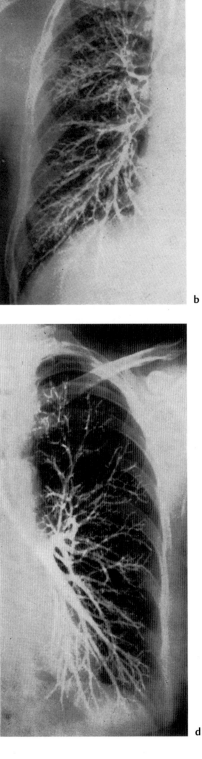

Fig. 1.**65 a–d**   Normal PA bronchogram (from Meschan 1981).

Magnetic Resonance Imaging

MRI yields multiplanar cross-sectional images (i.e., coronal, sagittal, and axial), as does computed tomography, but MRI allows for a greater degree of tissue characterization. When exposed to a strong external magnetic field, tissue protons realign along the plane of the magnetic gradient. From this position, they can be deflected momentarily by applying a radio frequency (RF) pulse. As they return to their original alignment, the protons emit a faint electromagnetic signal which is detected by a "receiving" radiofrequency coil. With suitable gradients along the magnetic field, signal detection can be confined to a preselected body plane. Processing of this data then yields a cross-sectional image of the plane of interest (Stark and Bradley 1999).

MRI is sometimes useful in the assessment of chest-wall and diaphragmatic lesions and, in selected cases, mediastinal pathology. It remains significantly inferior to CT for evaluation of the pulmonary parenchyma.

■ Normal Findings

See Figures 1.**66** and 1.**67**.

■ Cardiac MRI

MRI has emerged as a valuable tool in evaluation of the heart. It allows accurate evaluation of ventricular function and cardiac valve motion and allows for excellent depiction of cardiac and vascular anatomy in congenital heart disease. CMR also shows considerable promise in the field of myocardial first-pass perfusion and viability imaging.

CMR pulse sequences may be divided into dark/black blood and bright blood sequences. Black blood sequences include standard spin echo (SE), breath-hold turbo or fast spin echo (TSE and FSE) and half Fourier

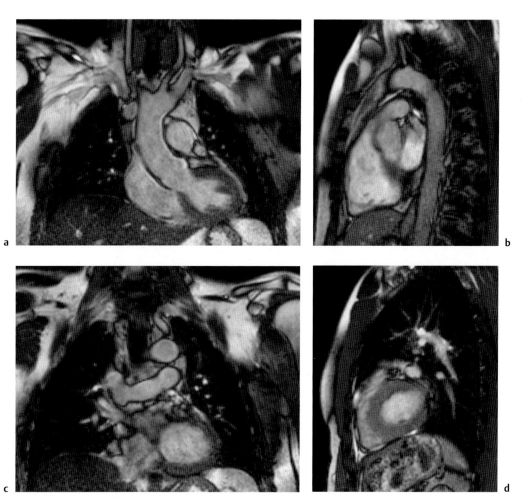

Fig. 1.**66 a–d** Coronal (**a, c**) and sagittal (**b, d**) MR images.

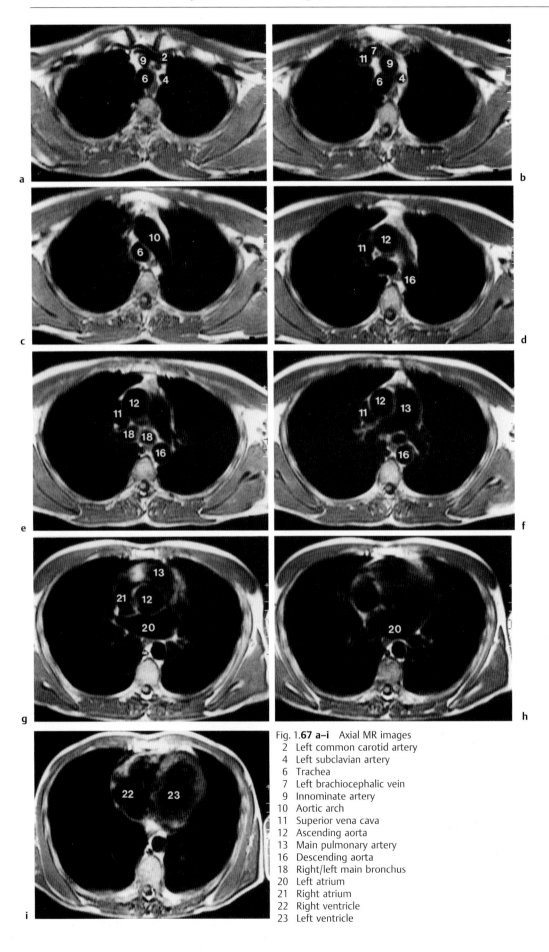

Fig. 1.**67 a–i**   Axial MR images
 2 Left common carotid artery
 4 Left subclavian artery
 6 Trachea
 7 Left brachiocephalic vein
 9 Innominate artery
10 Aortic arch
11 Superior vena cava
12 Ascending aorta
13 Main pulmonary artery
16 Descending aorta
18 Right/left main bronchus
20 Left atrium
21 Right atrium
22 Right ventricle
23 Left ventricle

turbo spin echo with double inversion recovery (HASTE, double-IR TSE/FSE). These allow excellent depiction of cardiac anatomy.

Bright blood sequences are gradient recalled echo (GRE) sequences and cine GRE is particularly useful. These allow evaluation of ventricular function and regional wall motion. GRE imaging using the segmented k-space technique and cardiac gating allows multiphase single slice or multislice single phase modes. Examples include TurboFLASH, fast SPGR, and TFE/FFE. Newer fast GRE sequences with completely refocused gradients include true FISP, balanced FFE, and FIESTA and these give excellent contrast between myocardium and blood pool (Poustchi-Amin et al. 2003).

Myocardial perfusion can be evaluated with gadolinium-enhanced dynamic "first pass" rest and stress studies, the latter during administration of a pharmacologic stress agent such as adenosine. Delayed imaging postgadolinium administration allows detection of regional myocardial hyperenhancement indicative of nonviable tissue. Dobutamine may also be used as a pharmacologic stress agent when resulting ventricular wall motion abnormalities may be assessed.

2 Malformations

Pulmonary malformations are rare and frequently associated with extrapulmonary anomalies.

Three main categories are recognized:
- Combined lung and vascular anomalies include bronchopulmonary sequestrations and hypogenetic lung (scimitar) syndrome.

- Bronchopulmonary anomalies include pulmonary agenesis and hypoplasia, bronchial atresia, bronchogenic cysts, congenital cystic adenomatoid malformations, and congenital lobar emphysema.
- Vascular malformations include pulmonary arteriovenous malformations and anomalous pulmonary venous drainage (Zylak et al. 2002).

Bronchopulmonary Sequestrations

■ Pathology

Bronchopulmonary sequestrations represent areas of nonfunctioning lung tissue that do not communicate with the tracheobronchial tree and have a systemic arterial blood supply. Embryologically, pulmonary sequestrations are due to anomalous ventral budding from the foregut or tracheobronchial tree. Occasionally, they have a fistulous connection to the esophagus or stomach. Sequestrations are classified as extra- or intralobar in type.

Extralobar Sequestration

Extralobar malformations constitute 25% of sequestrations. They are discrete accessory lobes of nonaerated lung invested within their own pleural covering (Rosado de Christensen et al. 1993). They are located most commonly between the lower lobe and the diaphragm. They

also may have an intradiaphragmatic, mediastinal, or intra-abdominal position. Extralobar sequestrations have a systemic arterial supply from branches of the aorta and a systemic venous drainage to the azygos veins or inferior vena cava. Associated anomalies including diaphragmatic hernia and bronchogenic cyst may be present in up to 60% of cases.

Intralobar Sequestration

Intralobar sequestrations usually have a systemic arterial supply and pulmonary venous drainage. Sixty percent of intralobar sequestrations are left-sided and they involve the lower lobes in 98% of cases. While extralobar sequestration is accepted as a congenital anomaly, substantial evidence suggests that intralobar sequestrations may have an acquired origin. Reports of intralobar sequestrations in infants are virtually absent and associated anomalies are relatively uncommon compared

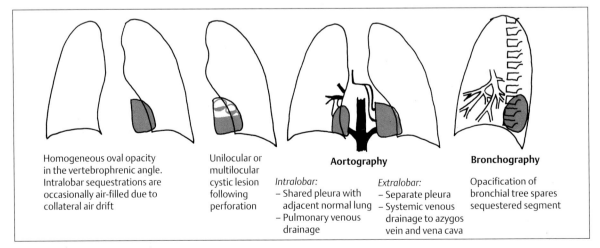

Homogeneous oval opacity in the vertebrophrenic angle. Intralobar sequestrations are occasionally air-filled due to collateral air drift

Unilocular or multilocular cystic lesion following perforation

Aortography

Intralobar:
– Shared pleura with adjacent normal lung
– Pulmonary venous drainage

Extralobar:
– Separate pleura
– Systemic venous drainage to azygos vein and vena cava

Bronchography

Opacification of bronchial tree spares sequestered segment

Fig. 2.1 Pulmonary sequestrations.

with their prevalence in association with other congenital thoracic anomalies (Stocker 1986, Frazier et al. 1997).

Accessory Lung

Like an extralobar sequestration, accessory lung has its own pleural covering. It also has a rudimentary bronchus, which may be patent and communicate with the trachea, the tracheal bifurcation, or the esophagus.

■ Clinical Features

Fifty percent of extralobar sequestrations present in the first 6 months of infancy. Clinical manifestations include dyspnea and cyanosis. The frequent association of other congenital anomalies also may lead to their detection.

Intralobar sequestrations present with productive cough and recurrent episodes of pneumonia. Up to 50% of patients will have become symptomatic by the age of 20 years.

■ Radiologic Findings

Chest Radiograph

The characteristic appearance of an extralobar sequestration is that of a well-defined round, oval, or triangular opacity located posteromedially at the lung base. Intralobar sequestrations are more variable in appearance. Findings include a well-defined homogeneous opacity, solitary pulmonary nodule, recurrent episodes of pneumonic consolidation, and an area of pulmonary hyperlucency. Infection with fistula formation to an adjacent bronchus may lead to formation of a multilocular cystic mass with air-fluid levels. This "cystic" transformation of an initially homogeneous mass in the left vertebrophrenic angle is strongly suggestive of the correct diagnosis (Fig. 2.1).

Sonography

Extralobar sequestrations may appear homogeneous and echogenic. If an intralobar sequestration becomes infected, a multicystic mass may be seen.

Computed Tomography (CT)

CT findings include a solid mass in both intra- and extralobar sequestrations. In addition, an area of homogeneous consolidation or a complex cystic mass may be seen in the intralobar variant. A peripheral zone of decreased lung attenuation is sometimes seen in intralobar sequestrations (Fig. 2.2) and has been attributed to collateral air drift through the incomplete, partially fibrous boundary between sequestrated and normal lung (Scully et al. 1981).

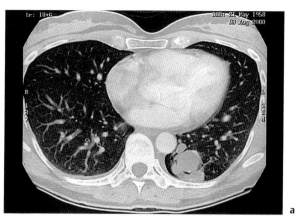
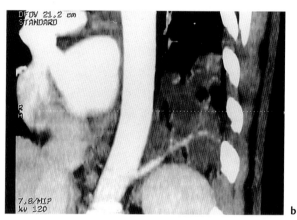
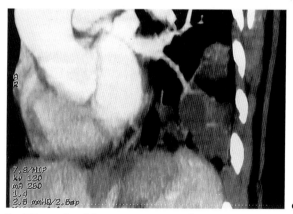

Fig. 2.**2a–c**   Intralobar sequestration. Axial CT image (**a**) shows a lobulated mass with a surrounding rim of decreased lung attenuation in the left lower lobe. Maximum intensity projection (MIP) reconstructions from CTA study show the systemic arterial supply from the thoracic aorta (**b**) and pulmonary venous drainage to the left atrium (**c**).

Occasionally, a focal area of decreased lung attenuation in the lower lobes may be the only parenchymal manifestation of intralobar sequestration (Ikezoe et al. 1990).

Dedicated thin-collimation helical CT with intravenous contrast medium allows demonstration of the systemic arterial supply and pulmonary/systemic venous drainage (Fig. 2.**3**)

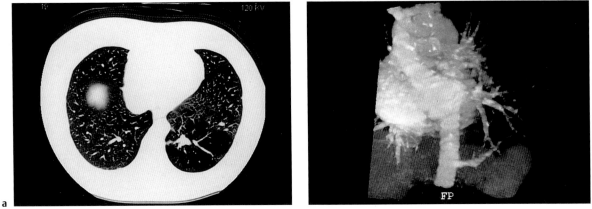

Fig. 2.**3 a, b**   Intralobar sequestration. CT shows a large area of decreased attenuation in the left lower lobe with a small central tubular opacity (**a**). Shaded surface display (SSD) 3D reconstruction demonstrates the systemic arterial supply and pulmonary venous drainage (**b**).

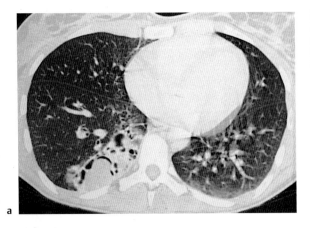

Fig. 2.**4 a–c**   Intralobar sequestration. CT shows a partly cystic lung lesion (**a**) which is supplied by a branch of the aorta and drained by pulmonary venous branches as seen at angiography (**b, c**). Pulmonary arteries (white) and pulmonary veins (black) as seen on DSA study (**c**).

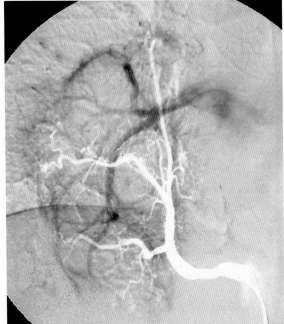

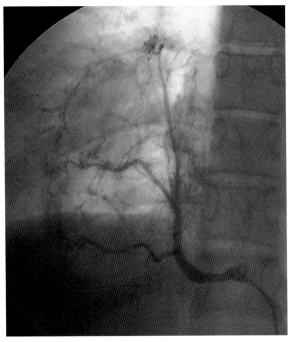

Angiography

CT has become the imaging modality of choice in investigation of sequestrations, and conventional angiography now is performed much less frequently. Aortography demonstrates a systemic arterial supply to the sequestration from the thoracic aorta in 70 % of cases, from the abdominal aorta in 20 %, and from an intercostal artery in 5 % (Ranniger and Valvassori 1964). An intralobar sequestration drains to the pulmonary veins; an extralobar sequestration drains to the vena cava, hemiazygos vein, azygos vein, or portal vein (Fig. 2.**4**).

Hypogenetic Lung Syndrome (Scimitar Syndrome)

■ Clinical Features

Hypogenetic lung syndrome almost always is seen on the right side. The right lung is hypoplastic, and both the right bronchial tree and pulmonary vessels show incomplete development. The hypoplastic lung therefore derives a significant proportion of its perfusion from the systemic circulation via branches of the aorta. The anomalous pulmonary vein runs inferiorly through the lung before curving medially to enter the inferior vena cava (IVC); it has the shape of a scimitar, thus accounting for the name of the syndrome. Congenital cardiac defects, usually septal defects, are present in 25 % of cases, and some patients also have bronchiectasis and tracheobronchial anomalies.

Clinically, patients may be asymptomatic or may suffer from recurrent infections. A significant left-to-right shunt may give rise to exertional dyspnea.

■ Radiologic Findings

The chest radiograph may show a small right lung and cardiac dextroposition. The "scimitar" vein descends vertically and then curves medially to join the IVC (Fig. 2.**5**). CT confirms the diagnosis and shows the scimitar vein draining to the IVC (Fig. 2.**6**) and the hypoplastic right pulmonary artery. It also may demonstrate associated bronchiectasis and tracheobronchial anomalies.

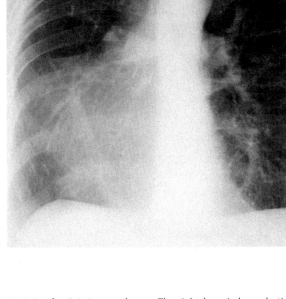
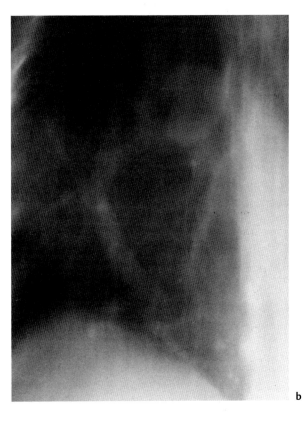

Fig. 2.**5 a, b** Scimitar syndrome. The right lung is hypoplastic and there is ipsilateral cardiac displacement. The right lower lobe vein drains to the vena cava (scimitar pattern), and the right upper lobe vein drains to the azygos vein.

a

b

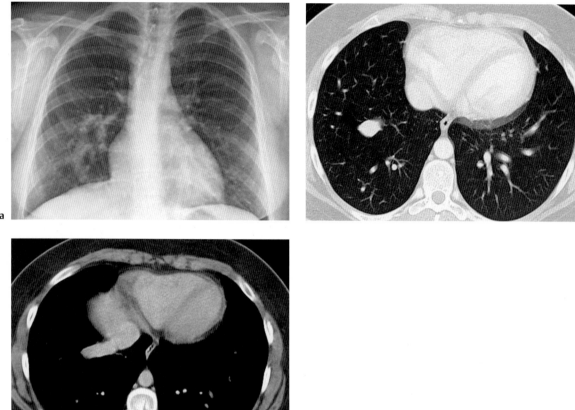

Fig. 2.**6a–c**   Scimitar CXR and CT. Chest radiograph (**a**) shows scimitar vein. Axial CT images (**b** and **c**) show vein traversing the right lower lobe and draining into the inferior vena cava.

Bronchogenic Cysts

■ Pathology

Both bronchogenic cysts and bronchopulmonary sequestrations embryologically are due to abnormal ventral budding from the foregut or tracheobronchial tree. However, in sequestration, there is subsequent induction of mesenchyme to form lung parenchyma. Bronchogenic cysts result from a failure in this induction process. Most bronchogenic cysts arise within the mediastinum or at the hilum; the remainder are intrapulmonary (Dee 1995c, Reed 1974).

Intrapulmonary Cysts

The central type of cyst occurs in the perihilar lung, is lined by respiratory epithelium, and contains viscous mucoid material. Peripheral lung cysts are usually multilocular and, when extensive, may be indistinguishable from congenital honeycomb lung.

Mediastinal Cysts

Bronchogenic cysts were described as mediastinal in 86, 77, and 65% of cases (Dee 1995, St-Georges 1991, Reed 1974, Di Lorenzo 1989). Most can be differentiated from esophageal duplications and enterogenic mediastinal cysts only by pathologic examination. The bronchogenic cyst is the most common congenital cyst of the mediastinum.

■ Clinical Features

Bronchogenic cysts may be an incidental radiographic finding in young adults. They become symptomatic if complicated by infection. Occasionally, a tension cyst develops through a check-valve mechanism and results in respiratory impairment (Fig. 2.**7**).

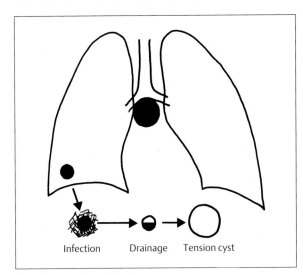

Fig. 2.**7** Bronchogenic cyst.

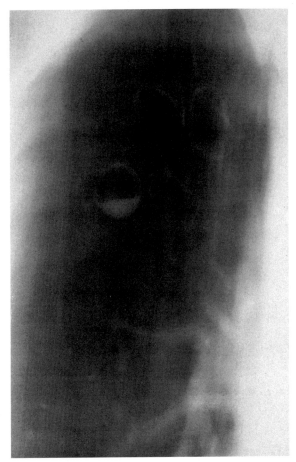

Fig. 2.**8** Multiple bronchogenic cysts. There is an air–fluid level in one cyst due to secondary infection.

■ Radiologic Findings

▒ Chest Radiograph

Two-thirds of intrapulmonary cysts occur in the lower lobes, appearing as well-defined homogeneous masses 2 to 4 cm in diameter. Mural calcification is rare. Cysts that have discharged their contents appear as thin ring shadows, which may contain an air-fluid level (Fig. 2.**8**). The rare tension cysts form a large air collection that displaces adjacent normal structures (Fig. 2.**9**).

Mediastinal cysts are smooth, round, homogeneous masses located adjacent to the trachea, carina, or main bronchi. They may compress the trachea or esophagus (Fig. 2.**10**).

▒ Computed Tomography

CT usually demonstrates a nonenhancing mass of variable attenuation molded to adjacent structures (Dee 1995). Mural calcification occasionally is seen.

▒ Magnetic Resonance Imaging

The MRI appearance of bronchogenic cysts has been described (Barakos 1989, Naidich 1988, Palmer 1991, Suen 1993). MRI signal intensity may be similar to water with low T1 and high T2 values. Bronchogenic cysts filled with blood, cholesterol, or proteinaceous material will be hyperintense on both T1- and T2-weighted sequences. Nonhomogeneous signal intensity may be due to hemorrhagic complications.

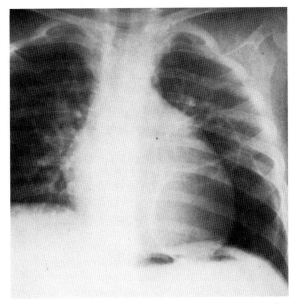

Fig. 2.**9** Tension cyst in the left lower lobe. Earlier studies showed a round homogeneous mass progressing to a small cyst.

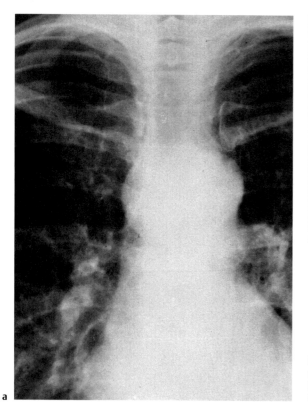

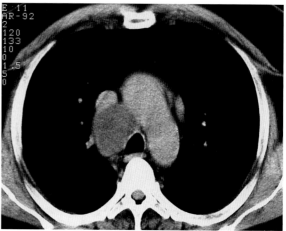

Fig. 2.**10a, b** Bronchogenic cyst. The chest radiograph (**a**) shows a round, sharply circumscribed mass in the right tracheobronchial angle. CT shows a round paratracheal mass of water attenuation (**b**).

Congenital Cystic Adenomatoid Malformation of the Lung (CCAM)

■ Pathology

This hamartomatous lesion accounts for 25% of all congenital pulmonary anomalies. It comprises fibrous tissue, smooth muscle, and back-to-back bronchiolar and duct-like structures of varying size. Cartilage is absent. This interconnecting system of clefts and cavities communicates with the adjacent parenchyma through the pores of Kohn. This permits collateral air drift and may account for the expansile nature of these lesions.

Congenital cystic adenomatoid malformation is classified into three types based on findings at microscopy.
- **Type 1 CCAM** contains large cysts lined by ciliated columnar epithelium.
- Multiple smaller cysts lined by columnar/cuboidal epithelium are found in **type II CCAM**. These have an association with other extrapulmonary congenital anomalies including renal agenesis.
- **Type III CCAM** contains bronchiolar and cleft-like structures which are lined by low cuboidal epithelium.

Both type II and III lesions are associated with a poor prognosis.

■ Clinical Features

Seventy to eighty percent of cases present in the neonatal period with symptoms of cough and dyspnea. Approximately 10% of cases present after the first year of life, usually with recurrent respiratory infections (Dee 1995).

■ Radiologic Findings

Type I CCAM is the most common (75%), and the chest radiograph may show an air-filled multicystic lesion with at least one dominant cyst greater than 2 cm in diameter. This produces local mass effect with displacement of adjacent pulmonary and mediastinal structures (Figs. 2.**11**, 2.**12**). There frequently is a degree of contralateral pulmonary hypoplasia. The size of the lesion may vary considerably on serial studies, and intercurrent mucus retention may produce granular and patchy opacities. Type II CCAM is composed of smaller, more uniform cysts, while type III lesions are solid masses composed of bronchoalveolar microcysts (Berrocal et al. 2003).

Antenatal sonographic diagnosis is possible, and a solid or cystic intrathoracic mass may be seen. There is frequently associated polyhydramnios and hydrops fetalis (Dee 1995).

The differential diagnosis includes congenital diaphragmatic hernia. This is associated with a "scaphoid" abdomen, whereas in CCAM the abdominal bowel gas pattern is normal.

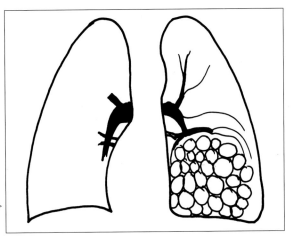

Fig. 2.**11** Congenital cystic adenomatoid malformation (CCAM), ▷ appearing as a hyperinflated cystic lesion with vascular displacement.

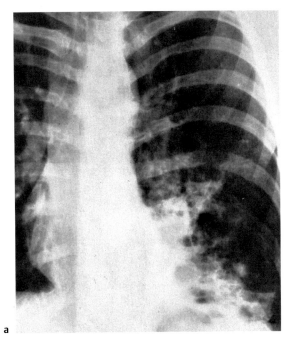

a

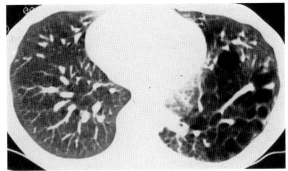

b

Fig. 2.**12 a, b** Congenital cystic adenomatoid malformation. Chest radiograph (**a**) shows increased left lung volume with mediastinal displacement to the right side and a pattern of cystic change and patchy opacification in the left lower zone. CT shows cystic transformation of the lower lobe with decreased vascularity (**b**).

Pulmonary Agenesis, Aplasia, and Hypoplasia

■ Pathology

Three degrees of severity are recognized in this failure of normal lung development (Fig. 2.**13**).

- *Pulmonary agenesis*, in which the lung and all associated structures are absent.
- *Pulmonary aplasia*, in which the lung parenchyma is absent but there is a rudimentary main bronchus which terminates blindly (Fig. 2.**14**).
- *Unilateral pulmonary hypoplasia*, in which a normally formed main bronchus terminates in a small, rudimentary lung with malformed lobes.

■ Clinical Features

Primary unilateral hypoplasia in the absence of scimitar syndrome is rare (Dee 1995). Patients may be asymptomatic, though affected children frequently are prone to bronchopulmonary infections. Some patients may have associated extrapulmonary anomalies.

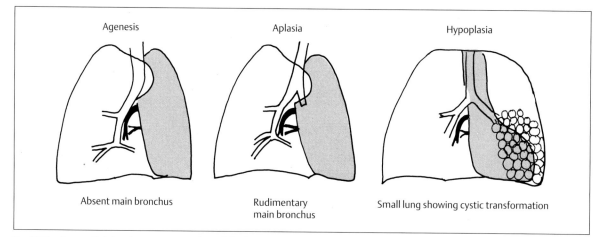

Fig. 2.**13**   Congenital development anomalies of the lung.

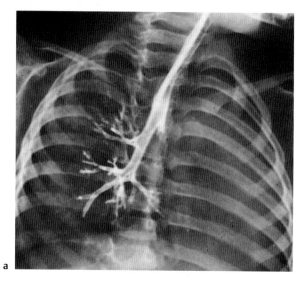

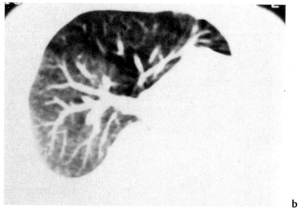

Fig. 2.**14 a, b**   Left lung aplasia. The stump of the left main bronchus is opacified at bronchography (**a**). Left-sided mediastinal displacement and right lung hyperinflation are seen (**b**).

■ Radiologic Findings

The affected hemithorax is small with narrow intercostal spaces, an elevated hemidiaphragm, and mediastinal displacement to the ipsilateral side. The contralateral lung shows compensatory hyperinflation with posterobasal and anteroapical herniation towards the affected side.

CT confirms pulmonary hypoplasia and accurately defines the extent of the herniation. The presence of a main bronchus serves to distinguish pulmonary aplasia from agenesis, although this distinction clinically is unimportant.

Pulmonary angiography shows large-caliber vessels in the opposite lung with an absent or rudimentary vascular system on the affected side.

■ Differential Diagnosis

The differential diagnosis includes pneumonectomy, congenital atelectasis, lobar emphysema, diaphragmatic hernia, fibrothorax, and MacLeod syndrome.

Congenital Lobar Emphysema

■ Pathology

Congenital lobar emphysema (CLE) is characterized by chronic hyperinflation of a lobe or one of its segments. Causes include congenital bronchial stenosis producing a check-valve obstruction and local mucous plugging. The etiology is unclear in 50% of cases. A polyalveolar variant of CLE also may occur, and in these cases the number of alveoli is increased. The left upper lobe is involved in 50%, the right middle lobe in 24%, and the right upper lobe in 18% of cases (Allen 1966, Kennedy 1991) (Fig. 2.15).

The lower lobes are involved in only 2% of cases (Dee 1995). There is an association with congenital heart disease (Hendren 1966).

■ Clinical Features

Patients present with tachypnea, tachycardia, and cyanosis in the first 2 to 4 weeks of life. In rare instances, a later manifestation may occur.

■ Radiologic Findings

In the first week of life, the affected lobe may present as an opaque mass due to retention of amniotic fluid distal to the obstruction. Later, the affected hemithorax is hyperlucent, the ipsilateral hemidiaphragm is depressed, and the mediastinum is shifted towards the contralateral side. The degree of mediastinal displacement increases in expiration (mediastinal flutter on fluoroscopy). Conventional and computed tomography demonstrate vascular markings in the hypertransradiant lung, a finding that excludes the presence of a pneumothorax or a tension cyst (Figs. 2.16, 2.17).

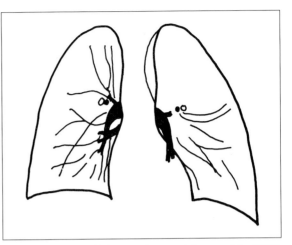

Fig. 2.**15**   Congenital lobar emphysema: left upper lobe (50%), right middle lobe (24%), right upper lobe (18%). Radiographs show localized hyperlucency with displacement of adjacent bronchovascular bundles.

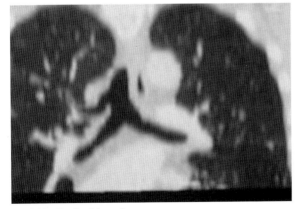

Fig. 2.**16**   Tracheal bronchus.

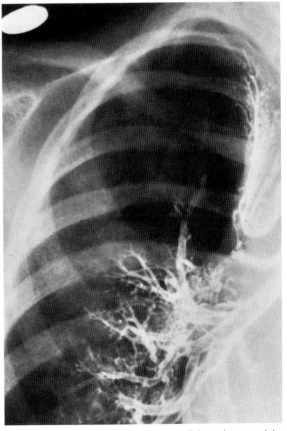

Fig. 2.**17**   Congenital lobar emphysema of the right upper lobe with bronchial displacement and crowding.

Congenital Bronchial Atresia

Congenital bronchial atresia frequently involves a segmental bronchus, and its functional effects usually are mild. The postatretic bronchi are structurally normal, although they may be ectatic and mucus filled (mucocele, mucoid impaction). The alveoli are aerated through

collateral air drift. The most common site is the apicoposterior segmental bronchus of the left upper lobe (Fig. 2.18).

■ Radiologic Findings

The chest radiograph shows an elongated, partially branched central opacity representing the mucocele. The affected lung segment may be hyperinflated and this combined with a degree of hypoperfusion results in hypertransradiancy.

Ventilation and perfusion scintigraphy confirm the absence of ventilation and diminished perfusion to the affected segment.

Helical computed tomography with reformats and three-dimensional reconstructions clearly depicts the mucocele, the focally decreased lung attenuation, and the hypoperfusion (Fig. 2.19).

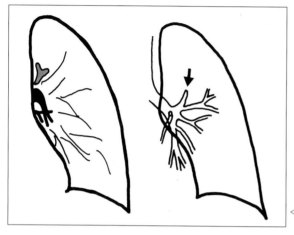

◁ Fig. 2.**18**   Bronchial atresia. The affected segment shows some degree of hyperinflation due to collateral air drift.

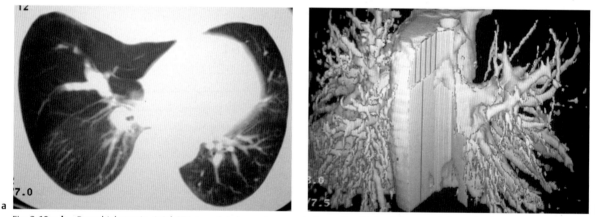

a   b

Fig. 2.**19 a, b**   Bronchial atresia. Axial CT image (**a**) shows decreased attenuation in the right upper lobe with a central tubular branching structure. SSD 3D reconstruction-posterior view (**b**) of pulmonary vasculature shows paucity of vessels to right upper lobe.

Vascular Malformations

Pulmonary Arteriovenous Malformations (AVM)

■ Clinical Features

Congenital pulmonary arteriovenous malformations may lead to cyanosis, polycythemia, and finger clubbing due to the presence of a right-to-left shunt. Hemoptysis, cardiac failure, and paradoxical emboli are uncommon. Some 50% of patients also have telangiectasia involving the buccal mucosa (Rendu–Osler–Weber telangiectasia), but only 15% of patients with Osler's disease have pulmonary AVMs.

■ Radiologic Findings

The chest radiograph frequently shows solitary (70%) or multiple (30%) well-circumscribed nodules in the lower zones (Fig. 2.**20**). These show active pulsations on fluoroscopy. Conventional pulmonary angiography (Fig. 2.**21**) has now been replaced by helical CT as the imaging modality of choice in the detection of pulmonary AVMs. CT angiography (CTA) is also useful in the pre-therapeutic evaluation of the angioarchitecture of these lesions as the number and orientation of feeding vessels are the most important factors in determining technical difficulty and duration of the embolization procedure (Remy-Jardin et al. 1999).

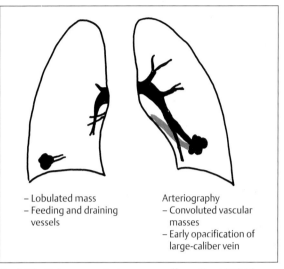

– Lobulated mass
– Feeding and draining vessels

Arteriography
– Convoluted vascular masses
– Early opacification of large-caliber vein

Fig. 2.**20**   Pulmonary arteriovenous malformations (AVMs).

Partial Anomalous Pulmonary Venous Drainage (PAPVD)

■ Clinical Features

Partial anomalous pulmonary venous drainage gives rise to a left-to-right shunt. PAPVDs are classified as supra-cardiac, cardiac, infradiaphragmatic, and mixed in type.

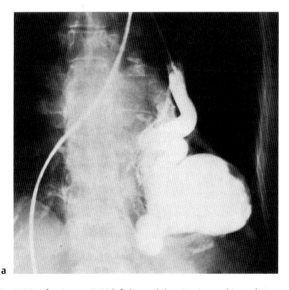

a

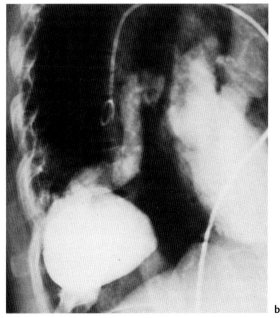

b

Fig. 2.**21 a, b**   Large AVM left lower lobe. Angiographic catheter is in the left lower lobar artery. There is early opacification of a markedly dilated left lower lobe vein.

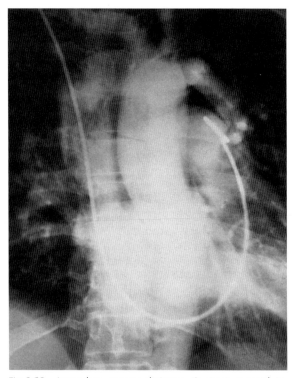

Fig. 2.**22** Anomalous venous drainage. Contrast material injected into the pulmonary artery opacifies the superior vena cava through a large-caliber left upper lobe vein (the aorta is also opacified).

A large shunt volume may result in right ventricular failure.

Scimitar syndrome is a specific example of PAPVD but with an associated lung bud anomaly.

■ Radiologic Findings

Occasionally, an anomalous vein is seen on the chest radiograph. These are recognized increasingly commonly at CT and may involve the left upper lobe with drainage of a vertical vein to the brachiocephalic vein (Alder et al. 1973) and the right upper lobe with drainage of a right superior pulmonary vein to the azygos vein (Thorsen et al. 1990). Careful evaluation of the CT study, however, is required to distinguish a persistent left superior vena cava (SVC) draining to the coronary sinus from left upper lobe PAPVD. The diagnosis may also be confirmed at angiography (Figs. 2.**22**, 2.**23**).

Hypoplasia and Atresia of the Pulmonary Artery

The pulmonary artery may be absent or atretic just past its origin. This entity is more commonly right-sided and when left-sided, there is an association with congenital cardiovascular anomalies. The affected lung and hilum are decreased in size and intrapulmonary vessels are decreased markedly in size and are systemic.

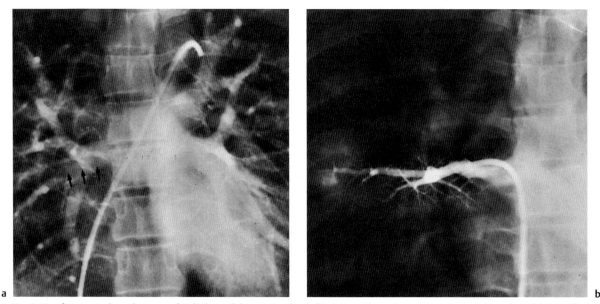

a   b

Fig. 2.**23 a, b**   Anomalous drainage of right lower lobe vein to the right atrium. The pulmonary angiogram is equivocal (**a**), but the anomalous drainage is confirmed by retrograde opacification of the vein from the right atrium (**b**).

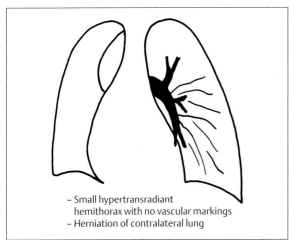

– Small hypertransradiant
  hemithorax with no vascular markings
– Herniation of contralateral lung

Fig. 2.**24** Pulmonary artery atresia.

■ Radiologic Findings

The chest radiograph shows a hypertransradiant lung which is reduced in size (Figs. 2.**24**, 2.**25**). There is no air trapping in contrast to the MacLeod syndrome of acquired constrictive bronchiolitis with secondary arterial hypoplasia.

Radionuclide perfusion scintigraphy demonstrates ventilation with no perfusion. CTA or MRI will confirm the diagnosis.

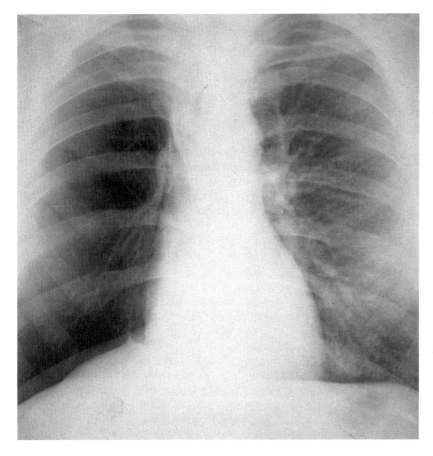

Fig. 2.**25** Congenital hypoplasia of the right pulmonary artery. Chest radiograph shows hypertransradiancy of the right lung with decreased vascularity. No air trapping was seen on the expiratory view.

3 Infection and Inflammatory Disorders

Pneumonia

Pneumonia is an infectious pulmonary process that may be caused by bacteria, mycoplasma, viruses, and other microorganisms. It is characterized by inflammatory exudate in both the alveoli and interstitium. Determination of the causative organism by sputum bacteriology or immunoserology may be helpful in initiation of therapy. Some textbooks classify pneumonias according to the causative organism (Murray 2000). However, given the similarity of the clinical manifestations and radiographic findings produced by different organisms, we shall focus our discussion on their morphologic features.

> **Goals of Diagnostic Imaging:**
>
> Confirm the presumptive clinical diagnosis; this frequently can be accomplished with frontal and lateral chest radiographs.
>
> Identify underlying predisposing factors such as bronchiectasis and bronchial neoplasia.
>
> Monitor the radiologic progression and resolution of disease.
>
> Detect complications such as cavitation, abscess formation, and development of empyema (Fig. 3.1).

■ Pathology

Morphologic classification distinguishes between lobar pneumonia, bronchopneumonia, and interstitial pneumonia. This classification depends on the nature and extent of inflammatory exudate in the alveoli and the degree of interstitial infiltration.

Lobar Pneumonia

Lobar pneumonia is an alveolar or airspace consolidation in which the causative organisms are inhaled. On reaching the alveoli, they proliferate and spread rapidly through the pores of Kohn across segmental boundaries until the entire lobe is involved. In lobar pneumonia there is relative sparing of the bronchi and interstitium.

The classic progression of lobar pneumonia through the stages of congestion (intra-alveolar edema), red hepatization (erythrocyte exudation), yellow hepatization (leukocyte exudation), gray hepatization (fibrinous change), and eventual lysis is rarely seen today. Effective antibiotic therapy also has led to a marked decrease in the incidence of lobar pneumonia.

Bronchopneumonia (Lobular Pneumonia)

Bronchopneumonia is acquired by inhalation or, less commonly, by hematogenous spread of the causative organism. On reaching the terminal and respiratory bronchioles, the organisms precipitate an inflammatory reaction which then spreads to adjacent alveoli. Further extension through the pores of Kohn results in involve-

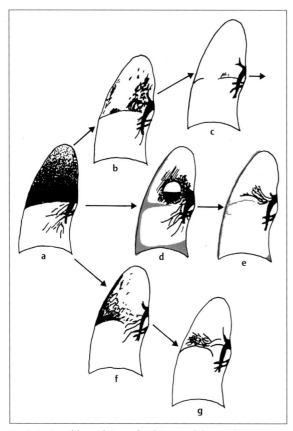

Fig. 3.1 Possible evolution of right upper lobar pneumonia. **a**, **b**, **c** Complete resolution. **a**, **d**, **e** Abscess formation with subsequent scarring and pleural thickening. **a**, **f**, **g** Pneumonia progressing to bronchiectasis (from Bohlig).

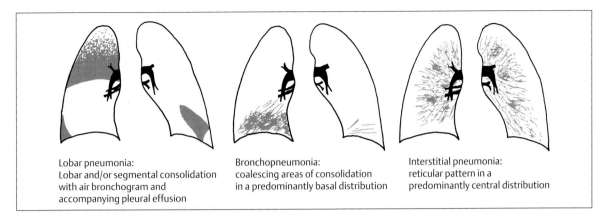

Lobar pneumonia:
Lobar and/or segmental consolidation
with air bronchogram and
accompanying pleural effusion

Bronchopneumonia:
coalescing areas of consolidation
in a predominantly basal distribution

Interstitial pneumonia:
reticular pattern in a
predominantly central distribution

Fig. 3.**2** Radiographic patterns of pneumonia.

ment of the entire secondary lobule. Bronchopneumonia tends to be multifocal and patchy in distribution, the infiltrated lobules being interspersed between areas of normally aerated lung. The most common causative organisms are *Staphylococcus aureus, Haemophilus influenzae, Pseudomonas* species, and anaerobes (Webb et al. 1992).

Interstitial Pneumonia

Inflammatory infiltration of the connective tissue framework of the lung is characteristic. Causative organisms include *Mycoplasma, Rickettsia,* and viruses. On reaching the bronchial wall via the airways, they destroy the ciliated epithelium, with resulting edema and lymphocytic infiltration of the bronchial mucosa. There is subsequent spread of the inflammatory process to the interlobular septa. There also is lymphocytic infiltration of the peribronchial alveoli and this appears similar to lobular pneumonia.

■ Clinical Features

Clinical manifestations include pyrexia, pleuritic chest pain, and cough productive of serous, purulent, or blood-stained sputum. Auscultatory findings of fine bubbling rales correlate with radiographic change in only 40% of cases. Leucocytosis with left shift and elevated antibody titers also may be present. Bacteriological diagnosis may be possible from sputum analysis with Gram stain and culture; serology may yield the diagnosis in atypical bacterial and viral pneumonia.

■ Radiologic Findings

The pathomorphologic classification of pneumonias may also be used to characterize their radiographic features, although differentiation is not always possible (Fig. 3.**2**).

Plain Chest Radiograph

Lobar Pneumonia

In classic lobar or segmental pneumonia, the radiographic features are characteristic with homogeneous opacification of the involved lobes or segments (Figs. 3.**3**–3.**5**). Segments often are incompletely opacified, and this makes their location difficult to determine except when the shadowing extends to a well-defined pleural/fissural margin. Patent bronchi within homogeneous consolidation appear as linear branching lucencies or, when seen end on, as rounded lucencies (air bronchogram). The volume of the affected segments may be diminished because of inflammatory narrowing of the airways and decreased surfactant production. Classic lobar pneumonia, caused by *Streptococcus pneumoniae* in 95% of cases, is extremely rare today. Segmental opacification, however, is quite common and very often represents confluent multifocal consolidation.

Bronchopneumonia

In bronchopneumonia, the radiologic pattern is that of multiple, ill-defined, confluent, nodular opacities, which represent multiple secondary lobules filled with inflammatory exudate (Figs. 3.**6**, 3.**7**). The nonhomogeneous pattern of ventilated and consolidated lobules results in a sponge-like pattern. Focal air trapping within secondary lobules due to check-valve obstruction of bronchioles may also contribute to this appearance. Poor aeration of the infected lung may lead to basal opaque bands similar to discoid atelectasis.

Interstitial Pneumonia

Inflammatory infiltration of the bronchial wall and interlobular septa leads to formation of linear and reticular opacities most marked in the perihilar lung. Simultaneously, focally confluent shadows are found which represent inflammatory exudate in the peribronchiolar alveoli (Fig. 3.**8**).

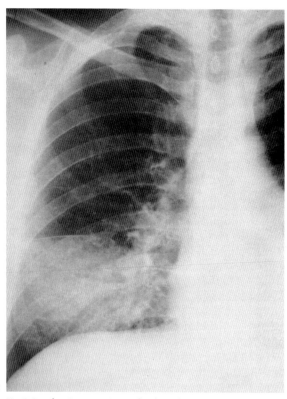

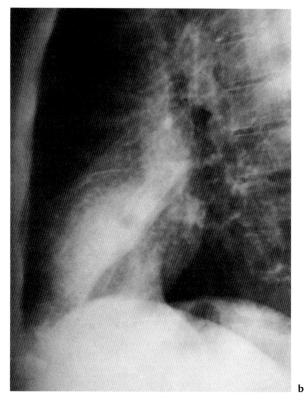

a

b

Fig. 3.**3 a, b** Pneumonia in the lateral segment of the right middle lobe: homogeneous consolidation with a sharp boundary anterosuperiorly at the minor fissure (**a**) and a well-defined poste-rior boundary at the major fissure (**b**). Patient presented clinically with pyrexia, productive cough, and leukocytosis.

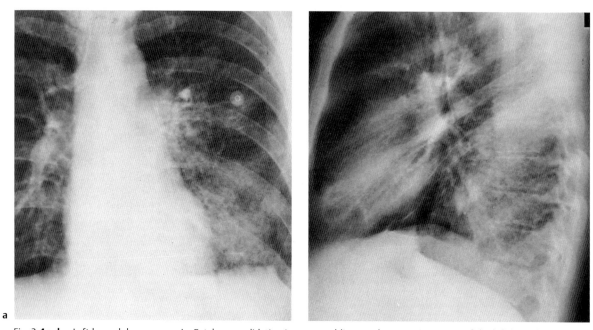

a

b

Fig. 3.**4 a, b**   Left lower lobe pneumonia. Patchy consolidation is seen to obliterate the posterior aspect of the left hemidiaphragm in the lateral view.

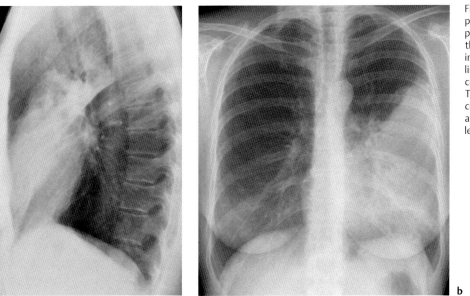

Fig. 3.**5a, b**   Lingular pneumonia. Note the posterior boundary of the major fissure (**a**), the indistinct cardiac outline, and the translucent costophrenic angle (**b**). There may be associated consolidation of the anterior segment of the left upper lobe.

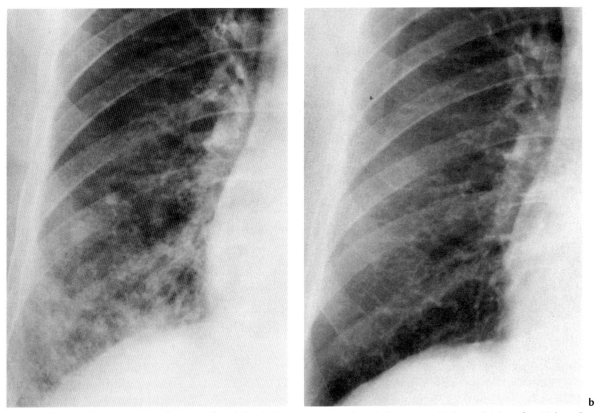

Fig. 3.**6a, b**   Bronchopneumonia. Diffuse reticulonodular shadowing is seen in the right lower zone. Radiograph taken after 10 days of antibiotic therapy shows complete resolution of change.

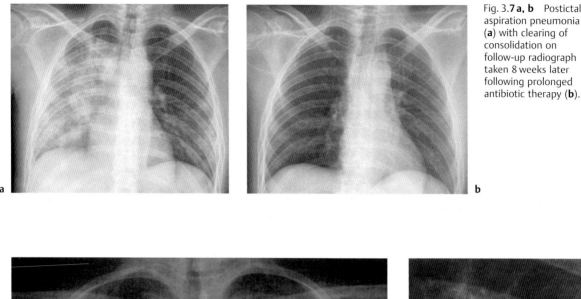

Fig. 3.**7 a, b**   Postictal aspiration pneumonia (**a**) with clearing of consolidation on follow-up radiograph taken 8 weeks later following prolonged antibiotic therapy (**b**).

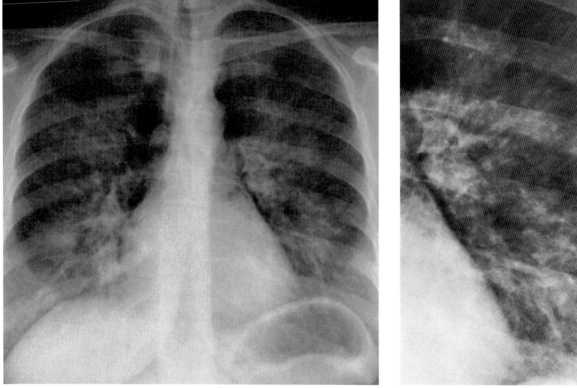

Fig. 3.**8 a, b**   Interstitial pneumonia. Radiograph shows increased perihilar linear markings in a patient who presented with cough, fever, hoarseness, and elevated mycoplasma antibody titers.

Parapneumonic Pleural Effusion

Pleural fluid usually collects adjacent to lobar pneumonia and causes homogeneous opacification of the pleural space. The effusion may form a spindle-shaped mass within the interlobar fissure, or it may be freely mobile and gravitate to the costophrenic sulcus, causing blunting of the costophrenic angle.

Computed Tomography (CT)

CT is rarely used in the investigation of community-acquired bacterial pneumonia; the diagnosis is usually based on clinical and plain radiographic findings. However, CT accurately demonstrates the extent of the pneumonia and allows for earlier detection than the plain radiograph. It also demonstrates complications such as pulmonary abscess formation and development of empyema.

Thin section/high resolution CT (HRCT) findings are similar to those found on the chest radiograph and include homogeneous consolidation with air bronchograms. Other manifestations of air space filling include ground-glass opacification and air space nodules.

Ground-glass opacification refers to a "hazy" increase in lung attenuation that does not obscure of pulmonary vessels. It may indicate interstitial thickening that is below the resolution of CT or partial filling of the alveoli.

Air space nodules range from 3 to 10 mm in diameter and probably represent peribronchiolar consolidation (Webb 1989, Murata 1986). They tend to be centrilobular in distribution but may spread and coalesce to give more extensive areas of patchy consolidation.

Lung Abscess and Septic Pulmonary Emboli

A lung abscess is a circumscribed area of inflammation with purulent liquefaction (Fig. 3.**9**). It may progress rapidly and erode into an adjacent bronchus or into the pleura. In this era of antibiotic therapy, abscess formation has become much less common though it remains a serious complication of pneumonia with reported mortality rates of 20–50%.

> **Goals of Diagnostic Imaging:**
> Detect abscess formation: this frequently is evident on the chest radiograph but CT may allow earlier detection and help to distinguish abscess from empyema formation.
>
> Detect predisposing factors such as aspirated foreign material, bronchial stenosis, and obstruction.

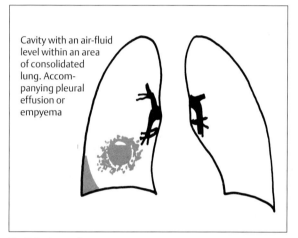

Cavity with an air-fluid level within an area of consolidated lung. Accompanying pleural effusion or empyema

Fig. 3.**9**   Lung abscess.

■ Pathology

Staphylococcal or *Klebsiella* pneumonia may be complicated by abscess formation. Abscesses also develop as a result of aspiration, as a complication of infarction, bronchiectasis, or distal to bronchial obstruction.

Multiple abscesses may also be a manifestation of septic lung emboli; this may be seen in the setting of a nidus of infection elsewhere (Fig. 3.**10**). Right-sided bacterial endocarditis including tricuspid valve infection in intravenous drug users, infected venous catheters, and bacterial pharyngitis/tonsillitis in the setting of Lemierre syndrome are recognized causes of septic pulmonary embolism (Fig. 3.**11**, 3.**12**).

The yellowish, purulent focus of the abscess is surrounded by a seropurulent exudate in the surrounding alveoli. In favorable cases the pus is expectorated and the process heals by scarring. In other cases residual cavities persist and may become colonized by *Aspergillus fumigatus* or other organisms. In severe cases the abscess may rupture into the pleural cavity, leading to formation of a pyopneumothorax.

In children, the residual lung cavity may hyperinflate via a check-valve mechanism, resulting in a pneumatocele which usually resolves in 4–6 weeks.

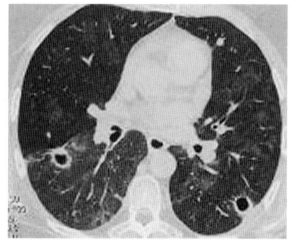

Fig. 3.**10**   Septic pulmonary emboli resulting from systemic sepsis in pyelonephritis.

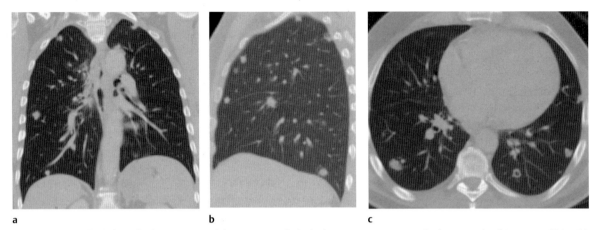

a   b   c

Fig. 3.**11 a–c**   Multiple foci of pulmonary consolidation, some of which show cavitation. Patient had an episode of acute tonsillitis with systemic sepsis.

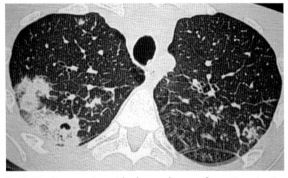

Fig. 3.**12**   Pneumonia with lung abscess formation in intravenous drug user. CT shows predominantly right-sided consolidation with areas of abscess formation.

■ Clinical Features

Symptomatology resembles that of acute pneumonia with fever, rigors, cough productive of purulent sputum, and leucocytosis. Patients with diabetes mellitus, alcoholism, and immunocompromised individuals are at increased risk of developing lung abscess.

■ Radiologic Findings

Plain Chest Radiograph

Most abscesses arise within areas of pneumonic consolidation and are marked by the development of a discrete area of low density necrosis and cavitation. The posterobasal segments of the lower lobes are most commonly involved (see Fig. 3.**9**).

Radiologic progression may be quite rapid. Rupture of an abscess into a draining bronchus produces a cavity with an air–fluid level (Fig. 3.**13**, 3.**14**). Multiple cavities developing within consolidated lung is known as necrotizing pneumonia.

Computed Tomography

CT allows earlier detection of abscess formation within areas of pulmonary consolidation than does the standard chest radiograph. CT is also superior in defining the relationship of the process to the pleural cavity, and the following features may help in differentiation from empyema:

Empyema tends to be lenticular in **shape**, and the angle of interface with the chest wall is usually obtuse. A lung abscess is usually spherical and produces an acute angle with the chest wall.

Empyema fluid lies between thickened parietal and visceral pleura (the split pleura sign; Fig. 3.**15**). This pleural thickening is relatively smooth in contrast to the wall of an abscess, which may be thickened, quite irregular, and contain locules of gas. Lung adjacent to an empyema is compressed with pulmonary vascular displacement. A lung abscess is associated with destruction of pulmonary parenchyma.

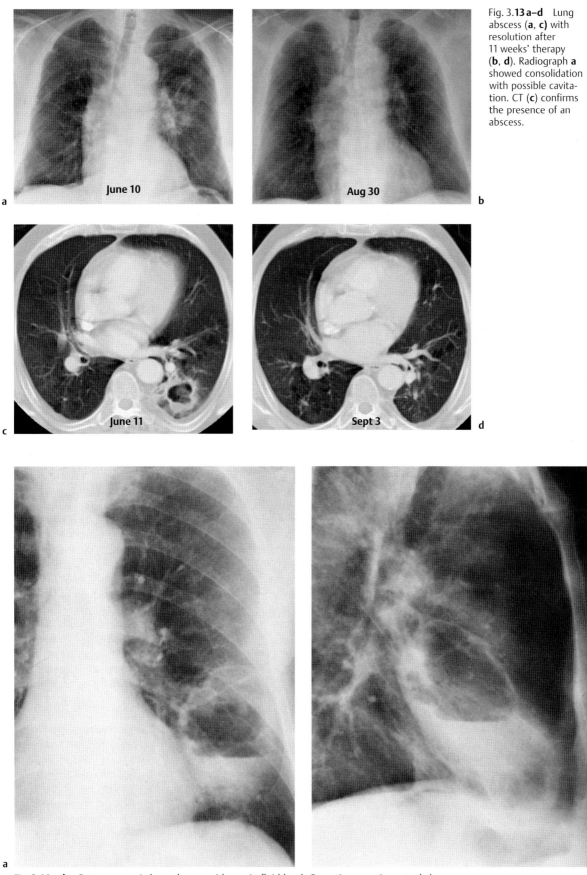

Fig. 3.**13 a–d**   Lung abscess (**a**, **c**) with resolution after 11 weeks' therapy (**b**, **d**). Radiograph **a** showed consolidation with possible cavitation. CT (**c**) confirms the presence of an abscess.

Fig. 3.**14 a, b**   Postpneumonic lung abscess with an air–fluid level. Causative organism: staphylococcus.

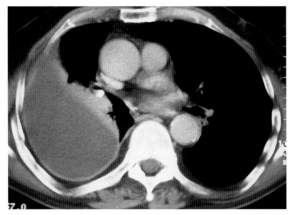

Fig. 3.**15** CT shows large right-sided empyema with "split pleura" sign.

Pulmonary Tuberculosis

Tuberculosis is an infectious disease which may affect any organ but shows a definite predilection for the lungs. In 95% of cases the causative organism is *Mycobacterium tuberculosis humanus*. A less common strain is *Mycobacterium bovis*. Atypical mycobacteria such as *M. kansasii* and *M. balnei* occur only sporadically. The incidence of another atypical mycobacterial infection, *mycobacterium avium complex* (MAC), increased markedly in the 1980s and 1990s mainly due to the increasing number of patients with acquired immunodeficiency syndrome (AIDS) and depleted helper T-lymphocyte CD4 counts (see p. 97).

In 1900, tuberculosis was still a worldwide epidemic with a mortality rate of approximately 250 per 100 000 per year. Effective antituberculous therapy and better socioeconomic conditions have substantially reduced the incidence and prevalence of tuberculosis, with a resulting decline in mortality rates. Mortality rates in Germany are less than 3 per 100 000 per year. In the United States, 1800 tuberculosis-related deaths are reported each year, corresponding to a mortality rate of less than 1 per 100 000 per year. There was a steady decline in the incidence of tuberculosis in industrialized countries during the second half of the 20th century until the mid 1980s. In Germany, the incidence had fallen from 174 new cases per 100 000 in 1942 to less than 32 new cases per 100 000 population in 1994 (1994 Report of the German Central Committee on Tuberculosis Control). However, in the late 1980s and early 1990s, this downward trend reversed, due mainly to the increasing numbers of cases in patients with AIDS (Im 1995). In the United States, there were approximately 20 000 new cases in 1985; this had increased to more than 25 000 new cases by 1990. More recently, the resurgence of tuberculosis in Western countries has also been attributed to immigration and the development of multidrug-resistant disease (MDR-TB; Faustini et al. 2006).

The incidence and prevalence of tuberculosis has always remained high in endemic regions and is the leading cause of death in patients with AIDS in developing countries.

The main factor determining whether tuberculous infection progresses to disease is the immune competence of the individual (Murray 1996). Today the disease most commonly is found in persons whose immune status is compromised by old age, alcohol abuse, diabetes mellitus, steroid therapy, or AIDS. There is also a relatively high incidence in certain ethnic groups, many of whom have recently immigrated to Western Europe and North America.

Tuberculosis is classically divided into primary and postprimary disease (Fig. 3.**16**). Some controversy exists as to whether the latter represents reactivation or reinfection (McAdams et al. 1995). Primary tuberculosis occurs in those not previously exposed to *M. tuberculosis*, is frequently asymptomatic, and therefore is not detected clinically. Postprimary or "cavitating" tuberculosis occurs in previously sensitized individuals; before the advent of antituberculosis chemotherapy, it was frequently fatal (*galloping consumption*). Today, fibrocirrhotic end-stage disease with severe ventilatory impairment may lead to eventual death from decompensated cor pulmonale.

The frontal chest radiograph remains the initial imaging investigation in tuberculosis. Some studies have emphasized the role of high-resolution CT, particularly in the detection of endobronchial spread (Lee 1991, Im et al. 1993, Hatipoglu et al. 1996). Bacteriological diagnosis is made from detection of acid-fast bacilli (AFB) in sputum, gastric washings, pleural fluid and, in patients proceeding to bronchoscopy, from bronchoalveolar lavage (BAL) fluid. Newer immunologic and nucleic acid-based techniques are also emerging (Furin and Johnson 2005).

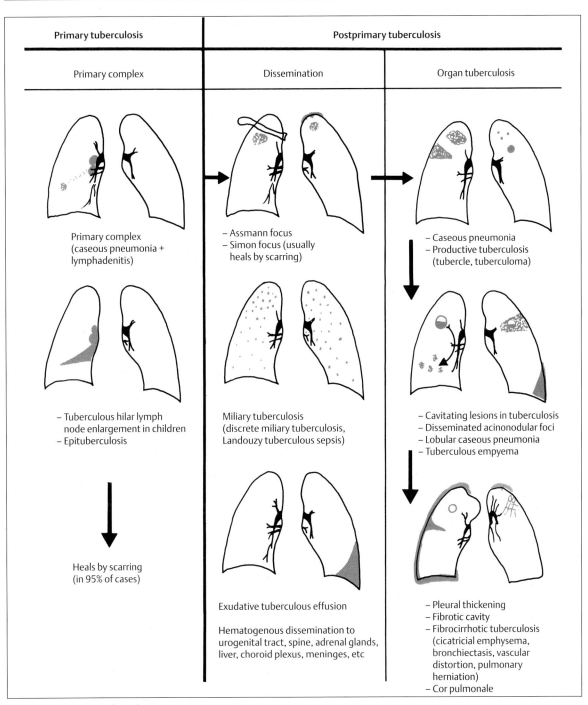

Primary tuberculosis	Postprimary tuberculosis	
Primary complex	Dissemination	Organ tuberculosis

Primary complex
(caseous pneumonia +
lymphadenitis)

– Assmann focus
– Simon focus (usually
  heals by scarring)

– Caseous pneumonia
– Productive tuberculosis
  (tubercle, tuberculoma)

– Tuberculous hilar lymph
  node enlargement in children
– Epituberculosis

Miliary tuberculosis
(discrete miliary tuberculosis,
Landouzy tuberculous sepsis)

– Cavitating lesions in tuberculosis
– Disseminated acinonodular foci
– Lobular caseous pneumonia
– Tuberculous empyema

Heals by scarring
(in 95% of cases)

Exudative tuberculous effusion

Hematogenous dissemination to
urogenital tract, spine, adrenal glands,
liver, choroid plexus, meninges, etc

– Pleural thickening
– Fibrotic cavity
– Fibrocirrhotic tuberculosis
  (cicatricial emphysema,
  bronchiectasis, vascular
  distortion, pulmonary
  herniation)
– Cor pulmonale

Fig. 3.**16**   Pulmonary tuberculosis.

Goals of Diagnostic Imaging:
Adequate screening programs to detect early disease particularly in high risk groups. In Germany, 30% of new infections are detected in this way.

Accurate interpretation of radiographic abnormalities with a relatively low threshold for suggesting tuberculosis in the differential diagnosis.

Monitoring the response to therapy with serial imaging.

Detecting the sequelae of healed tuberculosis such as cicatricial emphysema, bronchiectasis, and cor pulmonale.

■ Pathology

The German pathologist K. E. Ranke identified three stages in the evolution of tuberculosis. In modern nomenclature, the last two Ranke stages are included in the postprimary phase (Table 3.**1** and Fig. 3.**16**).

Table 3.**1** Stages of pulmonary tuberculosis (from Doerr, Schmidt, Schmincke)

A. Primary stage
Primary pulmonary focus (Ghon focus) and regional lymphadenitis = primary complex (dumbbell-shaped consolidation as described by K. E. Ranke)

B. Postprimary stage
I. Dissemination
    1. Early dissemination
        a) Simon foci
        b) Miliary tuberculosis
        c) Rarely in immunocompromised hosts: acute tuberculous sepsis (Landouzy)
    2. Late dissemination
        a) Subapical acinonodular disseminated foci
        b) Coarse granular dissemination (Aschoff–Puhl focus)
        c) Early infraclavicular consolidation (Assmann-Redeker-Simon)
II. Isolated organ tuberculosis
    1. Nodulation, fibrocirrhosis, cavitation
    2. Reticular lymphangitis

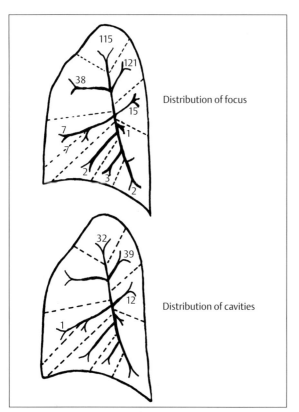

Fig. 3.**17** Frequency distribution of tuberculous lesions by lung segments (Doerr 1983).

Primary Complex

Inhaled tubercle bacilli initially evoke a focal, non-specific subpleural alveolitis which converts to a tuberculosis-specific inflammatory focus in about 10 days (Ghon focus). The latter is characterized by central colli-

quative necrosis, also termed caseous necrosis due to its grayish-yellow appearance. There is surrounding granulation tissue rich in lymphocytes, epitheloid cells, and Langerhans giant cells. Spread of tubercle via the lymphatics leads to a specific hilar lymphadenitis. In the great majority of cases, this primary complex (Ghon focus + regional lymphadenitis) heals with fibrosis and may calcify. Large infected lymph nodes may compress the bronchi, particularly the right middle lobe bronchus, with resulting distal atelectasis; this occurs almost exclusively in children (epituberculosis). In the severely immunocompromised patient, caseous lymphadenitis may erode into an airway resulting in tuberculous dissemination through primary endobronchial spread.

Hematogenous Dissemination

Mycobacteria entering the blood from the primary complex may become disseminated to numerous extrapulmonary sites (urogenital system, bones, meninges, adrenals, bowel, etc.).

- *Miliary tuberculosis*: Hematogenous dissemination appears as myriad small nodules (*millet seeds*) throughout the lung but displaying an upper zone predominance. These fine nodules are tubercles with a core of caseous necrosis and surrounding granulation tissue. Discrete miliary tuberculosis, characterized by fewer nodules, is associated with less severe degrees of immunocompromise. Disseminated tuberculosis with multiorgan involvement is associated with a high mortality rate.
- The most frequent pulmonary manifestation of hematogenous dissemination is the appearance of a *solitary tuberculous focus* at the lung apex (the Simon focus, Assmann infiltrate, subapical acinonodular focus). This predilection for the upper lobes is due to the higher tissue oxygen tension and relatively low perfusion in this region.
- *Exudative pleurisy*: Bacilli invade the pleura where they form tubercles; this is associated with development of a pleural effusion rich in lymphocytes.

Postprimary Organ Tuberculosis

This form of postprimary tuberculosis is characterized by cavitating lesions in the upper lobes or in the apical segments of the lower lobes (Fig. 3.**17**). Rupture of a parenchymal focus into an adjacent airway and subsequent endobronchial spread may lead to extensive pulmonary involvement.

- *Exudative tuberculosis* is characterized by a lobular, caseous pneumonia with relatively few epithelioid cells. Coalescence may occur to form larger foci of caseous pneumonia.
- *Productive tuberculosis* is characterized by well-defined solid nodules, 1–2 mm in diameter and rich in epithelioid cells; these correspond to the size of the primary lobule. If the immune response is weak,

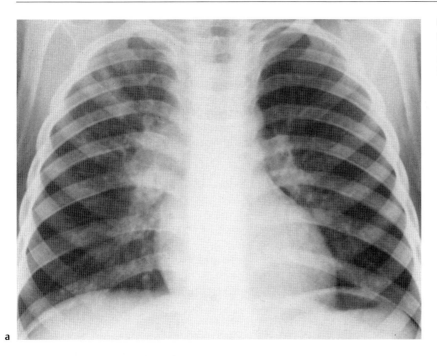

Fig. 3.**18 a, b** Acute primary complex. The hazy infiltrate in the right upper lobe, lymphatic stranding, and lymphadenitis form a dumbbell-shaped configuration.

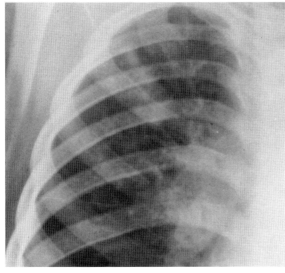

larger foci may develop (acinonodular form). Tuberculomas measuring 1–3 cm in diameter and comprising a caseous core surrounded by a mantle of granulation tissue are also found.

- *Cavitating tuberculosis*: Cavitation results from erosion of enlarging tubercles into the airway and associated liquefaction of caseous material. In active tuberculosis, the wall of the cavity contains infectious caseous material. Eventually, the cavity becomes fibrosed and may even acquire an epithelial lining.
- *Fibrocirrhotic tuberculosis*, in which the tuberculous process heals by fibrosis, is associated with fibrous contraction and distortion of the lung architecture leading to cicatricial emphysema and traction bronchiectasis.

■ Clinical Features

Primary tuberculosis usually is asymptomatic. Occasionally, low-grade pyrexia with night sweats, coughing, anorexia, and erythema nodosum develop. With progressive postprimary tuberculosis, the above clinical manifestations are present together with hemoptysis and dyspnea. The tuberculin skin test is positive, and acid-fast bacilli may be detected in the sputum, gastric washings, pleural and bronchoalveolar lavage fluid.

■ Radiologic Findings

Chest Radiograph

Primary tuberculosis is rarely detected on the chest radiograph. Positive radiographic findings are present in only about 20 % of children with a positive tuberculin skin test:

- The *Ghon focus* is a circumscribed, small, peripheral area of consolidation.
- *Hilar and mediastinal Lymphadenitis* presents as hilar enlargement and mediastinal widening. Occasionally, lymphangitic stranding connecting the primary focus with the hilar lymphadenitis forms a dumbbell-shaped opacity. This represents the primary complex (Fig. 3.**18**).
- *A segmental opacity* may be due to segmental atelectasis distal to bronchial compression by enlarged lymph nodes (epituberculosis).
- The *calcified healed primary complex* is a frequent incidental finding on chest radiographs and has no clinical significance (Fig. 3.**19**).

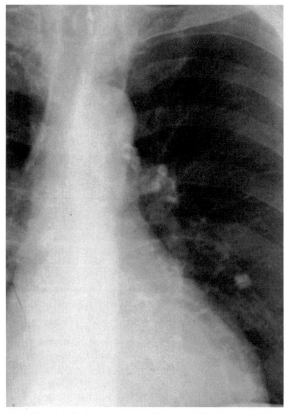

Fig. 3.**19** Calcified primary complex, considered a normal incidental finding.

Hematogenous Dissemination

- *Miliary tuberculosis* exhibits a finely mottled nodular pattern resulting from summation of individual nodules. The profusion of the mottling increases in an apicobasal direction. Occasionally, in advanced cases, miliary tuberculosis may produce a coarse granular or "snowstorm" pattern due to coalescence of the nodules (Fig. 3.**20**).
- *Exudative tuberculous pleuritis* radiographically resembles other effusions (Fig. 3.**21**).

Postprimary/secondary pulmonary tuberculosis produces a spectrum of radiographic manifestations; exudative, productive, cavitary, and fibrotic changes frequently occur simultaneously. Because of the predilection for the apical and posterior segments of the upper lobe and the apical segment of the lower lobe, parenchymal changes in these regions in the correct clinical setting should arouse suspicion of tuberculosis.

- *Exudative/productive tuberculosis* manifests as areas of confluent consolidation, or more discrete areas of nodular opacification may be seen. Fine nodular opacities may indicate bronchiolar involvement and endobronchial spread (Fig. 3.**22**).
- *Tuberculomas* form as pulmonary nodules or masses, 0.5–4 cm in diameter. They have smooth margins and a predilection for the upper zones (Fig. 3.**23**). In 80% of cases, conventional or computed tomography will show small satellite lesions and calcifications.

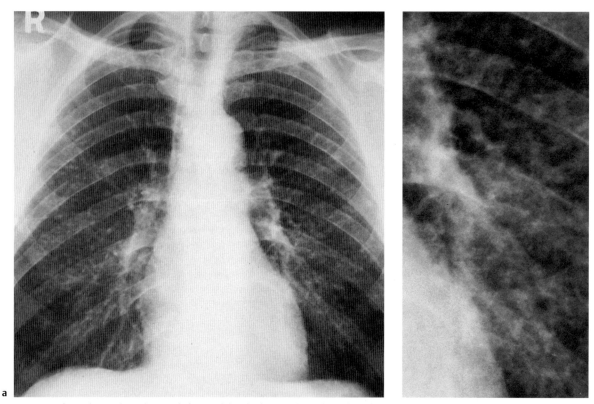

a   b

Fig. 3.**20 a, b** Miliary tuberculosis with fine nodular shadowing throughout both lungs.

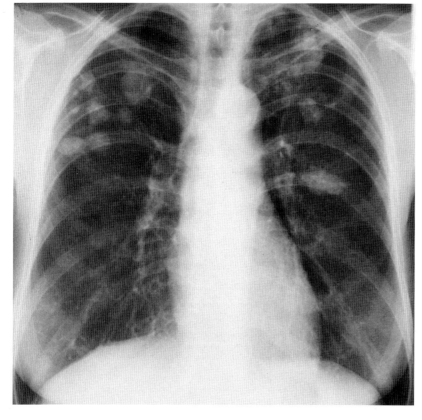

Fig. 3.**21** Tuberculous pleural effusion. Mycobacteria were cultured from the lymphocyte-rich pleural aspirate.

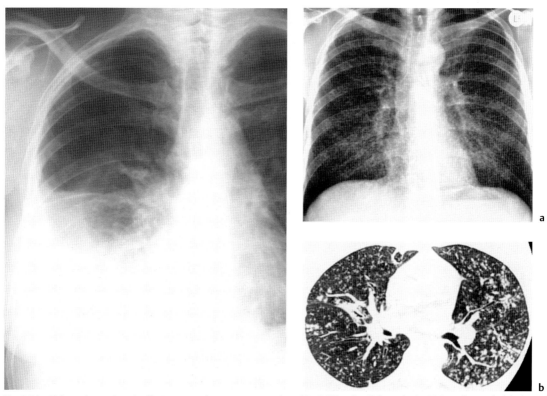

Fig. 3.**22 a, b** Tuberculosis. Plain radiograph (**a**) shows bilateral reticulonodular shadowing. CT (**b**) shows features of endobronchial spread.

Fig. 3.**23** Multiple tuberculomas.

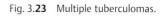

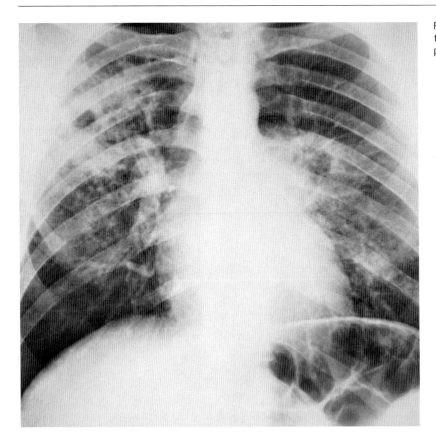

Fig. 3.**24** Exudative cavitating tuberculosis with areas of caseous pneumonia and liquefaction.

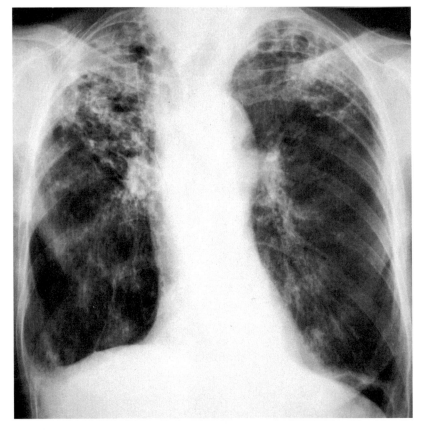

Fig. 3.**25** Fibrocirrhotic pulmonary tuberculosis. Upper lobe destruction and fibrosis are associated with elevation of the hila and compensatory emphysema in the lower zones.

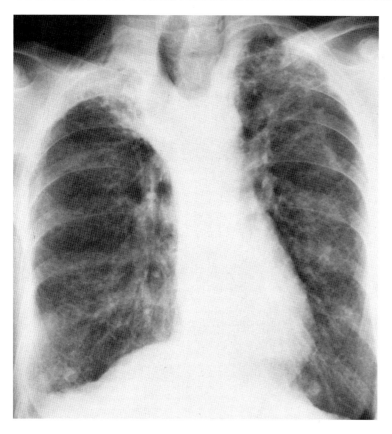

Fig. 3.**26**   Tuberculous pleural thickening and fibrocirrhotic pulmonary change.

- *Tuberculous cavities* are 5–10 cm in diameter and result from caseous necrosis of tuberculous pneumonia with subsequent expectoration of the contents. Cavities frequently are combined with disseminated acinar shadows due to endobronchial spread. Coalescence of the latter may occur (Fig. 3.**24**).
- Radiologic manifestations of *fibrotic tuberculosis* include apical pleural thickening, parenchymal scarring, calcification, and fibrotic bands radiating from the hilum to the apex. Cranial migration/elevation of hilar structures indicates fibrous contraction; eventually paracicatricial emphysema, bronchiectasis, and bronchovascular distortion may ensue (Fig. 3.**25**). A thick pleural peel may encase the residual lung and lead to thoracic deformity with kyphoscoliosis (Fig. 3.**26**).

Computed Tomography

CT manifestations of tuberculosis include:
- *Cavitation*: HRCT has been shown to be superior to the chest radiograph in demonstrating cavitation, particularly in cases complicated by fibrosis and architectural distortion (Im 1993, Naidich et al. 1984). Cavitation is frequently, but not invariably, an indicator of active disease (Fig. 3.**27**) as "healed" cavities may persist after antituberculous therapy (Webb et al. 1992).
- *Endobronchial spread*: Features of endobronchial spread are detected by HRCT in up to 98% of cases (Im 1993). These include centrilobular nodules or linear structures, "tree-in-bud" branching linear structures and poorly defined nodules (Fig. 3.**27**). Centrilobular nodules and tree-in-bud linear structures represent caseating material within the terminal and respiratory bronchioles (Im 1993). Poorly defined nodules probably represent peribronchiolar inflammation (Im 1993, Webb et al. 1992).
- *Miliary tuberculosis*: HRCT images show fine nodules that are distributed uniformly throughout the lungs (Fig. 3.**27**). These may be sharply or poorly defined and range in size from 1 to 4 mm in diameter (Oh 1994). These nodules are distributed randomly throughout the secondary lobule in contrast to the centrilobular nodules of endobronchial spread.
- *Fibrocirrhotic tuberculosis*: Findings indicating chronic parenchymal change include fibrotic bands, bronchovascular distortion, and cicatricial emphysema (Fig. 3.**27**).

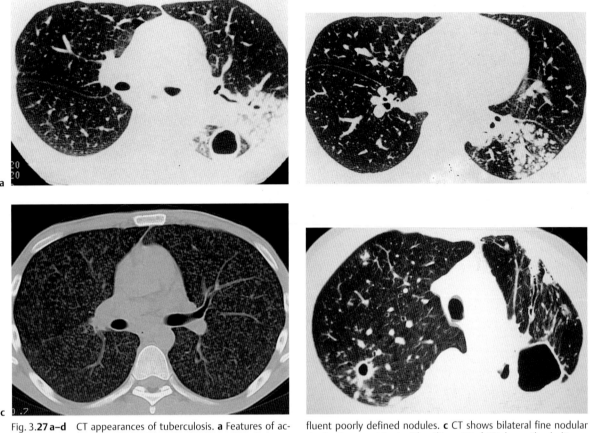

Fig. 3.**27 a–d**   CT appearances of tuberculosis. **a** Features of active postprimary tuberculosis with cavitating lesion in apical segment of left lower lobe and adjacent nodular shadowing in apicoposterior segment of left upper lobe. **b** Tuberculosis with features of endobronchial spread including centrilobular nodules, branching linear structures (*tree-in-bud* appearance), and confluent poorly defined nodules. **c** CT shows bilateral fine nodular shadowing consistent with miliary TB. **d** CT shows "healed" cavity with fibrosis in left upper lobe but with evidence of reactivated disease with cavitation and features of endobronchial spread in right upper lobe.

Fungal Diseases of the Lung

Fungal disease of the lung may be classified as endemic or opportunistic.

Endemic fungal diseases are caused by pathogenic fungi in an immunocompetent individual. They include histoplasmosis, coccidioidomycosis, blastomycosis, and sporotrichosis. These infections are endemic in the U.S., Africa, and Asia and are seen sporadically in Europe as a result of foreign travel.

Opportunistic fungal infection (aspergillosis, candidiasis) is caused by saprophytic fungi, which usually are present in the oral mucosa and become pathogenic in the immunocompromised host. These pneumomycoses have been encountered more frequently since the advent of antibiotics and chemotherapy. However, the overall incidence of pulmonary fungal infections remains low.

The clinical symptoms and radiographic findings of these diseases usually resemble those of bacterial pneumonia. Thin section/high resolution CT, in some cases, may be helpful in suggesting the diagnosis. Definitive diagnosis, however, is dependent on identification of the fungus at microscopy.

Candidiasis

■ Clinical Features

Candida albicans is part of the normal human microbial flora of the oral cavity. Pulmonary candidiasis occurs only in the immunocompromised individual.

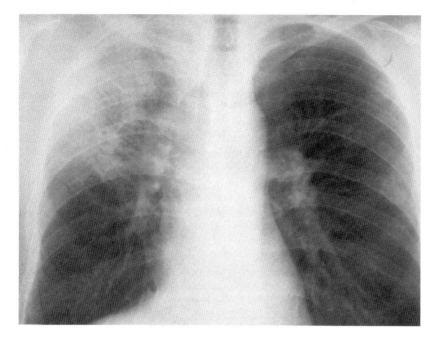

Fig. 3.**28** Candida pneumonia in a leukemic patient on chemotherapy, who presented with oral candidiasis. The right upper lobe continued to show patchy consolidation for several weeks, and two smaller cavitating foci developed on the left side.

Pulmonary candidiasis should be suspected in the presence of a pneumonia that is refractory to standard therapy or in the immunocompromised host with florid oral or esophageal candidiasis. The diagnosis may be established by demonstration of candida in transbronchial biopsy specimens. Sputum analysis is of no value because of the ubiquitous nature of the organism (Geary et al. 1980).

■ Radiologic Findings

A wide spectrum of radiographic findings has been described in candida pneumonia. Appearances may be indistinguishable from that of bacterial pneumonia with lobar or segmental consolidation (Fig. 3.**28**). Diffuse bilateral alveolar or mixed alveolar-interstitial shadowing may be seen (Buff et al. 1982; Fig. 3.**29**). Candida pneumonia may present as multiple small pulmonary abscesses; these may be randomly distributed if hematogenous spread has occurred or peribronchiolar when resulting from aspiration (Müller 1990). A miliary–nodular pattern has been described in pulmonary candidiasis (Pagani 1981), and diffuse pulmonary hemorrhage is also recognized as a manifestation (Müller 1991).

Aspergillosis

Aspergillus fumigatus, A. flavus, and *A. niger* are ubiquitous and flourish in substances such as cereal grains. They also constitute part of the flora of the healthy oral

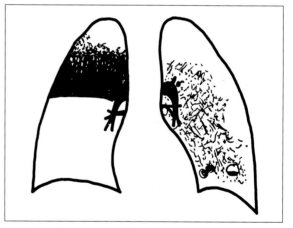

Fig. 3.**29** Pulmonary candidiasis may present as lobar pneumonia, interstitial pneumonia, or bronchopneumonia with cavitation.

cavity. The following are recognized manifestations of aspergillosis.

Primary invasive aspergillosis develops when massive amounts of fungal spores are inhaled, usually from cereal dust. The hosts have normal immunity.

Secondary angioinvasive aspergillosis occurs as an opportunistic infection in patients with severe debilitating illness, particularly leukemia and lymphoma, or in those undergoing prolonged therapy. Pathologically, this disease is characterized by mycotic vascular invasion, thrombosis, and hemorrhagic infarction with subsequent necrosis and cavitation. Invasive aspergillosis is associated with a mortality of 60 to 70%, and, in survivors, there is a 50% recurrence rate.

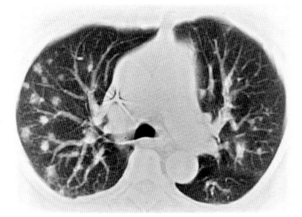

Fig. 3.**30**   Angiocentric invasive aspergillosis, confirmed at autopsy.

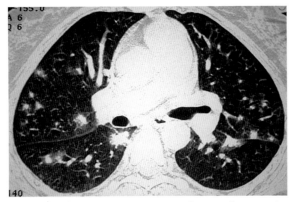

Fig. 3.**31**   Angiocentric invasive aspergillosis—early-stage disease with multiple areas of nodular consolidation some of which have a rim of ground-glass opacification highly suggestive of invasive fungal infection.

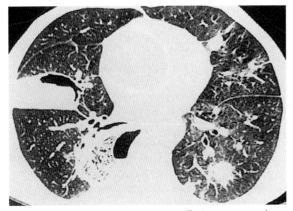

Fig. 3.**32**   Angiocentric invasive aspergillosis—recovery phase. Bilateral multifocal rounded consolidation with "air crescents" visible on the right side.

The initial *chest radiograph* may be normal. Multiple foci of consolidation may be present; these are frequently rounded in shape and probably represent infarcted parenchyma (Hruban et al. 1987). The characteristic "air crescent" sign develops late in the course of the disease and usually is associated with a recovering neutrophil count. It is seen in approximately 40% of cases and is associated with improved survival rates.

Computed tomography shows characteristic findings that strongly suggest the diagnosis early in the course of the disease (Kuhlman et al. 1988 and 1987). In early invasive aspergillosis, a "halo" of ground-glass opacification surrounds dense parenchymal foci (Fig. 3.**30**, Fig. 3.**31**). This represents a rim of hemorrhage or coagulation necrosis surrounding an area of infarction (Hruban et al. 1987). The halo sign precedes the air crescent sign (Fig. 3.**32**) by up to 2 weeks (Kuhlman et al. 1987).

Magnetic resonance imaging may also be helpful in early diagnosis of invasive aspergillosis (Herold 1989). On standard T1-weighted spin echo sequences, rounded consolidations have a target appearance with a hypointense center and hyperintense rim; the rim enhances on administration of intravenous gadolinium.

Invasive aspergillosis of the airways: Aspergillosis centered on the airways accounts for 14–34% of cases (Orr 1978, Young 1970) and also occurs in immunocompromised patients. Diagnosis is based on the presence of organisms deep to the basement membrane. CT findings include lobar consolidation, bilateral peribronchial consolidation, ground-glass attenuation, and centrilobular nodules less than 5 mm in diameter (Logan 1994).

Allergic bronchopulmonary aspergillosis (ABPA) represents a hypersensitivity reaction, usually in asthmatics, and manifestations include asthma, blood eosinophilia, precipitating antibodies to *Aspergillus* and elevated IgE titers. Pathologically, mycelial plugs develop in the proximal airways (Gefter et al. 1981), but, in contrast to invasive aspergillosis of the airways, tissue invasion is minimal or absent (Glimp and Bayer 1981).

The chest radiograph shows transient infiltrates in a lobar, segmental, or subsegmental distribution which predominantly involve the upper lobes. Atelectasis is less common, occurring in 3–46% of cases (Gefter et al. 1981, Malo et al. 1977). Bronchoceles also are a frequent radiographic manifestation of ABPA; these vary in shape but classically present a "gloved-finger" appearance. The lung distal to the bronchocele is aerated by collateral air drift. Eventually, central bronchiectasis involving the inner two-thirds of the bronchial tree and showing an upper lobe predominance may develop (Fig. 3.**33 a, b**).

Aspergilloma is the most common form of aspergillosis. It occurs in hosts with normal immunity, and the fungus colonizes preexisting cavities (cysts, tuberculous cavities, cystic bronchiectasis) and forms a fungus ball. This may erode the cavity wall both mechanically and through enzymatic action and lead to hemoptysis; this occurs in 50–80% of cases and may occasionally be life

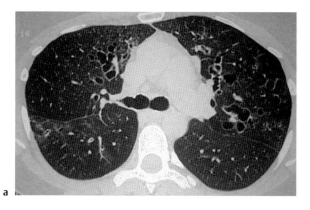

a

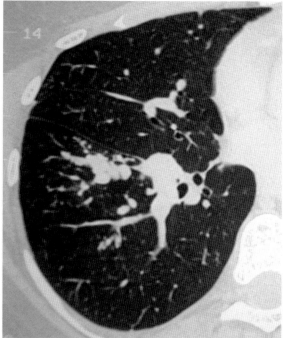

b

Fig. 3.**33a, b**   Allergic bronchopulmonary aspergillosis. Varicose bronchiectasis is seen in both upper lobes (**a**) with extensive mucoid impaction in the apical segment of the right lower lobe (**b**).

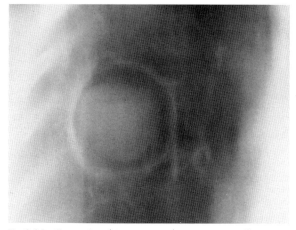

Fig. 3.**34**   Conventional tomogram shows an aspergilloma occupying an old tuberculous cavity.

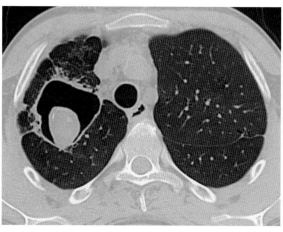

Fig. 3.**35**   CT of aspergilloma in an emphysematous bulla. The wall of the cavity is thickened due to recurrent episodes of inflammation. The aspergilloma is partially calcified.

threatening (Faulkner et al. 1978, Freundlich and Israel 1973, Jewkes et al. 1983).

The *chest radiograph* shows a round, homogeneous opacity which is mobile within the cavity. A circular or crescent-shaped air space may be visible between the mycetoma and the cavity wall (Fig. 3.**34**). Localized pleural thickening may be seen adjacent to the cavity, indicating superimposed aspergillus infection (Libshitz 1974).

CT will show the mycetoma of inhomogeneous attenuation and the surrounding crescent of air within the cavity (Figs. 3.**35**, 3.**36**). The mobility of the intracavitary

mass may be demonstrated by image acquisition in the prone position. The mycetoma has a characteristic sponge-like appearance and contains multiple foci of air (Armstrong et al. 1995, Roberts et al. 1987).

ABPA may be diagnosed by microscopic detection of *Aspergillus* mycelia in the bronchial aspirate. Aspergilloma may be largely a radiologic diagnosis. Both transbronchial and open lung biopsy may be hazardous in the immunocompromised with bone marrow suppression. Sputum analysis has no value because the sputum contains nonpathogenic fungi.

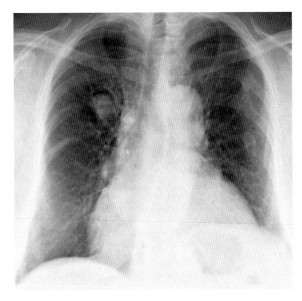

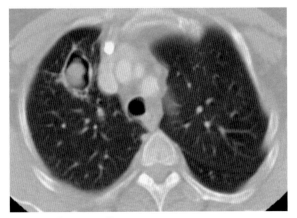

Fig. 3.**36 a, b**   Aspergilloma.

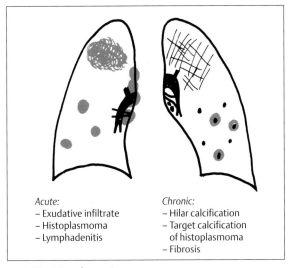

Acute:
– Exudative infiltrate
– Histoplasmoma
– Lymphadenitis

Chronic:
– Hilar calcification
– Target calcification
  of histoplasmoma
– Fibrosis

Fig. 3.**37**   Histoplasmosis.

Histoplasmosis

■ Clinical Features

Histoplasmosis is a fungal infection that occurs mainly in North America. Except for an endemic region in northern Italy, it occurs only sporadically in Europe. Pulmonary changes caused by *Histoplasma capsulatum* are comparable to tuberculosis in both primary and postprimary phases of development.

Acute histoplasmosis develops as a result of airborne primary infection. An incubation period of 2 weeks precedes the onset of pyrexia, malaise, dyspnea, productive cough, and hemoptysis; this infection may also run an asymptomatic course.

■ Radiologic Findings

- The *chest radiograph* shows multiple, ill-defined areas of consolidation throughout both lungs. There is accompanying hilar and mediastinal lymphadenopathy (Fig. 3.**37**). These pneumonic consolidations heal, leaving residual pulmonary granulomata that undergo central calcification to produce a target pattern (Connell and Muhm 1976; Fig. 3.**38**). When granulomata are multiple, calcification occurs in up to 75% of cases, but only 25% of solitary granulomata will calcify.
- *Chronic progressive histoplasmosis* is the consequence of reactivation and has a poor prognosis. Progressive cavitation with fibrosis may progress to complete lung destruction.

Coccidioidomycosis

■ Clinical Features

Coccidioidomycosis is endemic in the southwestern United States. It usually is asymptomatic and only the coccidioidin skin test is positive with elevated complement fixation. In those who become symptomatic, manifestations include severe pneumonia, pulmonary cavitation, pleurisy, and pericarditis. The development of pulmonary fibrosis represents end-stage disease (Bayer 1981, McGahan et al. 1981).

■ Radiologic Findings

The chest radiograph shows pneumonic consolidation and pulmonary nodules (coccidioidomas) that occasionally cavitate. In disseminated coccidioidomycosis, there is a generalized micronodular pattern (Fig. 3.**39**).

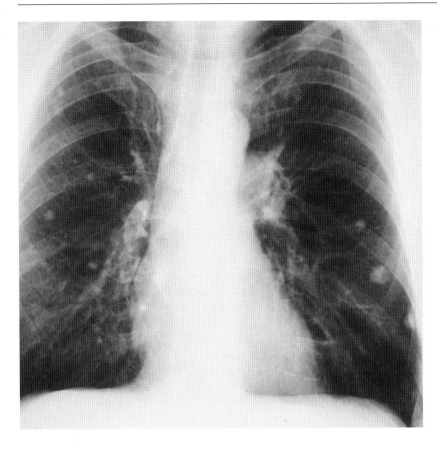

Fig. 3.**38** Histoplasmosis. Disseminated, calcified granulomas were
found in a North American male
who had a history of histoplasmosis
20 years earlier.

Changes of pulmonary fibrosis are associated with advanced disease.

Actinomycosis

■ Clinical Features

Actinomyces israelii is intermediate between mycelial fungi and bacteria and is a common saprophyte in the human mouth, especially in the presence of dental caries. This is a relatively rare disease entity and involves the cervicofacial region, the intestinal tract, and the lung. In the thorax, manifestations include chronic cavitating pneumonia, pleural empyema, and chest wall invasion (Fig. 3.**40**).

■ Radiologic Findings

The chest radiograph shows nonsegmental, predominantly peripheral consolidation that may cavitate. Consolidation typically crosses interlobar fissures. Pleuroesophageal and pleuropulmonary fistulae, pleural empyema, rib osteomyelitis, and inflammatory soft tissue masses of the chest wall may develop.

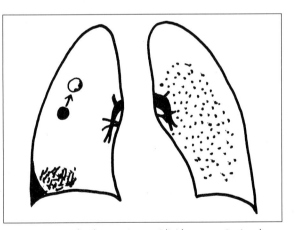

Fig. 3.**39** Coccidioidomycosis: coccidioidomas, cavitation, bronchopneumonia, pleural involvement, and widespread microgranulomas. Pulmonary fibrosis is present in end-stage disease.

Nocardiosis

Nocardia asteroides is a ubiquitous aerobic saprophyte found in the soil. It is a weakly acid-fast bacillus, which, after inhalation, may infect the lung sporadically. Pulmonary nocardiosis may be similar to actinomycosis in its radiographic appearance. Single or multiple

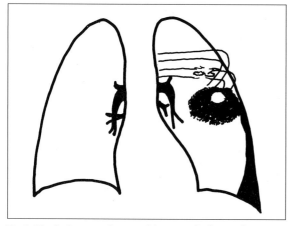

Fig. 3.**40** Actinomycosis: consolidation with abscess formation, pleural empyema, osteomyelitis, chest wall abscess.

Fig. 3.**41** Cryptococcosis: tumor-like masses with liquefaction, subpleural granulomas, and bronchopneumonia.

parenchymal abscesses frequently are seen, and pleural involvement is also common. There is an increased incidence of nocardiosis in the immunocompromised, in AIDS, and in alveolar proteinosis.

Cryptococcosis (Torulosis)

Cryptococcosis results from inhalation; the spores of *Cryptococcus neoformans* are found in dust and excreta (e. g., pigeon droppings) and cause pulmonary infection in immunocompromised hosts. The chest radiograph shows small, subpleural granulomas, foci of bronchopneumonia, and round masses (torulomas), which may cavitate (Fig. 3.**41**).

Other mycoses like North and South American blastomycosis, sporotrichosis, and mucormycosis are extremely rare and present radiologically as nonspecific pneumonic infiltrates. Diagnosis is based on demonstration of the fungus in tissue, smear, or culture.

Parasitic Infections

Parasitic infections are most prevalent in Asia, Africa, South America, and the Mediterranean basin. The causative organisms are protozoa (ameba, toxoplasma,) and helminths (echinococcus, schistosomes, ascarids, etc.). They induce hypersensitivity reactions in the lungs with formation of an eosinophilic "Loeffler" infiltrate. Parasites may colonize the lungs and form cysts, granulomata, and abscesses. Radiographic abnormalities together with blood eosinophilia should raise the suspicion of a parasitic pulmonary infection. Diagnosis is confirmed by identification of parasites in the sputum, stool, and urine, and if necessary by biopsy and histological assessment.

Amebiasis

■ Clinical Features

Amebae are found worldwide but are endemic in the Mediterranean region. They are ingested in contaminated food and initially induce colitis (amebic dysentery). They reach the liver via the bloodstream and form hepatic abscesses, which may extend through the diaphragm to infect the lung. Direct hematogenous spread from the liver to the lung is rare. Clinical manifestations include cough, blood eosinophilia, and expectoration of bile when a hepatobronchial fistula is present (Meng 1994).

■ Radiologic Findings

In 95 % of cases, the chest radiograph shows opacification of the right lower hemithorax due to pneumonic consolidation and an accompanying pleural effusion. The initially ill-defined infiltrate may form an abscess (Fig. 3.**42**).

Toxoplasmosis

■ Clinical Features

Infestation with *Toxoplasma gondii* is common but rarely leads to disease. Congenital toxoplasmosis due to transplacental infection is the most important form and presents with encephalitis and chorioretinitis. Adult toxoplasmosis is relatively uncommon except in patients with AIDS, in whom it is the most common cause of focal central nervous system lesions. In the HIV-negative population, it manifests as lymphadenitis and occasionally as interstitial pneumonia.

■ Radiologic Findings

Radiographs show focal reticular, linear, and ill-defined opacities resembling acute viral pneumonia. Associated hilar lymph node enlargement is frequent (Müller and Fraser 2001; Fig. 3.**43**).

Pneumocystis Jiroveci Pneumonia (Previously Known as Pneumocystis Carinii Pneumonia—PCP)

■ Clinical Features

Pneumocystis jiroveci/carinii pneumonia was originally described in premature infants. In adults, it is a frequent pathogen in the immunocompromised. The marked increase in the incidence of PCP has largely resulted from the acquired immunodeficiency syndrome epidemic; 60–70 % of patients with AIDS will develop PCP, and in the 1990s, it was the most frequent index disease for AIDS in industrialized countries (40 %) (Kuhlman 1996, Safrin 1993, Naidich and McGuinness 1991). It continues to be a significant cause of morbidity in HIV/AIDS and more recent studies have indicated that it is second only to bacterial pneumonia in the etiology of pulmonary complications (Benito Hernandez et al. 2005).

Initial growth of pneumocystis is in the alveoli where it becomes attached to Type 1 pneumocytes. Damage and death of these cells destroys the integrity of the

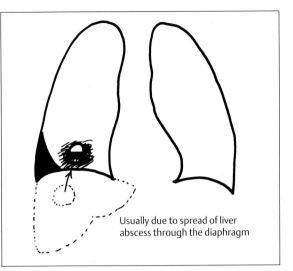

Fig. 3.**42** Amebiasis (amebic abscess): pleural effusion, basal pneumonia with cavitation.

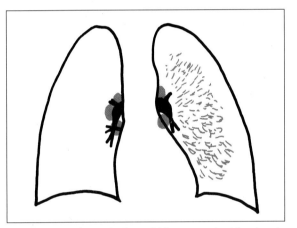

Fig. 3.**43** Toxoplasmosis: interstitial pneumonia, hilar lymphadenopathy.

alveolar-capillary membrane, and filling of the alveoli with eosinophilic exudate occurs. Concomitant activation of macrophages and plasma cells in the interstitium results in an interstitial pneumonitis (Kuhlman 1996).

In HIV-positive patients, the preferred method of diagnosis is induced sputum samples proceeding to bronchoalveolar lavage when necessary. Transbronchial biopsy is avoided because of the associated high mortality and risk of pneumothorax in these patients. In patients without AIDS, transbronchial or open lung biopsy is appropriate (Geary et al. 1980, Kuhlman 1996).

▓ Radiologic Findings

Chest Radiograph

The initial chest radiograph may be normal, but in 80 % of cases it shows diffuse, bilateral, granular, or reticular infiltrates (Kuhlman 1996, Safrin 1993, Naidich et al. 1991, Goodman 1991, DeLorenzo et al. 1987). These may involve the perihilar and lower zones or have an upper lobe distribution. Progression to diffuse air space consolidation may occur. Hilar lymph node enlargement and pleural effusions are unusual.

Computed Tomography

In acute PCP, the commonest HRCT finding is bilateral ground-glass opacification. Less commonly, a mosaic pattern with scattered foci of parenchymal involvement interspersed with normal lung is found (Fig. 3.**44**). In a

proportion of cases, thickened interlobular septa are found in association with ground-glass opacification (Bergin et al. 1990). Progression to diffuse homogeneous ground-glass opacification with sparing of the subpleural lung may occur (Kuhlman 1990, Scott 1991).

Recent years have seen a change in the pulmonary manifestations of pneumocystis infection. Cystic lung disease, spontaneous pneumothorax, and an upper lobe distribution of opacification are now seen more frequently (Figs. 3.**45**, 3.**46**). In the past, these were usually associated with aerosolized pentamidine prophylaxis but this has now been largely replaced by more effective chemoprophylaxis (Boiselle et al. 1999).

Schistosomiasis

▓ Clinical Features

Schistosomiasis hematobium is endemic in North Africa, *Schistosoma mansoni* in South America and the Caribbean, and *Schistosoma japonicum* in Japan. Cercariae, the infective larvae, penetrate the skin, enter the capillaries, and migrate through the systemic venous system to the right heart. From there they enter the pulmonary circulation and subsequently the systemic arterial system to reach the liver, kidneys, and urinary bladder. Diagnosis is based on identification of *Schistosoma* eggs in the stool and urine.

▓ Radiologic Findings

The chest radiograph shows transient pulmonary infiltrates representing an eosinophilic Loeffler-type pneumonia which is associated with passage of the larvae

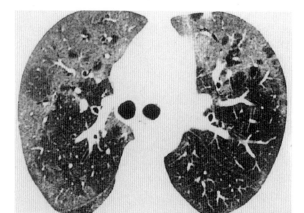

Fig. 3.**44**   Pneumocystis pneumonia. Ground-glass opacification involving both upper lobes. Some inhomogeneity is seen anteriorly with sparing of scattered secondary pulmonary lobules.

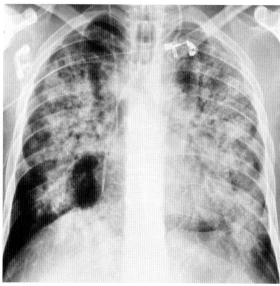

a

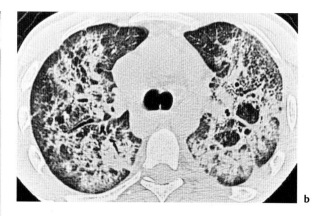

b

Fig. 3.**45 a, b**   Pneumocystis infection in a renal transplant patient. Extensive ground-glass opacification/consolidation, interstitial thickening, and some cystic change are seen.

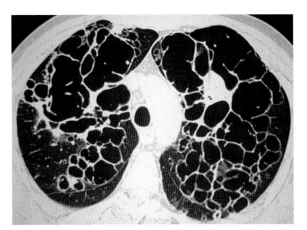

Fig. 3.**46**   Cystic lung disease in AIDS. CT through the upper zones shows extensive bilateral "cystic" change in a patient with advanced AIDS.

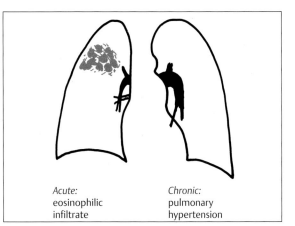

Fig. 3.**47**   Schistosomiasis.

Acute: eosinophilic infiltrate

Chronic: pulmonary hypertension

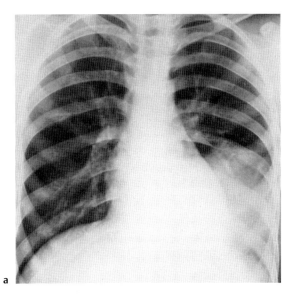

a

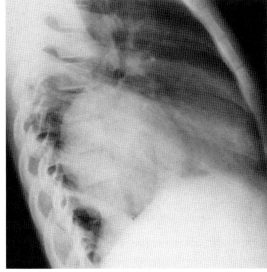

b

c

d

Fig. 3.**48 a–d**   Hydatid cysts in the left lower lobe and right liver of a 15-year-old Turkish male.

through the pulmonary capillaries. Occasionally the parasites lodge in the precapillary pulmonary arterioles and incite an obstructive endarteritis leading eventually to pulmonary hypertension and chronic cor pulmonale (Waldman 2001; Fig. 3.**47**).

Echinococciasis

■ Clinical Features

Hydatid disease is endemic in the Mediterranean basin and Africa. Humans ingest the ova of the dog tapeworm *Taenia echinococcus* in contaminated food. The larvae hatch in the intestine with subsequent hematogenous spread to the liver. Pulmonary, cerebral, and bone involvement occur in about 10% of cases. Larvae form fluid-containing hydatid cysts (endocyst and ectocyst) in the liver and lung. These are surrounded by a fibrotic capsule contributed by the host tissue (pericyst).

■ Radiologic Findings

The chest radiograph shows a solitary, smooth, round, homogeneous mass ranging from 1 to 10 cm in diameter (Fig. 3.**48**, 3.**49**). Multiple pulmonary hydatid cysts are

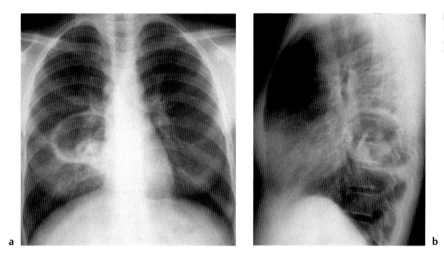

Fig. 3.**49 a, b** Hydatid cyst. Note the pericyst and the collapsed endocyst with subtle evidence of the "water lily" sign.

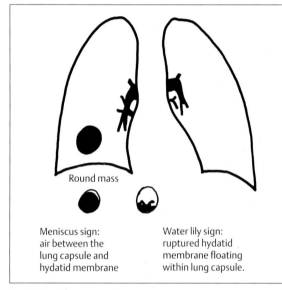

Round mass

Meniscus sign: air between the lung capsule and hydatid membrane

Water lily sign: ruptured hydatid membrane floating within lung capsule.

Fig. 3.**50** Echinococciasis.

rare. Occasionally a thin crescent of air is visible between the ectocyst and pericyst (meniscus sign); this is an indication of early rupture. Later, following cyst rupture, the chitin membrane of the endocyst may collapse and float on the residual fluid (water lily sign; Fig. 3.**50**).

Diagnosis is based on occasional demonstration of echinococcal scolices in the sputum and on serology or skin tests.

Paragonimiasis

■ Clinical Features

Infection with lung flukes of the genus *Paragonimus* is widespread in Southeast Asia and Central and South America. The metacercariae are ingested in seafood, penetrate the bowel wall, reach the peritoneal cavity, and pass through the diaphragm and pleura to enter the lungs. The parasites live in the lungs for many years, and the presence of eggs in the sputum may provide a diagnosis.

■ Radiologic Findings

The chest radiograph shows Loeffler-type eosinophilic infiltrates occasionally associated with pleural effusions. Later, predominantly basal nodules and cysts are seen. Calcification may occur in late cases.

Ascariasis

■ Clinical Features

The roundworm *Ascaris lumbricoides hominis* occurs throughout the world in areas inhabited by humans. The eggs are ingested with food. The larvae hatch in the small intestine and reach the lung capillaries via the lymphatics and bloodstream, where they penetrate the alveolar septa and are transported with bronchial secretions to the pharynx. Subsequently they are swallowed and reenter the intestine, where they mature into adult worms. This remarkable migration of *Ascaris* lasts approximately 2 weeks.

■ Radiologic Findings

Radiographs show regional, confluent infiltrates similar to eosinophilic Loeffler pneumonia. In atopic patients, asthma may be precipitated and results from a hypersensitivity reaction to the larvae (Fig. 3.**51**).

Diagnosis is based on identification of *Ascaris* in the stool together with a blood eosinophilia.

Strongyloidiasis and Ankylostomiasis

■ Clinical Features

Strongyloides stercoralis and *Ankylostoma duodenale* occur in warm, wet regions and inhabit warm mines in Europe. The larvae penetrate the skin, pass through the lungs and enter the intestine. Passage through the lung is associated with transient eosinophilic infiltrates, and, in atopic individuals, asthmatic episodes may be precipitated (Fig. 3.**51**). Clinical manifestations are usually less

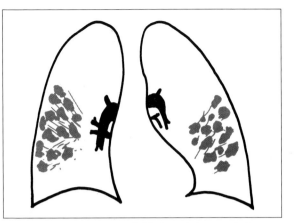

Fig. 3.**51** Ascariasis, strongyloidiasis, ankylostomatiasis: transient eosinophilic infiltrates.

severe than in ascariasis, but a massive *Strongyloides* infestation may be fatal. Miner's strongyloidiasis is an occupational disease. Diagnosis is made by identification of the worms in stool samples.

Sarcoidosis

Sarcoidosis is a generalized epithelioid cell granulomatosis. It frequently involves both the intrathoracic lymph nodes and the pulmonary parenchyma. The liver, spleen, skin, eyes, bones, salivary glands, and other organs also may be affected. Most patients have some immunologic abnormalities: a positive Kveim test, a negative tuberculin skin reaction, and elevated serum immunoglobulin levels. The etiology of sarcoidosis is unknown, but the frequency of pulmonary involvement may indicate an airborne agent (Murray 2000).

The incidence of sarcoidosis in Germany is 8–10 cases per 100 000 per year (Doerr 1983). In most cases, sarcoidosis runs a self-limiting course, sometimes extending over several years. However, pulmonary fibrosis will develop in 10%–20% of cases (Scadding 1970).

The typical radiologic findings of bilateral hilar lymph node enlargement (BHL) with or without pulmonary parenchymal involvement may suggest the diagnosis. Diagnosis may be established from transbronchial or lymph node biopsy.

■ Pathology

Granulomata 1–2 mm in diameter are found in involved lymph nodes and along the peribronchovascular, paraseptal, and subpleural lymph vessels. Histologically, these lesions are characterized by epithelioid cells, Langhans' giant cells, calcifying Schaumann bodies, and "asteroid bodies." In contrast to tuberculosis, sarcoid granulomata do not caseate. However, they are indistinguishable from other nonspecific granulomata such as those occurring in fungal infections, berylliosis, and brucellosis. These granulomatous foci may heal or may progress to pulmonary fibrosis. The latter, in severe cases, is associated with restrictive ventilatory impairment and eventual cor pulmonale.

■ Clinical Features

Clinical presentation is variable. Ocular symptoms such as iridocyclitis or Heerfordt syndrome (uveoparotid fever) may predominate. Cervical, axillary, and epitrochlear lymph node enlargement and cutaneous lesions (lupus pernio) also occur. Lofgren syndrome, an acute form of sarcoidosis, is seen mainly in Scandinavia and presents with fever, arthralgia, and erythema nodosum. It is found almost exclusively in females.

Up to 50% of cases are asymptomatic and are detected incidentally on routine chest radiographs. Pulmonary symptoms include dyspnea and dry cough. Restrictive ventilatory impairment may be evident on pulmonary function tests.

The tuberculin skin test is negative. Serum immuno-globulin levels may be elevated and there is increased activity of angiotensin I converting enzyme (ACE), which is released by activated macrophages. Bronchoalveolar lavage demonstrates an increase in activated T lymphocytes. Seventy-five percent of patients have a positive Kveim test, i. e., a sarcoid nodule forms at the site of the subcutaneous injection of a saline suspension of sarcoid granulomata.

■ Radiologic Findings

Chest Radiograph

Three stages of the disease are described (Fig. 3.**52**):

Stage I (Intrathoracic Adenopathy)
- *Bilateral hilar lymph node enlargement*: The hilar lymph nodes show bilateral symmetrical enlargement. Enlarged hilar shadows are well-defined with scalloped lateral borders (Fig. 3.**53**). A thin stripe of lung tissue is often visible between the hilar and mediastinal contours; this is in contrast to lymphoma and bronchial carcinoma, which extend from the hilum to the mediastinum without interruption.
- *Unilateral hilar lymph node enlargement* and calcified lymph nodes are found infrequently in sarcoidosis, accounting for less than 5 % of cases (Armstrong et al. 1995).

- *Mediastinal lymph node enlargement*. Mediastinal lymph node enlargement may lead to widening and lateral scalloping of the mediastinum, usually more pronounced on the right side. Subcarinal lymph node enlargement may cause splaying of the tracheal carina. In most cases of stage I sarcoidosis, pulmonary granulomata are detectable histologically, but parenchymal change may not be evident radiologically (Murray 2000). Stage I disease usually resolves spontaneously over a variable time period (3–24 months), but it may persist for many years or progress to stage II disease.

Stage II (Miliary Stage)
While the stage I adenopathies gradually regress, pulmonary granulomas enlarge. However, lung involvement is twice as frequent with simultaneous lymph node enlargement as in isolation. Pulmonary parenchymal disease is most pronounced in the midzone and in the perihilar regions. An interstitial pattern with reticulonodular shadowing predominates (Figs. 3.**54**, 3.**55**). Less commonly, acinar shadows up to 7 mm in diameter, segmental infiltrates, round masses, or atelectasis distal to obstruction by endobronchial granulomatous lesions are seen. Today the diagnosis is usually established by analysis of bronchoalveolar lavage fluid and by histological confirmation from transbronchial biopsy.

Fig. 3.**52** Sarcoidosis.

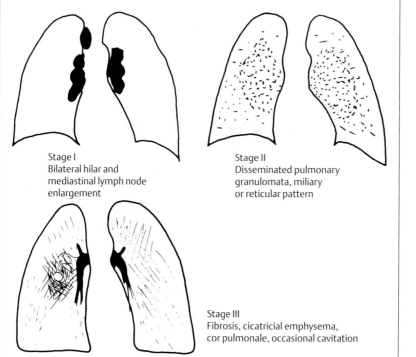

Stage I
Bilateral hilar and
mediastinal lymph node
enlargement

Stage II
Disseminated pulmonary
granulomata, miliary
or reticular pattern

Stage III
Fibrosis, cicatricial emphysema,
cor pulmonale, occasional cavitation

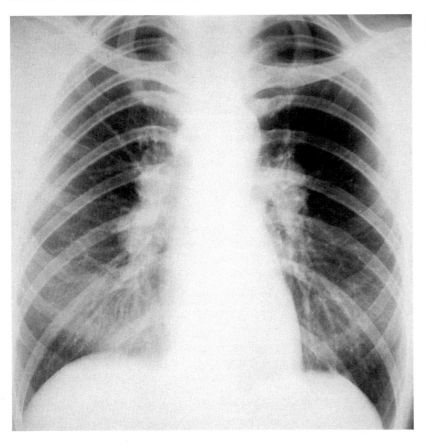

Fig. 3.**53**   Stage I sarcoidosis with bilateral hilar lymph node enlargement. Clinical examination identified erythema nodosum.

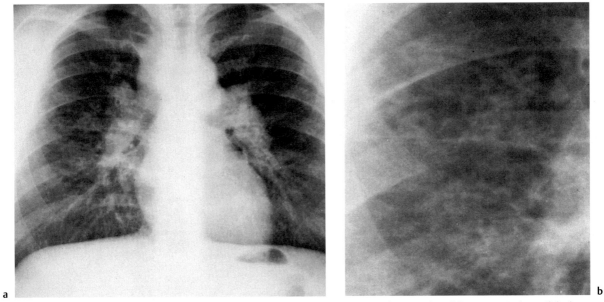

a

b

Fig. 3.**54 a, b**   Stage I/II sarcoidosis: mediastinal and hilar lymph node enlargement with a reticulonodular pattern in the perihilar lung.

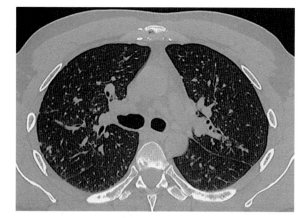

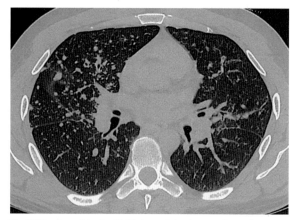

Fig. 3.**55**   **Sarcoidosis**. Multiple nodules in a peribronchovascular distribution. Precarinal lymph node enlargement is also present.

Stage III (Pulmonary Fibrosis)

Stage II disease may progress to pulmonary fibrosis, frequently without a discrete transition between stages. Linear opacities radiate from the hila into the lung. This is accompanied by coarse reticular markings and a honeycomb pattern. These changes are most marked in the mid and upper zones (Fig. 3.**56**). End-stage disease is associated with paracicatricial emphysema, traction bronchiectasis, and eventual pulmonary hypertension with cor pulmonale (Schermuly 1977).

Computed Tomography

The characteristic findings of bilateral hilar and paratracheal lymph node enlargement with or without pulmonary change are seen in 60–70% of cases (Webb et al. 1992, Hillerdal et al. 1984, Scadding 1985).

Pulmonary parenchymal features of sarcoidosis include:

- **Small well-defined nodules**, 2–10 mm in diameter, which are found intimately related to the parahilar bronchi and vessels in the lobular core, within the interlobular septa, adjacent to the fissures and in the subpleural lung (Webb et al. 1992; Fig. 3.**55**). Pathologically, these nodules represent coalescent granulomata (Lynch 1989).
- **Irregular or nodular thickening of bronchovascular bundles and interlobular septa** (Webb et al. 1992, Dawson 1990).
- **Areas of ground-glass opacification** may represent active alveolitis (Lynch 1989) or widespread intersti-

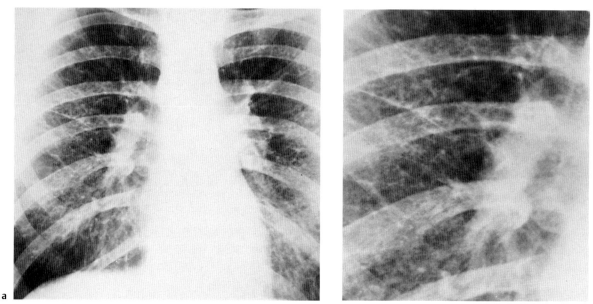

a   b

Fig. 3.**56 a, b**   Stage II/III sarcoidosis: Reticular shadowing and a honeycomb pattern.

tial granulomata below the resolution of HRCT. The former is favored by resolution of ground-glass change following steroid therapy (Lynch 1989, Webb et al. 1992).

- Appearances suggesting **alveolar sarcoidosis** occur in 4 to 27 % of cases (Wilson 1995). The typical appearance is of bilateral, poorly defined opacities, peripheral in distribution (Berkmen 1985, Rubinowitz et al. 1974, Shigematsu et al. 1978; Fig. 3.**57**). Lesions may also have a fine nodular pattern creating the appearance of acinar rosettes (Ziskind 1963).
- Patchy **air trapping at the level of the secondary lobule** in keeping with small-airway disease has been described (Gleeson et al. 1996). Images acquired in inspiration show the affected parenchyma to be of decreased attenuation relative to normal lung; this results in a mosaic pattern. Changes due to air trapping are accentuated in expiration.
- **Developing fibrosis** is associated with the appearance of irregular reticular opacities, including irregular septal thickening, and these frequently are seen along the perihilar bronchovascular bundles (Webb et al. 1992). Central conglomerations along perihilar vessels and bronchi and traction bronchiectasis develop with progression. Changes tend to be most marked in the upper lobes and central perihilar lung.

Radionuclide Imaging

In active disease, intense gallium uptake is frequently observed in the enlarged hilar and mediastinal lymph nodes.

Idiopathic Interstitial Pneumonias

The idiopathic interstitial pneumonias are a heterogeneous group of lung diseases characterized by differing degrees of interstitial and alveolar inflammation and fibrosis.

The initial Liebow classification in 1969 (Liebow and Carrington 1969) recognized five entities:
- Usual interstitial pneumonia (UIP)
- Desquamative interstitial pneumonia (DIP)
- Lymphocytic interstitial pneumonia (LIP)
- Giant cell interstitial pneumonia (GIP)
- Bronchiolitis and interstitial pneumonia (BIP)

GIP is now recognized as a pneumoconiosis and LIP is accepted as a lymphoproliferative disorder. Bronchiolitis and interstitial pneumonia subsequently termed bronchiolitis obliterans organizing pneumonia (BOOP) and then organizing pneumonia (OP) is now considered a disease of small airways and airspaces and no longer as an interstitial pneumonia.

The current classification recognizes the following entities:

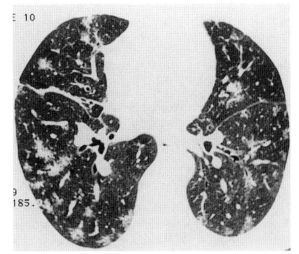

Fig. 3.**57** HRCT: Sarcoidosis. CT shows foci of alveolar opacification in a predominantly peripheral distribution (*starburst pattern*).

- Usual interstitial pneumonia
- Desquamative interstitial pneumonia–respiratory bronchiolitis interstitial lung disease (DIP-RBILD)
- Acute interstitial pneumonia (AIP)
- Nonspecific interstitial pneumonia (NSIP)

Usual Interstitial Pneumonia

UIP is a disease of middle-aged adults. Onset may be gradual with dry cough and progressive dyspnea. Prognosis is poor with reported mean survivals of 2.8–6 years (Bjoraker et al. 1998, Carrington et al. 1978).

UIP is characterized histologically by a variegated pattern with foci of normal lung, interstitial cellular infiltrates, and zones of active fibrosis.

The chest radiograph shows a reticular pattern predominantly in a peripheral and subpleural distribution.

HRCT shows a subpleural and predominantly basal distribution of intralobular septal thickening and honeycombing. Bronchovascular distortion and traction bronchiectasis are seen (Fig. 3.**58**). Areas of ground-glass opacification may reflect patchy septal fibrosis rather than active alveolitis (Nishimura et al. 1992) and this correlates with the relative lack of response of this entity to steroid therapy. HRCT findings frequently are diagnostic to the extent that histological confirmation is not considered necessary.

Desquamative Interstitial Pneumonia—Respiratory Bronchiolitis Interstitial Lung Disease

Desquamative interstitial pneumonia was included in Liebow's original classification and, for a period, was considered by some to represent the early cellular phase of UIP. This concept now has been largely abandoned (Reynolds and Hansell 2000). Respiratory bronchiolitis (RB) is an incidental finding in asymptomatic smokers and is

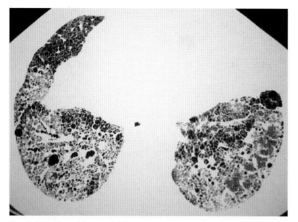

Fig. 3.**58** Usual interstitial pneumonia: HRCT shows extensive honeycombing with traction bronchiectasis.

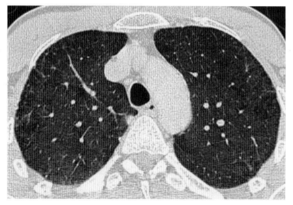

Fig. 3.**59** Respiratory bronchiolitis-interstitial lung disease. HRCT through the upper lobes shows extensive ground-glass opacification in a heavy smoker.

characterized by pigmented macrophages within the respiratory bronchioles with minor peribronchiolar inflammation. In RBILD, the inflammatory change is more extensive and these individuals tend to be symptomatic with a restrictive pattern at pulmonary function tests.

DIP shows very significant histologic overlap with RBILD and 90% of patients with DIP and RBILD are heavy smokers. This suggests a histologic spectrum of small airways and parenchymal reactions to cigarette smoke. Both entities are characterized by the presence of intra-alveolar macrophages but in DIP the distribution is more diffuse and less bronchiolocentric than in RBILD.

The chest radiograph may be normal, show a reticulonodular pattern or ground-glass opacification sometimes with a nodular or granular texture (Reynolds and Hansell 2000).

Heyneman et al. (1999) looked at HRCT findings in respiratory bronchiolitis (RB), RBILD, and DIP. RBILD was characterized by centrilobular nodules (38%), ground-glass opacification (50%; Fig. 3.**59**), and a fine reticular pattern (25%). DIP was characterized by ground-glass opacification (100%) and a fine reticular pattern (63%).

This is consistent with the concept of a spectrum of disease ranging from bronchiolocentric RBILD to more diffuse involvement of the secondary lobule in DIP.

Nonspecific Interstitial Pneumonia

NSIP initially was used by Katzenstein and Fiorelli in 1994 to denote cases of interstitial pneumonia in which histology did not conform to any of the recognized patterns. These cases were characterized histologically by spatially uniform interstitial inflammation with a variable amount of fibrosis.

The concept of NSIP as a specific clinicopathologic entity subsequently has begun to emerge. This is strengthened by the finding that the prognosis for histologically proven NSIP is very much better than for UIP, with a 10 year survival of 60% versus 10% (Nagai et al. 1998, Tukiainen et al. 1983).

The chest radiograph is abnormal in over 90% of cases but findings tend to be nonspecific (Reynolds and Hansell 2000).

Hartman et al. have described the HRCT findings in NSIP (Hartman et al. 2000). They described ground-glass opacification (GGO) in 76%, irregular linear opacities in 46%, honeycombing in 30%, consolidation in 16%, and nodular opacities in 14% of cases and concluded that CT findings in NSIP were variable. However, all studies on NSIP suggest that it predominates in the mid to lower lung zones and that GGO is the salient feature (Lynch 2001).

The differentiation of NSIP from DIP is likely to be less important than distinguishing either entity from UIP, since both NSIP and DIP tend to be steroid-responsive and both have a much better prognosis than UIP.

Acute Interstitial Pneumonia

Acute interstitial pneumonia is rare and is characterized by sudden onset of severe and progressive dyspnea in previously fit individuals with rapid progression to respiratory failure with requirement for mechanical ventilation. This is the interstitial pneumonia which equates most closely to that described by Hamman and Rich, although this syndrome may also have included some cases of rapidly progressive UIP (Hollingsworth and Mark 2001). This essentially is the idiopathic form of adult respiratory distress syndrome (ARDS) and has three distinct histological stages. These acute exudative, subacute proliferative (Fig. 3.**60**) and chronic fibrosing stages are characterized by alveolar edema and hyaline membrane formation progressing to fibroblast proliferation but with little mature collagen formation.

Both the chest radiograph and HRCT show a combination of bilateral symmetric air space consolidation, ground-glass opacification, traction bronchiectasis, and architectural distortion most commonly in a mid to lower lung zone distribution. Johkoh et al. (1999) found that the extent of ground-glass opacification and traction bronchiectasis increased with disease duration.

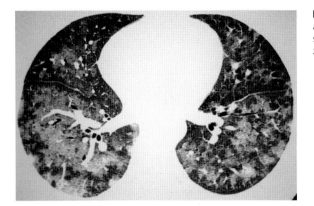

Fig. 3.**60**   Biopsy-proven acute interstitial pneumonia. CT shows a nonhomogeneous pattern of ground-glass opacification/consolidation with some intralobular septal thickening in a mid-lower zone distribution.

Acquired Immunodeficiency Syndrome

Acquired immunodeficiency syndrome (AIDS) results from infection with the human immunodeficiency virus (HIV). Groups at high risk of exposure include the male homosexual population, intravenous drug users, and, in the past, those in receipt of regular blood transfusions or blood products (Abrams 1985, Bessen 1988). HIV-positive individuals may remain healthy for several years before the onset of AIDS.

Since its recognition as a disease entity in the industrialized world in the early 1980s (Gottlieb 1981 a, Gottlieb 1981 b), the incidence of both HIV positivity and AIDS have increased quite dramatically but rates now show a degree of stabilization in Western countries. However, the spread of HIV infection has been alarming in developing countries, particularly in sub-Saharan Africa and Southeast Asia (Von Overbeck 2005).

Intrathoracic disease is common in patients with AIDS and is associated with significant morbidity and mortality (Hartman et al. 1994). The main intrathoracic manifestations of AIDS are infections, neoplasia, and lymphoproliferative disorders.

Infections

Organisms causing intrathoracic infection in AIDS include bacteria, typical and atypical mycobacteria, protozoa, viruses, and fungi.

Mycobacteria

There is increased susceptibility to infection with both typical and atypical mycobacteria. *Mycobacterium tuberculosis* may cause disease in individuals in whom resistance to atypical mycobacteria, *Pneumocystis*, and fungal infections is preserved (Goedert et al. 1987). Radiologic manifestations of tuberculosis, however, depend on the degree of host immune impairment. Classic features of postprimary organ tuberculosis including endobronchial spread and cavitation are seen in the mildly immunocompromised. Tuberculosis in advanced AIDS is frequently aggressive and manifestations may be those of primary or miliary tuberculosis. Cavitation is unusual in the severely immunocompromised.

Mycobacterium avium complex is found in up to 20 % of AIDS patients and is associated with severe degrees of immunocompromise. Pulmonary manifestations are less common than in infection with *Mycobacterium tuberculosis*. When present, they include parenchymal nodules, masses, and consolidation in association with mediastinal lymph node enlargement (Hartman et al. 1994).

Mycobacterium tuberculosis and MAC are the organisms most frequently responsible for mediastinal adenopathy in AIDS (Kuhlman 1989, Sider 1993). These nodes may have low-attenuation centers (Pastores 1993) with evidence of rim enhancement on iodinated contrast-enhanced images (Kuhlman 1996; Fig. 3.**61**).

Many patients with AIDS now receive highly active antiretroviral therapy. This therapy leads to some degree of restoration of cell-mediated immunity. However, its initiation has been reported to be associated with transient worsening of radiographic abnormalities in AIDS patients with tuberculosis. New or increased pulmonary parenchymal disease, lymphadenopathy, and pleural effusions have been described (Fishman et al. 1998).

Pneumocystis Jiroveci/Carinii Pneumonia

See p. 87

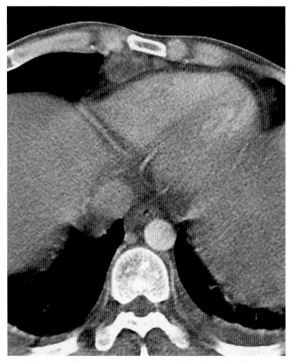

Fig. 3.**61** Mycobacterium avium complex (MAC) infection in patient with AIDS. Enlarged right paracardiac lymph node shows peripheral enhancement with low density center.

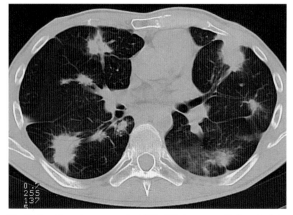

Fig. 3.**62** Kaposi sarcoma in AIDS. CT shows multiple spiculate masses of Kaposi sarcoma. Diagnosis was confirmed at autopsy.

Viruses

Cytomegalovirus (CMV) is ubiquitous in patients with AIDS. It may cause severe esophagitis and colitis. All viruses, especially CMV, are an infrequent cause of pneumonia in AIDS. Radiographic manifestations include diffuse parenchymal infiltration which may be indistinguishable from noncardiogenic pulmonary edema. Pleural effusions and adenopathy are absent.

Fungi

Pulmonary fungal infection is usually a manifestation of disseminated disease. Cryptococcosis is the most common pulmonary fungal infection in AIDS and frequently coexists with cryptococcal meningitis (Chuck 1989). Intrathoracic manifestations include mediastinal lymph node enlargement, pleural effusions, and focal alveolar and diffuse reticulonodular shadowing (Dee 1995 b, Chechani and Kamholz 1990, Katz et al. 1989).

Some infections, such as invasive aspergillosis, are relatively rare in AIDS as the neutrophil count is preserved. However, neutropenia resulting from AZT and ganciclovir therapy occasionally may result in its development.

Intrathoracic Malignancy

Kaposi Sarcoma

Kaposi sarcoma is a common intrathoracic malignancy in the patient with AIDS, occurring in approximately 25% of cases. It is found almost exclusively in homosexual and bisexual men, suggesting a cofactor in the homosexual population (Des Jarlais et al. 1987), and its incidence appears to be on the decline. Pulmonary involvement develops in approximately 20% of patients with Kaposi sarcoma (Kuhlman 1996, Meduri et al. 1986) and is rare in the absence of cutaneous lesions.

Findings on the chest radiograph may be nonspecific, particularly as there frequently is coexisting opportunistic infection (Dee 1995 b, Ognibene et al. 1985). Characteristic features on HRCT are bilateral irregular nodules or areas of consolidation in a peribronchovascular distribution (Figs. 3.**62**, 3.**63**, 3.**64**). Interlobular septal thickening, lymph node enlargement, and pleural effusions are also common (Hartman et al. 1994).

Lymphoma

Pulmonary lymphoma is the second most common malignancy linked to HIV positivity (Dee 1995 b, Kaplan et al. 1987). All types of lymphoma have an increased incidence in AIDS (Kuhlman 1996), and while non-Hodgkins lymphoma (NHL) constitutes an AIDS-defining illness, Hodgkin lymphoma does not (Dee 1995 b, Boring et al. 1985). B cell non-Hodgkin type is the most common AIDS-related lymphoma. These are aggressive tumors with a predilection for extranodal sites, including the pulmonary parenchyma and the gastrointestinal tract (Kuhlman 1996, Sider et al. 1989, Ziegler et al. 1984).

AIDS-related lymphoma (ARL) uncommonly involves the chest as a major site of disease. Blunt et al. (1995) found this to be the case in 15 of 116 patients with ARL (12%). In this series, pleural and intrapulmonary masses, frequently peripheral and sometimes cavitating, were the most frequent imaging finding.

Pleural effusions and mediastinal lymph node enlargement also were common.

Lymphoproliferative Disorders

A number of lymphoproliferative disorders are found in AIDS. These include:

Lymphocytic Interstitial Pneumonia

LIP is an AIDS-defining index disease in children (Centers for Disease Control 1985); such an association in HIV-positive adults is controversial (McGuinness et al. 1995). Pathologically, there is infiltration of the peribronchial interstitium by polyclonal lymphocytes, plasma cells, and immunoblasts. Alveolar air-space obliteration may be due to distal atelectasis, and coalescence of these areas of air-space obliteration may lead to development of nodular masses (Dee 1995b).

The chest radiograph may show diffuse reticular shadowing and reticulonodular infiltrates with or without patchy alveolar infiltration. These changes are usually most marked at the lung bases (Dee 1995b, Oldham 1989). In patients with HIV infection, however, nodular shadowing may predominate (Bragg 1994). CT patterns in LIP in adult patients with AIDS have been described (McGuinness et al. 1995); nodules 2–4 mm in diameter were the predominant finding. Bronchiectasis, bronchiolectasis, and bronchial-wall thickening were also seen.

Mucosa-Associated Lymphoid Tissue Lymphoma (MALTOMA)

MALTOMA is defined as multiple, small (less than 5 mm in diameter) nodular infiltrates of lymphoid cells with a primarily peribronchial distribution. The lymphocytes have a proportion of atypical cells which may infiltrate the bronchial epithelium in clusters to produce lymphoepithelial lesions (McGuinness et al. 1995, Harris 1991, Herbert et al. 1985). The predominant CT findings in the series by McGuinness et al. (1995) were nodules 5–6 mm in diameter, in a peribronchovascular distribution.

Atypical Lymphoproliferative Disorder (ALD)

ALD is defined as diffuse infiltration of the interstitium by a mixed population of atypical lymphoid cells. CT findings include parenchymal nodules 2–4 mm in diameter, air-space consolidation, and ground-glass opacification (McGuinness et al. 1995).

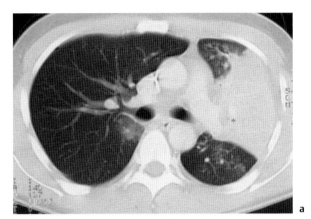

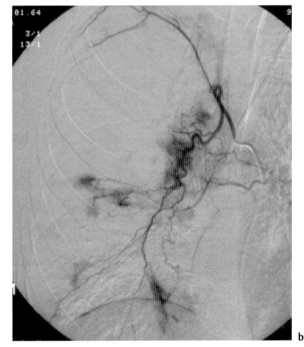

Fig. 3.**63a, b**   Bacterial pneumonia in patient with AIDS (**a**). Lesions of Kaposi sarcoma are visible and show "tumor blush" on bronchial artery injection (**b**).

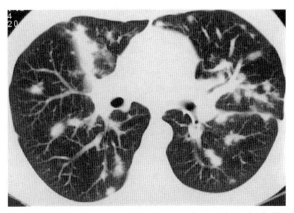

Fig. 3.**64**   Kaposi sarcoma. CT shows multiple bilateral "fluffy" nodules in a peribronchovascular distribution.

Autoimmune Disorders/Connective Tissue Diseases

Autoimmune disorders are pathologic processes in which the immune system develops antibodies that react with endogenous tissues. Antibodies frequently can be detected in the patient's blood. There is usually multiorgan involvement. The collagen vascular diseases affect connective tissue, the ubiquity of which accounts for the varied clinical picture.

Pulmonary manifestations are common and connective tissue disease-associated interstitial pneumonia may progress to fibrosis. Pleural inflammation, pericarditis, and myocarditis may also be seen.

Systemic Lupus Erythematosus

■ Clinical Features

Systemic lupus erythematosus (SLE) is a chronic disease with acute exacerbations that primarily affects premenopausal females. The principal manifestations are polyarthritis, glomerulonephritis with nephrotic syndrome, pleurisy, and pancarditis. Clinical features of pneumonitis and pulmonary fibrosis are unusual, although pulmonary involvement may be demonstrated histologically in 70% of patients (Baum 1974). Diagnosis is based on detection of lupus (LE) cells in the blood, elevated serum antinuclear factor (ANF), anti double-stranded DNA and anticardiolipin antibodies.

■ Radiologic Findings

Pleuropulmonary involvement has been reported in SLE with an incidence ranging from 7 to 100% (Orens 1994).

Pleural involvement is common and the chest radiograph may show bilateral pleural effusions or thickening. In the lungs, there may be evidence of acute lupus pneumonitis, pulmonary edema, pulmonary vasculitis with hemorrhage, interstitial pneumonia, and occasionally an organizing pneumonia. Some pulmonary parenchymal changes may regress with steroid therapy. In advanced disease, there may be evidence of pulmonary fibrosis with reticular and honeycomb shadowing (Fig. 3.**65**).

The HRCT findings in SLE have been described (Fenlon 1996). Interstitial changes including thickened interlobular septa were present in 44% of cases, while airway changes of bronchiectasis and bronchial-wall thickening were seen in 21% of patients. Mediastinal lymph node enlargement was also a frequent finding (18%), HRCT features of interstitial and airway disease were frequently seen in asymptomatic individuals with both normal chest radiographs and normal pulmonary function tests.

Rheumatoid Arthritis

■ Clinical Features

Some degree of pulmonary fibrosis is present histologically in the majority of patients with rheumatoid arthritis (RA). Approximately 20% of all cases of pulmonary fibrosis are attributed to rheumatoid disease (Cervantes-Perez et al. 1980). Most of these changes are subclinical, and positive radiographic findings may be expected in only 1–2% of cases. Other thoracic manifestations include intrapulmonary necrobiotic nodules, which histologically resemble subcutaneous rheumatoid nodules, pleural and pericardial effusions (Fig. 3.**66**).

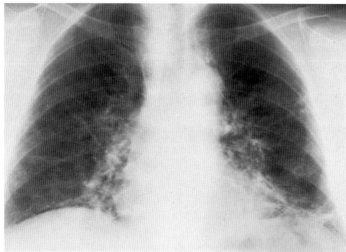

Fig. 3.**65** Lupus erythematosus. Frontal radiograph shows perihilar and basal linear shadowing in a patient with SLE.

■ Radiologic Findings

Pleural effusion is the most common intrathoracic manifestation of rheumatoid arthritis. HRCT may show interstitial pneumonia with either a UIP or NSIP pattern (Tanaka et al. 2004; Fig. 3.**67**). Occasionally, multiple necrobiotic nodules are present. They range from 3 mm to 7 cm in diameter, are usually subpleural, and may cavitate (Fig. 3.**66**). They are found in association with subcutaneous rheumatoid nodules and may pursue a similar course. A continuum exists from these lesions to the Caplan syndrome. The latter occurs in anthracosilicosis and may represent a hypersensitivity reaction in a patient with underlying rheumatoid disease.

Bronchiectasis and changes of small airway disease have been described in patients with RA (Remy-Jardin et al. 1994, Tanaka et al. 2004).

Small airway changes of centrilobular nodules and branching linear structures in RA may also be a manifestation of follicular bronchiolitis (Howling et al. 1999; Fig. 3.**68**).

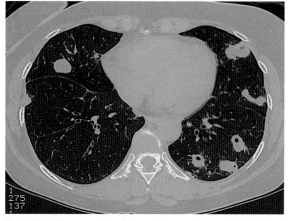

Fig. 3.**66**   Rheumatoid nodules with central necrosis (**a**). Pleural change is also present. Rheumatoid arthritis (**b**).

Progressive Systemic Sclerosis (PSS)

■ Clinical Features

This collagen vascular disease leads to atrophy and induration of the skin and sclerosis of the gastrointestinal tract. Pulmonary fibrosis is present histologically in 90% of cases, but no more than 20% of these cases manifest clinical symptoms and radiographic abnormalities (Gürtler et al. 1979, Kauffmann et al. 1983a, Otto and Reinhard 1970).

■ Radiologic Findings

The chest radiograph and HRCT may show characteristic basal interstitial changes of interstitial pneumonia (Fig. 3.**69**). It has been noted that interstitial pneumonia found in association with systemic sclerosis has a better prognosis than "lone cryptogenic fibrosing alveolitis" (Wells et al. 1994). It has been postulated that this may be due to a NSIP-type entity being commoner than UIP-type pneumonitis in these patients (Fig. 3.**70**).

Esophageal dysmotility with dilatation is also seen in PSS and may be associated with episodes of aspiration pneumonia.

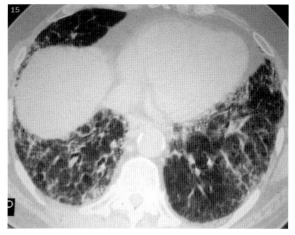

Fig. 3.**67**   "NSIP" pattern in rheumatoid arthritis. CT through the lower zones shows patchy ground-glass opacification with fine reticular change and some traction bronchiectasis.

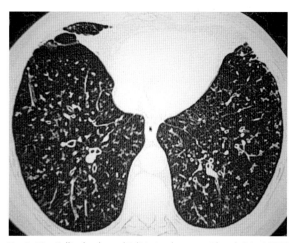

Fig. 3.**68**   Follicular bronchiolitis in rheumatoid arthritis. HRCT shows bronchial wall thickening with features of a "cellular bronchiolitis." Histology was consistent with follicular bronchiolitis.

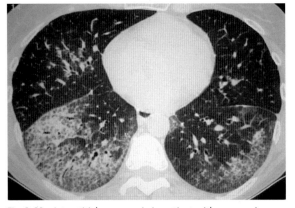

Fig. 3.**69**   Interstitial pneumonia in patient with progressive systemic sclerosis. HRCT shows bilateral ground-glass opacification, consolidation, and some interstitial thickening.

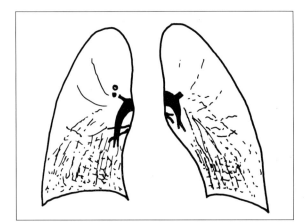

Fig. 3.**70**   Progressive systemic sclerosis: predominantly basal pulmonary fibrosis.

Sjögren Syndrome

Sjögren syndrome (sicca syndrome) is characterized by the triad of keratoconjunctivitis sicca, parotitis sicca, and polyarthritis. There is an association with LIP. HRCT findings include ground-glass opacification (Fig. 3.**71**), focal areas of consolidation, ill-defined nodules, and pulmonary cysts (Fig. 3.**72**; Honda et al. 1999).

Dermatomyositis

Mino et al. (1997) have described CT findings in poly- and dermatomyositis. These include consolidation in a subpleural and patchy distribution, ground-glass opacification, parenchymal bands, and irregular bronchovascular thickening (Fig. 3.**73**). These were seen to be reversible with corticosteroid and immunosuppressant therapy.

Chest wall involvement with muscular weakness may lead to restricted ventilation.

Ankylosing Spondylitis (AS)

Upper lobe fibrosis and bullous emphysema are sometimes found in association with ankylosing spondylitis. In chronic cases, radiographic findings may be indistinguishable from healed postprimary tuberculosis. Cavitation may also occur, and the upper lobes may then be colonized by aspergillus to form mycetomata. Diagnosis is facilitated by the typical radiographic findings in the axial skeleton and the occurrence of the human leuko-

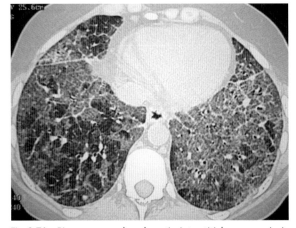

Fig. 3.**71**   Biopsy-proven lymphocytic interstitial pneumonia in Sjögren syndrome. HRCT through the lower lobes shows bilateral ground-glass opacification with interlobular septal thickening.

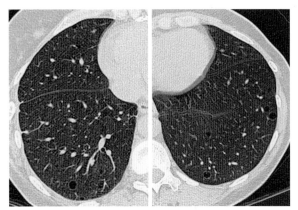

Fig. 3.**72**   Lymphocytic interstitial pneumonia in Sjögren syndrome. HRCT shows scattered bilateral lung cysts.

cyte antigen (HLA)-B27 antigen in approximately 90% of patients with AS.

Wegener Granulomatosis (WG)

Wegener granulomatosis is classified as a form of angiitis and granulomatosis. It is characterized by upper airway ulceration, cavitating pulmonary nodules, a disseminated vasculitis, and glomerulonephritis (De-Remee et al. 1980). Histologic findings include geographic basophilic necrosis, an inflammatory background with scattered giant cells, and absence of sarcoid-like granulomata. Eccentric mononuclear cell vasculitis that may evolve into a necrotic granuloma within the vessel wall is also found (Colby 1996).

Diagnosis may be made from biopsy, but findings are frequently those of nonspecific inflammatory change. A positive ANCA (antineutrophil cytoplasmic antibody) test may then be helpful in establishing the diagnosis.

Traditionally, untreated WG was associated with a high mortality, death occurring within months from renal failure. The prognosis now is much improved and chemotherapeutic regimes encompassing cyclophosphamide together with steroid therapy can induce and maintain remission in the majority of patients, giving 5-year survival rates of 90 to 95% (Wilson 1995, Fauci et al. 1983, Thurlbeck and Müller 1989).

■ Radiologic Findings

Eighty-five to ninety percent of patients with WG will develop pulmonary involvement during the course of their illness (Wilson 1995, Maguire et al. 1978). Multiple pulmonary nodules with or without cavitation are common. Focal infiltrates, which may be fleeting, are also seen (Fig. 3.**74**). Bilateral diffuse alveolar consolidation is usually a manifestation of diffuse pulmonary hemorrhage (Fig. 3.**75 a**).

HRCT findings in WG include multiple pulmonary nodules frequently cavitating (Fig. 3.**76**), diffuse bilateral consolidation consistent with pulmonary hemorrhage (Fig. 3.**75 b**), and pleurally based wedge-shaped opacities resembling pulmonary infarcts (Wilson 1995, Maskell et al. 1993). Maskell found a high incidence of bronchial abnormalities in WG; these included bronchiectasis and bronchial-wall thickening. Peripheral reticular change was also seen in a percentage of cases in this series, and the authors suggest that interstitial fibrosis may be part of the pathologic spectrum of WG (Fig. 3.**77**).

Subglottic tracheal narrowing is an infrequent but important complication of WG (Wilson 1995). In the Mayo series (McDonald et al. 1982) it was found in approximately 15% of cases, and some 50% of these required tracheostomy. CT will show abnormal soft tissue

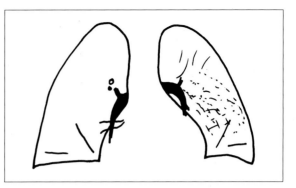

Fig. 3.**73** Dermatomyositis, diaphragmatic paralysis, discoid atelectasis, and pulmonary fibrosis (rare).

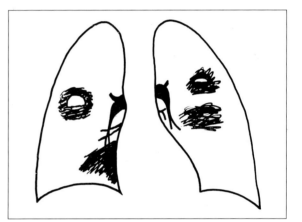

Fig. 3.**74** Wegener Granulomatosis: pulmonary infiltrates, cavitating masses, atelectasis, and subglottic tracheal stenosis.

within the proximal trachea and associated thickening and calcification of tracheal rings (Stein et al. 1986). Mainstem and lobar bronchial stenoses are also a feature of WG and may be demonstrated by multi-detector computed tomography (MDCT).

Allergic Angiitis and Granulomatosis (Churg−Strauss Disease)

■ Clinical Features

Intrathoracic manifestations of this systemic necrotizing vasculitis include bronchial asthma, recurrent pulmonary infiltrates, and pleural and pericardial effusions. An

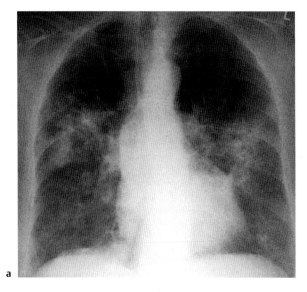

a

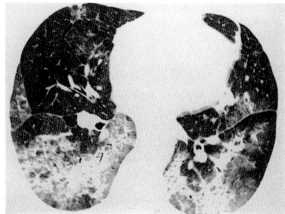

b

Fig. 3.**75 a, b** Wegener's granulomatosis: Chest radiograph and HRCT show bilateral airspace consolidation consistent with diffuse pulmonary hemorrhage.

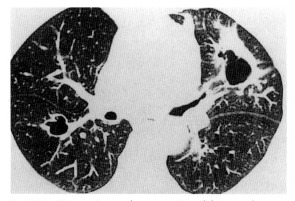

Fig. 3.**76** Wegener's granulomatosis: Consolidation with cavitation in left upper lobe with a thin-walled cavity in the apical segment of the right lower lobe.

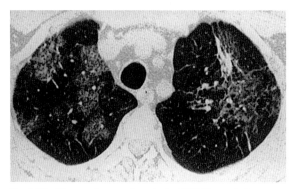

Fig. 3.**77** Wegener's granulomatosis: HRCT through the upper lobes in a patient with resolving pulmonary hemorrhage shows multifocal reticular shadowing with soft tissue stranding in the left upper lobe.

associated peripheral blood eosinophilia invariably is present.

The disease may evolve in three stages; asthmatic, eosinophilic, and vasculitic (Wilson 1995).

■ Radiologic Findings

Radiographic changes are found in the eosinophilic and vasculitic stages of disease. Chest radiographs may show transient, recurrent nonsegmental infiltrates, accentuated interstitial markings, and noncavitating pulmonary nodules. Pleural effusions may be found in up to 29% of cases (Lanham et al. 1984), and cardiomegaly may result from pericarditis or myocarditis (Wilson 1995, Armstrong et al. 1995).

CT findings have been described. These include ground-glass opacification and consolidation, centrilobular nodules, interlobular septal thickening, hilar and mediastinal lymph node enlargement, pleural and pericardial effusions (Fig. 3.**78**).

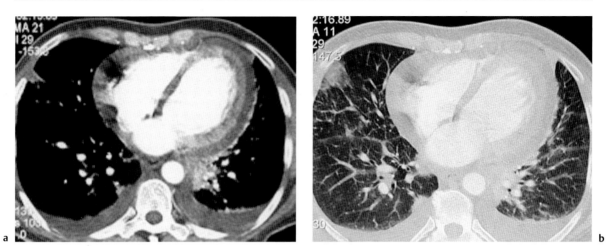

Fig. 3.**78 a, b**   Churg–Strauss disease. Pericardial and bilateral pleural effusions with anterobasal infiltrate in the right lung.

Antiglomerular Basement Membrane Disease (AGBMD)

■ Clinical Features

AGBMD or Goodpasture syndrome is characterized by glomerulonephritis, recurrent episodes of diffuse pulmonary hemorrhage, and antiglomerular basement membrane antibody. It usually affects young men with clinical manifestations that include hemoptysis, hematuria, renal failure, and arterial hypertension. Diagnosis usually is established by renal biopsy and detection of linear deposits of IgG on glomerular basement membranes (Müller 1991).

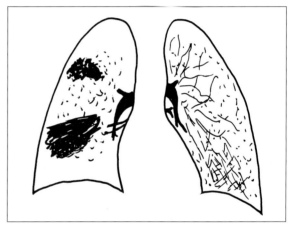

Fig. 3.**79**   Antiglomerular basement membrane disease. Pulmonary hemorrhage, hemosiderosis, and eventual fibrosis.

■ Radiologic Findings

The chest radiograph and HRCT show diffuse unilateral or bilateral alveolar shadowing consistent with pulmonary hemorrhage (Figs. 3.**79** and 3.**80**). As the alveolar shadowing clears, it is replaced by an interstitial pattern of irregular linear opacities and interlobular septal thickening (Müller 1991).

Idiopathic Pulmonary Hemosiderosis (IPH)

■ Clinical Features

The etiology of this disorder which gives rise to episodic pulmonary hemorrhage is unknown. A disease of children and young adults, IPH is characterized by anemia and pulmonary infiltrates but with no demonstrable renal or immunologic abnormality (Müller 1991). Open lung biopsy usually is required for diagnosis and shows alveolar hemorrhage, hemosiderin-laden macrophages, and fraying of elastin fibers.

■ Radiologic Findings

Pulmonary parenchymal changes resemble those of AGBMD (Fig. 3.**79**). Hilar and mediastinal lymph node enlargement have been reported in the childhood variant (Case Records of Massachusetts General Hospital 1988).

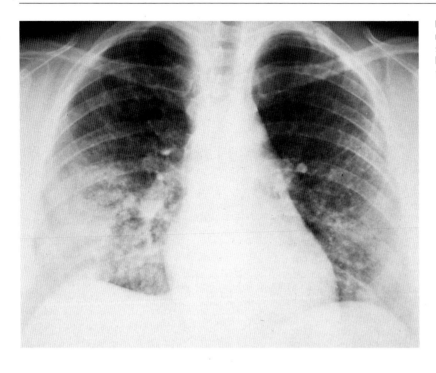

Fig. 3.**80** Antiglomerular basement membrane disease: confluent airspace shadowing in the right lower lobe. Patient had presented clinically with hemoptysis and renal failure.

Pulmonary Eosinophilia (Eosinophilic Lung Disease)

These disorders are characterized by blood and tissue eosinophilia usually in association with an abnormal chest radiograph. Eosinophilic lung disease is usually classified according to etiology (Table 3.**2**). The pulmonary histologic response depends on the route by which the organism enters the lung. Allergic bronchopulmonary aspergillosis caused by inhalation of fungal spores is associated with a bronchocentric reaction, while the pulmonary eosinophilia associated with drugs and parasites tends to be angiocentric.

Known causes of pulmonary eosinophilia are drugs, parasites, and fungal spores: see allergic bronchopulmonary aspergillosis (p. 82), parasitic infections (p. 86), and drug-induced lung disease (p. 108).

In approximately 25 % of cases, etiology is unknown and these are labeled cryptogenic pulmonary eosinophilia. Characteristic findings include a pulmonary eosinophilic infiltrate, granuloma formation, and a vasculitis. The individual diseases are classified according to the relative amounts of each pathological change (Flower 1995).

Cryptogenic pulmonary eosinophilia may present in acute or chronic forms:

Acute Eosinophilic Pneumonia (Löffler Syndrome)

This disorder is characterized by nonpersistent, usually peripheral consolidation (Figs. 3.**81** and 3.**82**).

Chronic Eosinophilic Pneumonia

In chronic eosinophilic pneumonia, the consolidation is persistent lasting for four or more weeks and tends to be quite extensive. In 50 % of cases the chest radiograph

Table 3.**2**   Pulmonary eosinophilia (from Carrington and Reeder)

Idiopathic eosinophilic pneumonia, acute (Löffler syndrome)
- Chronic eosinophilic lung diseases of known etiology
  - Drug allergy (nitrofurantoin, penicillin, sulfonamides, imipramine, PAS, diclofenac, ibuprofen, aspirin, phenytoin, cocaine, tamoxifen, bleomycin, methotrexate, etc.)
  - Asthma
  - Fungal allergy (bronchopulmonary aspergillosis, candidiasis, coccidioidomycosis)
  - Parasitic diseases (ascariasis, echinococciasis, strongyloidiasis, ankylostomiasis, tropical pulmonary eosinophilia, filariae, larva migrans, schistosomiasis)
  - Collagen diseases (polyarteritis nodosa, Wegener granulomatosis, antiglomerular basement membrane disease, Churg–Strauss allergic granulomatosis, rheumatoid arthritis)
  - Eosinophilic leukemia
  - Hodgkin's disease
  - Paraneoplasia (e. g., in bronchial carcinoma)
  - Brucellosis

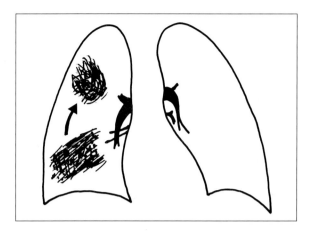

shows nonsegmental airspace consolidation confined to the outer third of the lung, the "photographic negative of pulmonary edema" (Jederlinic et al. 1988, Gaensler 1977). CT is useful in demonstrating the peripheral nature of the consolidation when the chest radiograph is not characteristic (Flower 1995). Associated mediastinal lymph node enlargement may be evident at CT in up to 50% of cases (Mayo et al. 1989).

Fig. 3.**81** Löffler syndrome: transient pulmonary infiltrates with blood eosinophilia.

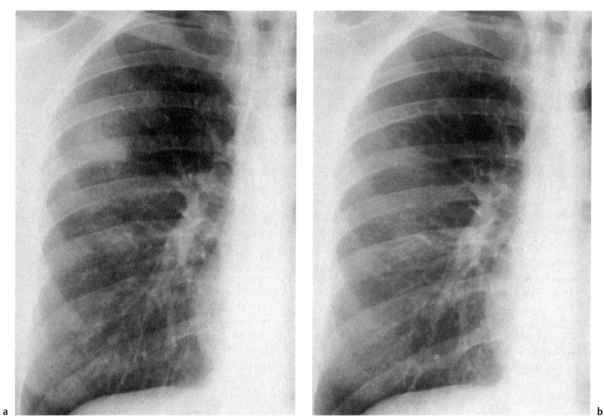

a   b

Fig. 3.**82 a, b** Eosinophilic Löffler infiltrate. Scattered patchy infiltrates in the upper and midzones cleared within 1 week. Blood eosinophilia was 42%. Ascariasis was confirmed.

Radiation-Induced Lung Disease

■ Pathology

The radiation dose required for treatment of primary lung cancer almost invariably causes some damage to the surrounding lung parenchyma. The reproductive capacity of both capillary endothelial cells and pneumo-cytes is reduced, and eventually this imbalance in cell turnover becomes significant.

Radiation pneumonitis occurs 1 to 6 months after commencing therapy and may eventually progress to fibrosis.

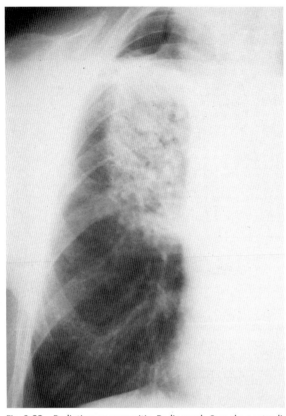

Fig. 3.**83**   Radiation pneumonitis. Radiograph 6 weeks postradiotherapy (56 Gy for bronchial carcinoma) shows densely confluent consolidation with air bronchogram conforming to the radiation portal.

■ Clinical Features

Clinical manifestations of acute radiation pneumonitis include nonproductive cough, dyspnea, and malaise. The erythrocyte sedimentation rate (ESR) is elevated, and pulmonary function tests may show restrictive ventilatory impairment. Hypoxemia may be present in severe cases.

■ Radiologic Findings

Chest radiographs initially show homogeneous consolidation with an air bronchogram conforming to the shape of the radiation portal (Fig. 3.**83**). Pathologically, these changes of pneumonitis represent thickening of alveolar septa, hyperplasia, and desquamation of pneumocytes, intra-alveolar exudate, endothelial cell damage, and thrombus formation (Dee 1995 a). Eventually, the opacities progress to reticular and linear shadowing and finally to fibrosis with streaky opacities and loss of lung volume (Teates 1980).

CT is superior to the chest radiograph in detection of postirradiation lung change. Pneumonitis is manifest as consolidation of geographic distribution (Bell et al. 1988). Transition to fibrosis is gradual and is characterized by fibrous bands, loss of volume, bronchovascular distortion, and traction bronchiectasis.

Drug-Induced Lung Disease

A number of drugs may cause pulmonary change. The following radiographic patterns are recognized:

Hypersensitivity Reactions

Drugs may evoke a hypersensitivity reaction; this sometimes occurs in patients with a history of atopia. Onset of symptoms may be acute, and the reaction is unrelated to the cumulative dose. A peripheral eosinophilia may be present in 40 % of cases (Cooper and Matthey 1987). Histologically, hypersensitivity reactions are characterized by pulmonary eosinophilia and alveolitis. Methotrexate is frequently implicated in these reactions (Cooper and Matthey 1987, Searles and McKendry 1987).

The chest radiograph may show a diffuse interstitial pattern, sometimes in association with airspace shadowing. These changes may regress within days. Ground-glass opacification is the most common HRCT finding in hypersensitivity alveolitis (Padley et al. 1992).

Pneumonitis and fibrosis are the most common type of drug-induced lung damage and frequently result from administration of cytotoxic chemotherapy and, in particular, bleomycin (Figs 3.**84 a**, **b**) (Padley et al. 1992, Kuhlman 1991, Lien et al. 1985). HRCT findings may be similar to those found in usual or nonspecific interstitial pneumonia with a predominantly basal and subpleural distribution.

Adult Respiratory Distress Syndrome

Pulmonary change may develop within days of chemotherapy administration (Cooper and Matthey 1987). One chemotherapeutic agent, in particular bleomycin, has been implicated. HRCT shows diffuse alveolar consolidation, which may have a dependent distribution (Padley et al. 1992). Drug-induced ARDS is associated with a better prognosis than ARDS of other etiology.

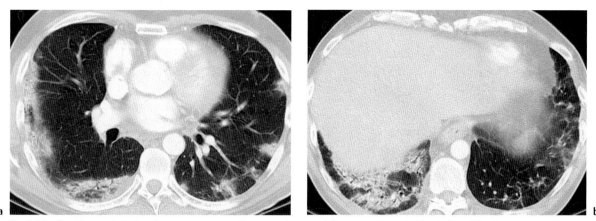

Fig. 3.**84 a, b**   Bleomycin-induced pneumonitis. CT shows patchy consolidation in a peripheral subpleural distribution.

Organizing Pneumonia/Bronchiolitis Obliterans Organizing Pneumonia (BOOP)

BOOP-type reactions have been described particularly in association with amiodarone therapy for cardiac arrhythmias and with nitrofurantoin. HRCT shows patchy, bilateral ground-glass opacification/consolidation in a subpleural and peripheral distribution (Ellis et al. 2000).

Bronchiolitis obliterans has been described in association with penicillamine therapy for rheumatoid arthritis (Geddes et al. 1977), although its role in development of pulmonary change is somewhat controversial. HRCT findings include bronchial-wall thickening and areas of decreased lung attenuation (Padley et al. 1992) with air trapping in expiration.

4 Chronic Obstructive Pulmonary Disease and Diseases of the Airways

Chronic obstructive pulmonary disease (COPD) is very common and has been reported as being second only to arteriosclerosis as a cause of disability and absence from work (Heitzman 1993, Hofner et al. 1977).

COPD is characterized by increased airway resistance and obstructive-type ventilatory impairment. The term has a strong correlation with a smoking history and encompasses two main disorders:

- Emphysema
- Chronic bronchitis

Diseases of the airways are characterized by increased airway resistance, sputum production, obstructive type ventilatory impairment, and air trapping.

Diseases of the airways include:

- Bronchiectasis
- Small airway disease/bronchiolitis
- Bronchial asthma

Emphysema

Emphysema is common in the elderly. Mild degrees of emphysematous change are found in two-thirds of all autopsies while more severe forms are present in approximately 10% of cases (Otto 1976, Thurlbeck and Müller 1994).

The word emphysema means "lung overinflation" (*emphysein* = to inflate). We define this entity as "a chronic and irreversible dilatation of the airspaces distal to the terminal bronchiole with associated destruction of their walls" (World Health Organization 1961).

Emphysema may lead to significant respiratory impairment with resulting dyspnea, cyanosis, and eventual cor pulmonale.

The classification of emphysema most commonly used today is based on the anatomical distribution of lung destruction. This subdivision into three main groups is as follows: centrilobular (centriacinar, proximal acinar), panlobular (panacinar), and paraseptal (distal acinar). This "pathological" classification of emphysema is useful as it correlates with findings on high-resolution computed tomography (HRCT).

In practice, the diagnosis of emphysema usually is based on the appropriate clinical history, abnormal pulmonary function tests, reduced diffusing capacity, and a chest radiograph showing pulmonary hyperinflation. However, as both standard chest radiographs and pulmonary function tests are relatively insensitive to the presence of early disease, HRCT is useful when there is diagnostic uncertainty (Webb et al. 1992).

Goals of Diagnostic Imaging:

Classification of emphysema together with documentation of the distribution and severity of change.

Detection of any coexisting pulmonary diseases that may complicate emphysema.

Evaluation of regional perfusion and ventilation disturbances with radionuclide ventilation/perfusion scintigraphy.

■ Pathology

Destruction of alveolar septa reduces both the surface area available for gas exchange and the total cross-sectional area of the pulmonary vessels. This leads to increased vascular resistance and pulmonary hypertension. A further pathophysiologic phenomenon is ventilation-perfusion mismatch: in normal individuals the von Euler–Liljestrand reflex, also known as hypoxic vasoconstriction, regulates regional perfusion and matches it to ventilation. In emphysema, this control mechanism is lost and very poorly ventilated regions continue to be perfused. This results in an effective venoarterial shunt with systemic arterial hypoxemia.

Macroscopically, the lungs are large and hyperinflated. Emphysematous change may be patchy in distribution and interspersed between areas of normal lung. The lungs do not collapse when the chest is opened as elastic recoil is diminished. The diaphragm is depressed and hypertrophic, sagittally oriented muscle fibers may indent the surface of the liver.

Dilated confluent airspaces result from destruction of both alveolar and lobular septa. They may form bullae, which are air-containing cystic cavities greater than 1 cm in diameter (bullous emphysema). Bullae occupying more than one-third of the lung are known as giant bullae.

The resulting pulmonary arterial hypertension leads to ectasia and sclerosis of the pulmonary arteries and right ventricular hypertrophy. Eventually, right ventricular decompensation may supervene (cor pulmonale).

■ Clinical Features

Manifestations of emphysema include dyspnea and cyanosis. Transitional forms are common but sometimes it is possible to identify specific clinical patterns:

- *"Pink puffer":* These individuals usually are thin and dyspneic. However, they are not cyanosed and clinical features indicating the presence of associated chronic bronchitis are absent.
- *"Blue bloater":* These are "heavy-set" individuals who are cyanosed and have concomitant chronic bronchitis.

Physical examination reveals a barrel chest, relatively shallow respirations, and hyperresonance to percussion. Spirometry shows increased FVC, diminished FEV1, and decreased FEV1/FVC ratio. Blood gas analysis reveals arterial hypoxemia and hypercapnia particularly in blue bloaters. Arterial oxygen and carbon dioxide levels may be relatively normal in pink puffers.

■ Radiologic Findings

▣ Chest Radiograph

Findings on the chest radiograph are secondary to pulmonary hyperinflation with subsequent deformity and/or displacement of the chest wall, heart, and diaphragm. There is also attenuation and disorganization of the pulmonary vasculature with features of oligemia and pulmonary hypertension (Figs. 4.**1** and 4.**2**).

- *Barrel chest*: Sagittal chest diameter is increased, the posterior ribs have a horizontal orientation, and the intercostal spaces are widened.
- *Diaphragmatic depression*: Findings include flattening of the domes of the diaphragm and a costophrenic angle of approximately 90° (so-called "pseudoblunting"). On the lateral view, the diaphragm may show inferior convexity. Respiratory diaphragmatic excursion is also restricted (< 3 cm in emphysema vs. normal values of 5–10 cm).
- *Small, vertically orientated cardiac shadow*: In the presence of a relatively low diaphragm, the heart assumes a vertical orientation and cardiothoracic ratio decreases on the frontal radiograph. There may also be a degree of left ventricular atrophy as left heart filling and left ventricular output sometimes are reduced in patients with emphysema, especially in cases complicated by cor pulmonale.
- *Increased retrosternal space*: On the lateral radiograph, the retrosternal space is widened due to both the increased sagittal diameter of the chest and the relatively "small" heart.
- *Dilatation of the central pulmonary arteries*: Increased pulmonary vascular resistance and subsequent pulmonary arterial hypertension lead to dilatation of the central pulmonary arteries. This is manifest as bilateral symmetric hilar enlargement on the chest radiograph.

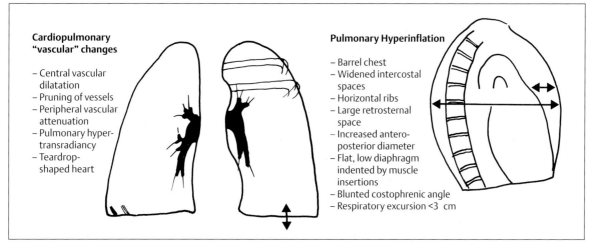

Cardiopulmonary "vascular" changes

– Central vascular dilatation
– Pruning of vessels
– Peripheral vascular attenuation
– Pulmonary hyper-transradiancy
– Teardrop-shaped heart

Pulmonary Hyperinflation

– Barrel chest
– Widened intercostal spaces
– Horizontal ribs
– Large retrosternal space
– Increased antero-posterior diameter
– Flat, low diaphragm indented by muscle insertions
– Blunted costophrenic angle
– Respiratory excursion <3 cm

Fig. 4.**1** Pulmonary emphysema.

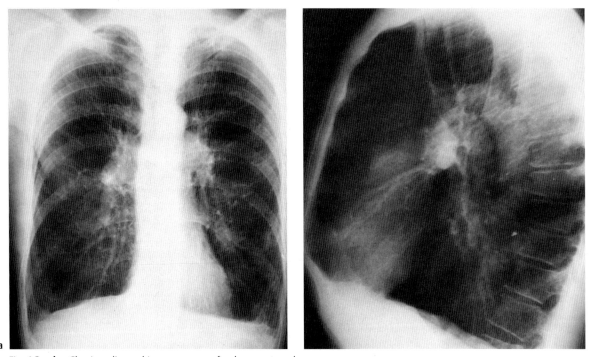

Fig. 4.**2 a, b**   Classic radiographic appearance of pulmonary emphysema.

- *Rapid tapering of pulmonary vessels*: The dilated central vessels decrease markedly in caliber at the segmental level. This may occasionally give the appearance of an "amputated hilum."
- *Attenuation of peripheral pulmonary vessels*: The combination of pulmonary hyperinflation together with attenuation of peripheral vessels results in increased lucency in the lung periphery.
- *Marker vessels*: Emphysema is often focal in distribution. In these cases, pulmonary blood flow will be redistributed to areas of relatively normal lung and result in regional vascular dilatation. In addition, emphysematous bullae may compress adjacent normal lung and cause crowding, displacement, and draping of vessels. These findings are best appreciated on conventional and computed tomography (CT).
- *Bullae*: Thin-walled emphysematous spaces greater than 1 cm in diameter sometimes are visible on the chest radiograph. However, CT will show these thin-walled, air-filled cysts much more convincingly.
- *Increased bronchovascular markings*: Emphysema often is found in association with chronic bronchitis. Peribronchovascular fibrosis is found in the latter and is manifest as tortuosity, poor definition, and segmentation of vascular shadows (increased pulmonary markings, "dirty chest," Thurlbeck and Müller 1994).
- *Atypical appearance of pneumonia and pulmonary edema*: Emphysema may alter the radiographic appearance of other pulmonary diseases. Conversely,

emphysema frequently becomes apparent on the chest radiograph only when common disorders such as pneumonia and pulmonary edema supervene (Fig. 4.3). Pneumonic consolidation and cardiogenic edema develop with relative sparing of regions of avascularity. Therefore, emphysematous lung that is devoid of capillaries tends to be spared. This results in nonhomogeneous, relatively coarse infiltration. Pulmonary edema may be asymmetrical or localized depending on the distribution of emphysematous involvement.

Computed Tomography

Correlation between CT and spirometric data has been reported to be relatively poor (Miller 1989). HRCT, however, is valuable in detection of early disease. It is also possible to classify emphysema on the basis of findings on HRCT:

- *Centrilobular emphysema*: Centrilobular emphysema classically develops in the setting of chronic bronchitis and shows a predilection for the upper lobes. Alveolar destruction is mainly around the respiratory bronchioles at the center of the pulmonary acinus and therefore involves the center of the secondary pulmonary lobule (Webb et al. 1992). HRCT shows centrilobular areas of low attenuation, sometimes several millimeters in diameter. These foci have imperceptible walls, which helps in differentiating them from cysts, bronchiectasis, and the honeycombing of pulmonary fibrosis (Figs. 4.**4**, 4.**5**).

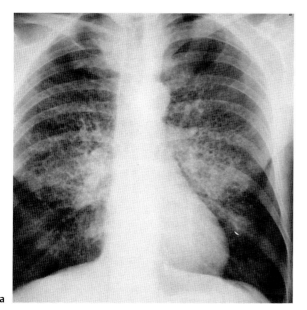

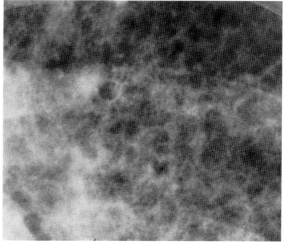

Fig. 4.**3a, b**   Pulmonary edema in emphysema. Coarse reticular shadowing is seen in the perihilar lung with sparing of areas of emphysematous lung.

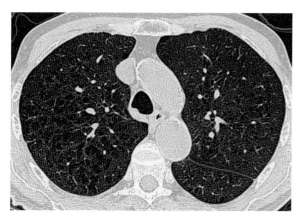

Fig. 4.**4**   Centrilobular emphysema. HRCT shows areas of decreased lung attenuation lying centrally within the secondary pulmonary lobule.

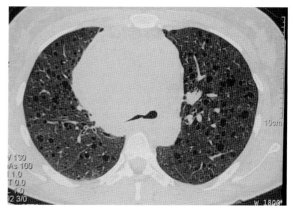

Fig. 4.**5**   Centrilobular emphysema.

- *Panlobular emphysema*: This is characterized by destruction of alveoli throughout the lobule. Panlobular emphysema is associated with α_1-antitrypsin deficiency and has a predilection for the lower lobes. This is an autosomal recessive disease associated with low serum levels of α_1-antitrypsin. Homozygotes have 20% of normal enzyme activity. This deficiency allows leucocyte proteases to attack and destroy the lung parenchyma with changes most marked in regions of maximal perfusion (i.e. the basal zones). Clinical presentation is most common in the fourth decade of life. HRCT shows panlobular low attenuation which persists on expiratory views (Fig. 4.**6**).
- *Paraseptal emphysema*, a form of bullous emphysema with a familial tendency, is characterized by subpleural bullae (Fig. 4.**7**). It usually is asymptomatic unless complicated by a spontaneous pneumothorax.

- HRCT will show subpleural and perifissural bullae and CT studies have shown a high incidence of apical paraseptal emphysema in young adults presenting with spontaneous pneumothorax (Lesur 1990).

Quantification of abnormally low lung attenuation due to emphysema is possible with volumetric CT acquisition and three-dimensional reconstructions using a threshold for inspiratory studies of approximately –900 Hounsfield units. This method has been reported as showing good correlation with pulmonary function tests (Mergo et al. 1998).

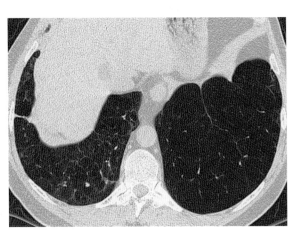

Fig. 4.**6**   Panlobular emphysema. HRCT image through the lower zones shows panlobular emphysema with diffuse decreased lung attenuation particularly in the left lower lobe.

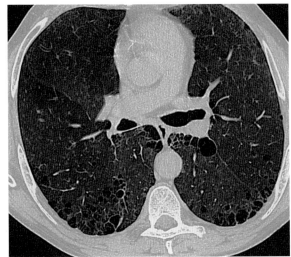

Fig. 4.**7**   Paraseptal emphysema.

Other Forms of Emphysema

Cicatricial Emphysema

Cicatricial or "scar" emphysema is seen when areas of developing fibrosis retract and cause distortion of surrounding pulmonary parenchyma. These retractile forces together with bronchial narrowing may lead to areas of pulmonary hyperinflation. The most common causes of cicatricial emphysema are fibrocirrhotic tuberculosis and progressive massive fibrosis in pneumoconiosis.

The chest radiograph shows coarse reticular shadowing, vascular distortion, and foci of increased lucency (Fig. 4.**8**).

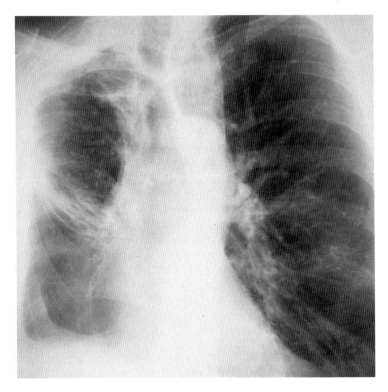

Fig. 4.**8**   Cicatricial emphysema in a patient with healed pulmonary tuberculosis and fibrothorax. Note the left upper lobe herniation and the absence of vascular markings in the right lower zone.

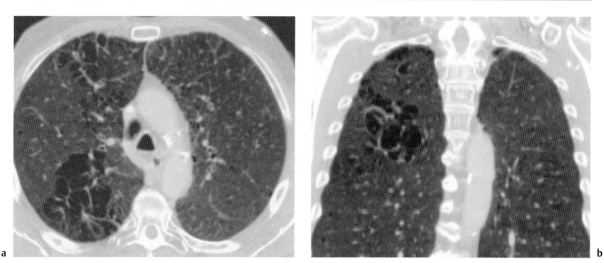

a   b

Fig. 4.**9 a, b**   Localized bullous emphysema. Axial CT image and coronal reformat show change involving the posterior segment of the right upper lobe.

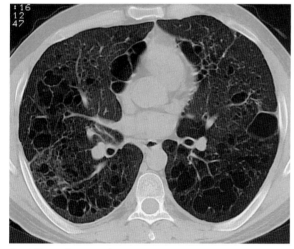

Fig. 4.**10**   Bullous emphysema.

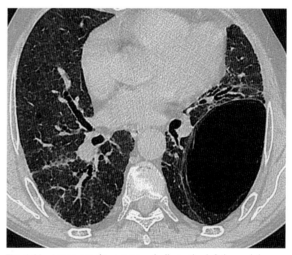

Fig. 4.**11**   Large emphysematous bulla in the left lower lobe.

Bullous Emphysema

Bullae are defined as air-containing spaces greater than 1 cm in diameter, but they may reach a considerably larger size (Müller and Fraser 2001). Giant bullae occupy up to one-third of total lung volume and may be recognized by their space-occupying effect. Bullae may be solitary or, when multiple, tend to occur in clusters. Their predilection for the upper lobes may be due to greater gravitational stresses in that region. "Vanishing lung" is a form of bullous emphysema which develops following recurrent episodes of bronchitis and it may gradually lead to lobar or lung destruction. Bullae appear as local, well-circumscribed, thin-walled lesions of increased lucency and absent vascularity (Figs. 4.**9**, 4.**10**).

Bullae may become more visible on expiratory views as they do not empty on expiration. CT will show the exact volume of the bulla, define its relationship to surrounding structures, and demonstrate the extent and severity of surrounding emphysematous change (Fig. 4.**11**).

Compensatory Emphysema

Compensatory emphysema occurs as a physiologic response to adjacent volume loss whether it is due to lobar atelectasis or lobectomy.

The chest radiograph shows hyperlucent areas with attenuated vascular markings. There may be associated displacement of interlobar fissures and hilar structures.

Chronic Bronchitis

Chronic bronchitis is defined as increased sputum production for at least 3 months in each of two consecutive years. It therefore is a clinical diagnosis, but imaging is important in detection of coexisting conditions such as emphysema and bronchiectasis.

■ Pathology

The mucus-secreting glands of the bronchial mucosa are hypertrophied, hyperplastic, and secrete very viscous mucus. Inflammatory change is evident in both the bronchial wall and surrounding peribronchial connective tissue. Severe bronchitis is associated with airway obstruction and development of emphysema.

■ Clinical Features

Clinical manifestations include dyspnea and cough productive of mucoid sputum. Characteristically, an obstructive pattern is seen on pulmonary function tests.

■ Radiologic Findings

The *chest radiograph* may be normal or may show the following changes (Fig. 4.**12**):
- Increased lung markings throughout both lungs. This "dirty-chest" pattern is believed to be due to peribronchial and perivascular fibrosis (Müller and Fraser 2001).
- *Tramlines* are parallel lines spaced approximately 3 mm apart. They probably represent bronchial wall thickening and are seen most clearly in the right paracardiac lung.
- *Thick-walled ring shadows* at the superior poles of the hila. These represent the anterior and posterior segmental bronchi of the upper lobe.
- *Transient, functional tracheal narrowing.* Fluoroscopy shows partial collapse of the tracheal lumen on forced expiration, coughing, or sniffing. This is attributed to inflammatory weakening of the tracheal wall together with increased transmural pressure. Eventually, this may lead to a fixed stenosis and a saber-sheath trachea (coronal narrowing and sagittal widening of the intrathoracic trachea, in which the ratio of coronal to sagittal dimensions is less than 0.6). The cervical trachea is not affected.

HRCT may show bronchial wall thickening, the presence of concomitant emphysema, superimposed infective consolidation, or development of bronchial neoplasia.

Ventilation-perfusion scintigraphy shows nonhomogeneous tracer distribution due to ventilation-perfusion mismatch. Inhaled radionuclide aerosols show delayed clearance from the airways due to destruction of the mucociliary escalator.

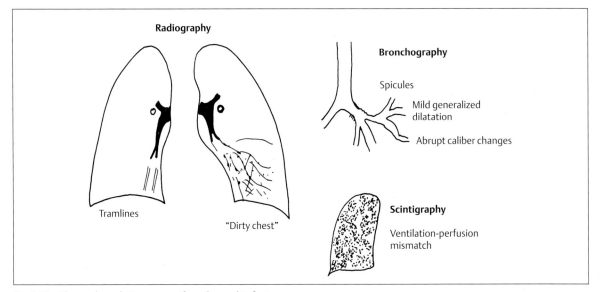

Fig. 4.**12**   Chronic bronchitis: nonspecific radiographic features.

Bronchiectasis

Bronchiectasis refers to an irreversible dilatation of the bronchial tree. Changes may be localized or widespread in distribution. Bronchiectasis is associated with an obstructive pattern on pulmonary function tests and predisposes to recurrent episodes of bronchopneumonia.

> **Goals of Diagnostic Imaging:**
> To establish the diagnosis: HRCT has replaced bronchography as the investigation of choice in suspected bronchiectasis.
>
> To identify the presence of associated small airway change.

Bronchiectasis may be secondary to early childhood infection. Other causes are listed in Table 4.1. Today, with prompt antibiotic therapy and the availability of vaccines against measles and whooping cough, there has been a marked decline in the incidence of bronchiectasis. Other sources suggest that the true incidence of bronchiectasis may have been underestimated in the past when diagnosis was based on findings at bronchography. HRCT has revealed increasing numbers of mild cases (Webb et al. 1992). The incidence of severe symptomatic bronchiectasis, however, certainly appears to be on the decline.

■ Pathology

Bronchiectasis most commonly occurs in the posterobasal segments of the lower lobes. The Reid Classification (1950) identifies:

Cylindrical Bronchiectasis

The bronchi show cylindrical dilatation most marked from the 6–10th bronchial generations. They retain a smooth contour, and they terminate abruptly where the smaller bronchi and bronchioles become plugged with mucus. The bronchial tree, however, has a structurally normal branching pattern dividing into 17–20 generations.

Varicose Bronchiectasis

The bronchial lumen shows irregular dilatation with a "beaded" wall contour. There are only 3–11 generations of patent airways with obliteration of the more distal airways.

Table 4.1 Etiologic classification of bronchiectasis (modified from Huzly 1973 b)

Congenital bronchiectasis
- Bronchiectatic honeycomb lung: a dysgenetic anomaly in which numerous dilated bronchi terminate blindly in fibrous tissue.
- Mounier–Kuhn tracheobronchomegaly: cystic dilatation of the tracheobronchial tree, tracheal diameter greater than 3 cm, wavy outlines of trachea and large bronchi (tracheal diverticulosis); familial incidence, related to Ehlers–Danlos syndrome (Fig. 4.13).
- Kartagener syndrome: autosomal recessive disorder marked by triad of bronchiectasis, situs inversus, and chronic sinusitis.
- Ciliary dyskinesia syndrome: autosomal recessive disorder marked by impaired mucociliary clearance, sperm immotility, and bronchiectasis; often combined with Kartagener syndrome.
- Turpin syndrome: thoracic malformation syndrome characterized by megaesophagus, tracheoesophageal fistula, rib deformity, and bronchiectasis.
- Cystic fibrosis: congenital glandular disorder with viscous secretions leading to bronchiectasis, cystic pancreatic fibrosis, meconium ileus, and abnormal electrolyte levels in sweat and saliva (Wood 1997).
- Alpha$_1$-antitrypsin deficiency syndrome: like congenital immunodeficiencies, predisposes to recurrent inflammations leading to bronchiectasis.

Primary bronchiectasis
- These are acquired in early childhood and usually are secondary to bronchiolitis.

Secondary bronchiectasis
- Postobstructive bronchiectasis: caused by inflammatory bronchial strictures, a slow-growing bronchial tumor, or scarring of the lung parenchyma.
- Toxic bronchiectasis: toxic gas inhalation may incite a bronchiolitis leading to secondary bronchiectasis.

Saccular Bronchiectasis

In saccular or cystic bronchiectasis, bronchial divisions are greatly reduced in number with only 3–5 bronchial generations remaining. Medium-sized bronchi terminate in clusters of cystic cavities which may extend to the pleural surface. Saccular bronchiectasis is found most commonly in older patients and may be associated with a degree of proximal bronchial stenosis. Over 50 % of these patients have histological evidence of an associated constrictive bronchiolitis. Hemoptysis may be due to erosion of inflammatory granulation tissue in the peripheral bronchi or dilatation of bronchial arteries and bronchopulmonary anastomoses.

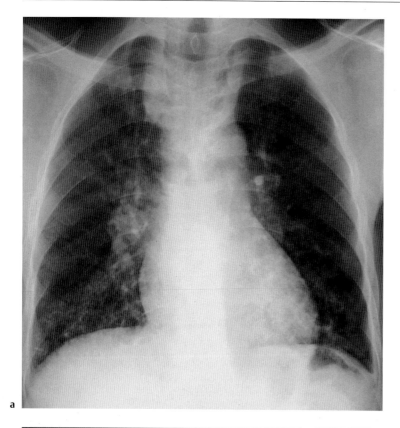

a

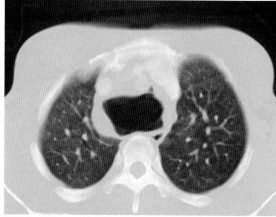

b

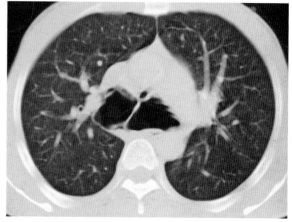

c

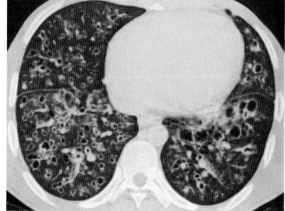

d

Fig. 4.**13 a–d**   Mounier–Kuhn tracheobronchomegaly characterized by tracheomegaly and bronchiectasis.

■ Clinical Features

Features of bronchiectasis detected in asymptomatic individuals may not be significant. However, most patients with significant abnormality suffer recurrent episodes of infection with purulent sputum and hemoptysis. In advanced disease, severe dyspnea and finger clubbing may also be present.

■ Radiologic Findings

Findings on the chest radiograph frequently are nonspecific. The following features, however, are suggestive of bronchiectasis (Figs. 4.**14** and 4.**15**):
- *Coarse linear shadowing* probably represents peribronchial fibrosis.
- *Crowding of linear markings* may represent subsegmental atelectasis.

- *Parallel line shadows (tramlines)* represent thick-walled, cylindrically dilated bronchi.
- *Cystic cavities* 1–3 cm in diameter: These ring shadows, usually in clusters, correspond to areas of saccular bronchiectasis. Fluid levels are due to mucus and purulent exudate lying dependently within these focal dilatations of the airways.
- *Areas of nodular shadowing* may reflect associated cellular bronchiolitis (see p. 122)
- *Regions of increased pulmonary transradiancy* may reflect air trapping and indicate an associated constrictive bronchiolitis.

High resolution/thin collimation CT may show:
- *Cylindrical bronchiectasis*: Dilated bronchi running in the plane of section have roughly parallel walls. Those bronchi running perpendicular to the plane of section are seen as ring shadows (Figs. 4.**16**, 4.**17**, 4.**18**):

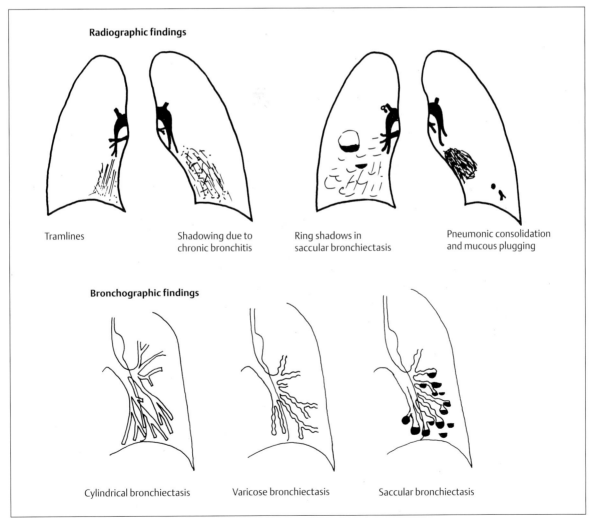

Fig. 4.**14** Radiographic appearances of bronchiectasis.

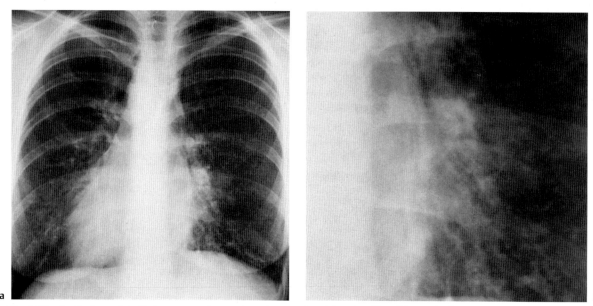

a
b

Fig. 4.**15 a, b** Radiograph in Kartagener syndrome shows increased peripheral and basal linear shadowing. Bronchography showed cylindrical and saccular bronchiectasis. Situs inversus is also present.

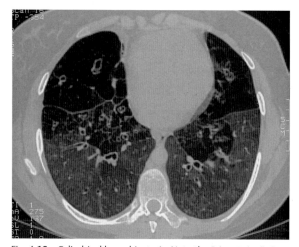

Fig. 4.**16** Cylindrical bronchiectasis. Note the "signet ring" signs and areas of air trapping consistent with a degree of associated "constrictive bronchiolitis."

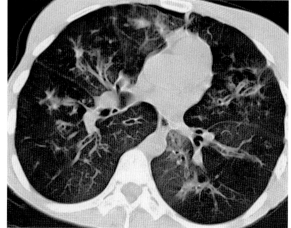

Fig. 4.**17** CT image in patient with cystic fibrosis shows widespread bronchiectasis and small right-sided anterior pneumothorax.

- There is bronchial wall thickening.
- Bronchial cross-sectional diameter is greater than that of the accompanying artery, thus producing the classic "signet ring" sign.
- These dilated bronchi fail to taper as they reach the lung periphery.
- *Cystic and varicose bronchiectases*: Bronchi running in the plane of section have a beaded contour ("string of cysts"). In the perihilar regions, bronchiectatic airways are sometimes crowded together due to adjacent pulmonary atelectasis. On axial CT sections, this gives rise to the so-called "bunch of grapes" pattern (Figs. 4.**19**, 4.**20**).

- *Mucus-filled bronchi.* These are easily recognized when the lumen is partially fluid-filled and the characteristic air–fluid level is present. Dilated bronchi that are completely filled with mucus (mucoceles) may occasionally resemble vascular structures. Differentiation is usually aided by observing that these bronchi are considerably dilated relative to adjacent vessels. The presence of surrounding air-filled, dilated, thick-walled bronchi may also be helpful. If diagnostic difficulty persists, then contrast-enhanced images may be useful.
- *Features of associated "small airway" disease/bronchiolitis (see p. 122).*

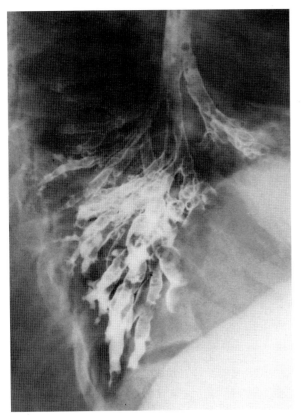

Fig. 4.**18**   Cylindrical bronchiectasis.

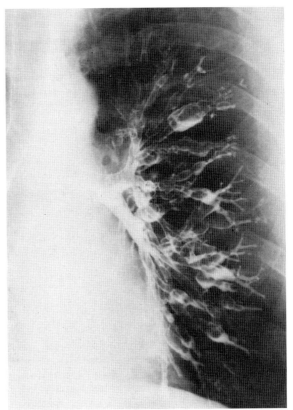

Fig. 4.**20**   Saccular bronchiectasis.

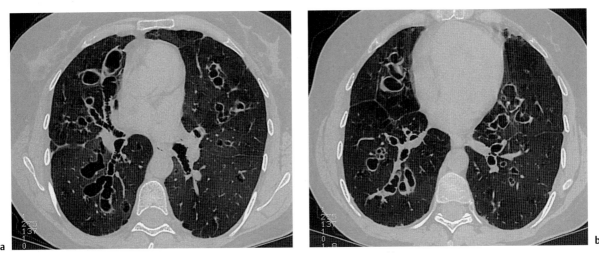

a   b

Fig. 4.**19 a, b**   Varicose bronchiectasis with bronchial wall thickening and "varicose" dilatation.

Radionuclide Scintigraphy

Ventilation scintigraphy shows radiolabeled aerosol (particle size 2 μm) accumulating in the central bronchi due to turbulence in the dilated airways. Clearance of the collected particles from the airways via the mucociliary escalator is delayed as the cilia have been destroyed.

Bronchiolitis–Small Airway Disease

The current classification of bronchiolitis/small airway disease includes:

- Cellular bronchiolitis
- Organizing pneumonia [also known as bronchiolitis obliterans organizing pneumonia (BOOP) and cryptogenic organizing pneumonia (COP)]
- Constrictive bronchiolitis.

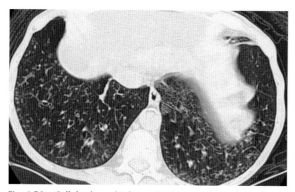

Fig. 4.**21**   Cellular bronchiolitis: HRCT image through the lower zones shows bronchiectasis with centrilobular change consistent with an associated cellular bronchiolitis.

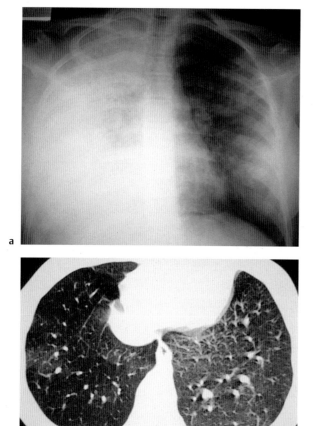

Cellular Bronchiolitis

Cellular bronchiolitis comprises inflammatory cells in the walls of the airways and exudate in the lumen. The commonest cause is *acute infectious bronchiolitis*. This is seen most commonly in young children. Causative organisms include respiratory syncytial virus (RSV), adenovirus, and mycoplasma and this entity usually resolves without sequelae. Cellular bronchiolitis is frequently seen in association with bronchial diseases and particularly with bronchiectasis. Other causes of cellular bronchiolitis include endobronchial spread of tuberculosis (see p. 303) and Japanese diffuse panbronchiolitis.

The *chest radiograph* may show areas of nodular shadowing. HRCT features include centrilobular nodules and centrilobular branching linear structures (the so-called "tree-in-bud" appearance, Fig. 4.21).

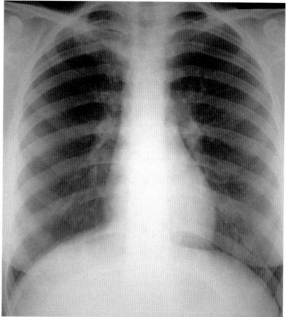

Fig. 4.**22 a–c**   Postinfectious bronchiolitis (**a–c**). Initial chest radiograph (**a**) shows bilateral pulmonary consolidation more extensive on the right side. Patient represented some weeks later with progressive dyspnea. Further radiograph (**b**) shows resolution of consolidation but pulmonary hypertransradiancy on the right side. HRCT shows mosaic pattern of lung attenuation consistent with air trapping (**c**).

Constrictive Bronchiolitis

Constrictive bronchiolitis is the pathologic correlate of the clinical entity "bronchiolitis obliterans." Constrictive narrowing of the bronchioles by submucosal and peribronchiolar fibrosis is seen and this leads to chronic airway obstruction.

This entity may be idiopathic or represent the irreversible sequel of childhood viral/mycoplasma infection (see Swyer–James–McLeod syndrome). It may be secondary to toxic fume inhalation and is seen as a complication of both bone marrow and lung transplantation. In bone marrow transplantation, it is a manifestation of graft-vs.-host disease whereas in lung transplantation, it reflects chronic rejection. There is also an association with rheumatoid arthritis and in the past penicillamine therapy has been implicated in its development. It is occasionally seen in the setting of inflammatory bowel disease (Mahadeva et al. 2000).

HRCT very occasionally may show "direct signs" of centrilobular change. However, "indirect" signs are much more frequent and include (Figs. 4.22, 4.23):
- Mosaic lung attenuation on inspiration
- Air trapping in expiration
- Associated central bronchial dilatation

Swyer–James–Macleod Syndrome

This entity is believed to represent a variant of postinfectious constrictive bronchiolitis.

The *chest radiograph* may show unilateral hyperlucency with attenuated vascular markings. The affected lung is small on inspiration but does not deflate normally on expiration (air trapping, Fig. 4.24).

Radionuclide imaging shows diminished perfusion in the affected lung.

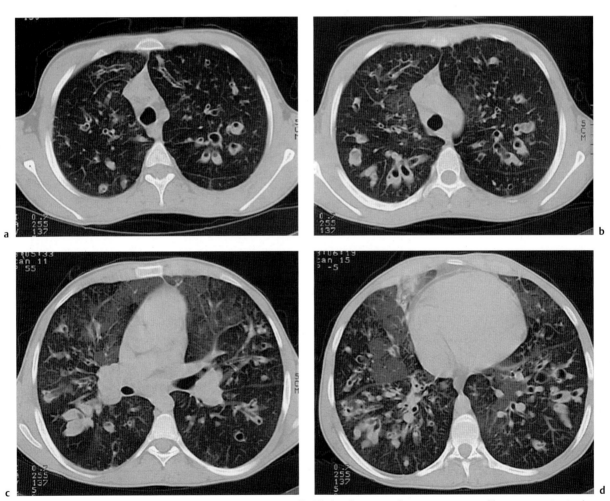

Fig. 4.**23 a–d** Cystic fibrosis. Dilated bronchial lumina are partially filled with mucus. The mosaic pattern of lung attenuation in the lower zones probably reflects air trapping.

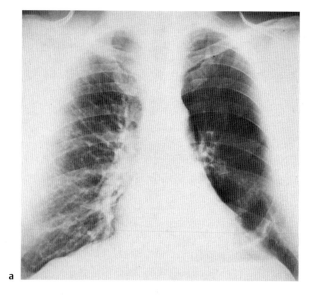

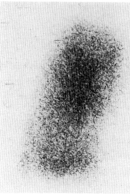

Fig. 4.**24 a, b** Swyer–James–Macleod syndrome. Frontal radiograph (**a**) shows a hypertransradiant left lung with decreased vascular markings. The perfusion study (**b**) shows absence of radionuclide uptake in the affected lung. These changes had been known to exist for more than 30 years in this 42-year-old man.

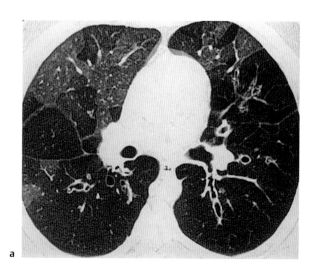

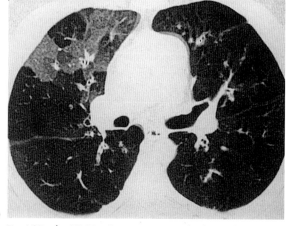

Fig. 4.**25 a, b** HRCT: Swyer–James–Macleod syndrome. CT image acquired in inspiration (**a**) shows mosaic pattern; areas of low attenuation are interspersed with areas of normal lung. Central bronchiectasis is also present. Image acquired in expiration (**b**) shows air trapping.

High-resolution CT: HRCT findings in Swyer–James–Macleod syndrome have been described (Marti-Bonmati 1989, Moore et al. 1992) and include areas of decreased attenuation. Changes may be unilateral, although, more frequently, bilateral abnormalities are evident. These tend to be patchy in distribution, giving a mosaic pattern. Regions of low attenuation are interspersed with areas of normal lung. Air trapping is seen on expiratory images (Wilson 1995, Fig. 4.**25 a, b**).

Associated bronchiectasis, central in distribution, may be present.

Organizing Pneumonia/Cryptogenic Organizing Pneumonia (also known as Bronchiolitis Obliterans Organizing Pneumonia)

Organizing pneumonia or cryptogenic organizing pneumonia represents an organizing pneumonia and a "proliferative" bronchiolitis. Pathologically, the bronchiolitis is characterized by epithelial denudation with proliferation of granulation tissue polyps that contain characteristic Masson inclusion bodies. This entity was also known as BOOP, but recently there has been a tendency to abandon this term as it potentially may cause confusion with the clinical entity of bronchiolitis obliterans (see Constrictive Bronchiolitis, p. 123).

HRCT shows areas of consolidation and ground-glass opacification in a peripheral subpleural distribution (Fig. 4.**26**). The differential diagnosis includes infection, chronic eosinophilic pneumonia, bronchioloalveolar cell carcinoma, and pulmonary lymphoma. Occasionally the "bronchiolar component" is visible radiologically and this is characterized by small centrilobular nodules.

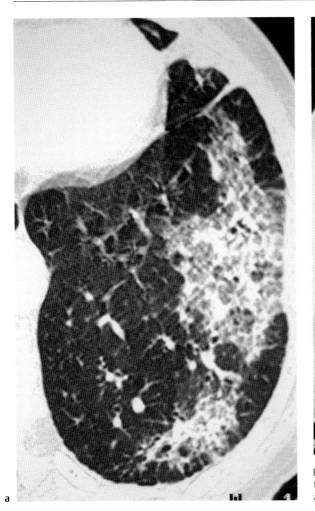

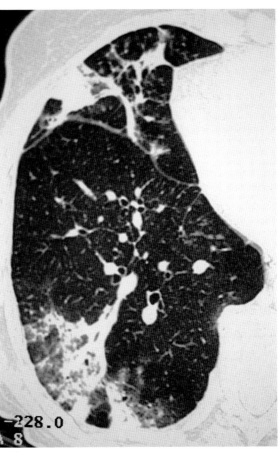

Fig. 4.**26a, b** Organizing pneumonia (BOOP). HRCT images through the lower zones show areas of ground glass opacification and consolidation in a peripheral subpleural distribution.

Bronchial Asthma

Bronchial asthma is characterized by hyperreactivity of the airways to a variety of allergic, infectious, toxic, and psychic stimuli. There is airway inflammation and reversible obstruction, the latter responding to bronchodilator therapy.

Up to 75 % of all asthmatic patients have a normal chest radiograph (Simon and Pride 1973). Other studies have described bronchial wall thickening as the most common plain radiographic finding, being present in 48 % (Paganin et al. 1992) to 71 % (Lynch et al. 1993) of patients. However, this is a relatively nonspecific finding and may also be seen in bronchitis.

Pulmonary hyperinflation may be seen in patients with asthma but it is unusual to see marked hyperinflation in patients who do not have co-existing emphysema (Lynch 1998).

HRCT may be performed to detect bronchiectasis when ABPA (allergic bronchopulmonary aspergillosis) is suspected in asthmatic patients (see Fig. 3.33) or to detect emphysema in smokers with asthma. It may also be performed to exclude entities such as hypersensitivity pneumonitis which may mimic asthma.

The true prevalence of bronchiectasis in patients with chronic uncomplicated asthma remains unclear (Lynch 1998). Mild elevations in bronchoarterial ratio may be seen in patients with asthma but may be due to hypoxic vasoconstriction in areas of air trapping rather than true bronchial dilatation. Bronchial wall thickening is seen in 16–92 % of patients (Grenier et al. 1996, Paganin et al. 1992) and probably reflects a combination of submucosal thickening due to inflammation, thickening of the muscularis mucosae due to muscle hypertrophy and peribronchial fibrosis. Mucoid impaction and decreased lung attenuation may also be seen.

5 Inhalational Lung Diseases and Pneumoconioses

Foreign Body Aspiration

Foreign body aspiration is typically seen in early child-hood. Much less frequently, adults may inhale tooth fragments or dental fillings. Aspirated foreign bodies usually pass down the right main bronchus, which has a more vertical orientation than the left main bronchus. Radiographic features may indicate the presence and lo-cation of the foreign body (Figs. 5.1, 5.2). This can then be confirmed and removed at bronchoscopy or com-puted tomography (CT) may be performed prior to bron-choscopy.

■ Clinical Features

Aspiration material leads to tracheal/bronchial irritation with symptoms of cough and dyspnea. If the foreign body is not detected promptly, it becomes surrounded by fibrous tissue and patients then may be asympto-matic or have minimal symptoms for many years.

■ Radiologic Findings

▓ Chest Radiograph

Radiopaque foreign bodies such as coins, marbles, and teeth are visible on standard radiographs. Indirect signs indicating the presence of a nonopaque foreign body in-clude: (Figs. 5.3 and 5.4):
- *Unilateral pulmonary lucency*: This results from hy-perinflation due to a check-valve obstruction and from reflex oligemia due to hypoventilation.
- *Mediastinal shift*: Air trapping in the affected lung leads to mediastinal shift to the contralateral side in expiration and a return to its normal position in in-spiration.
- *Lobar atelectasis and distal pneumonia* develop when bronchial obstruction persists for at least several hours.

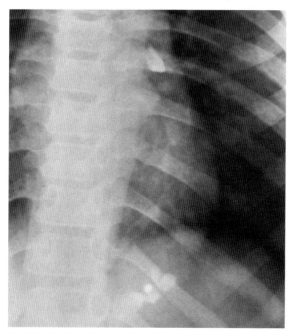

Fig. 5.**1** Swallowed and aspirated teeth.

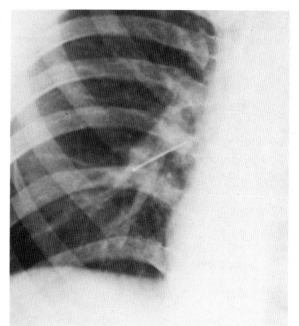

Fig. 5.**2** Aspirated pin.

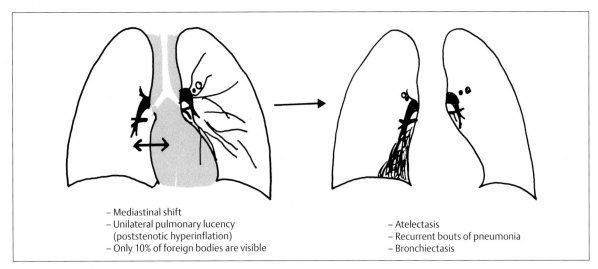

- Mediastinal shift
- Unilateral pulmonary lucency
  (poststenotic hyperinflation)
- Only 10% of foreign bodies are visible

- Atelectasis
- Recurrent bouts of pneumonia
- Bronchiectasis

Fig. 5.**3**   Foreign body aspiration.

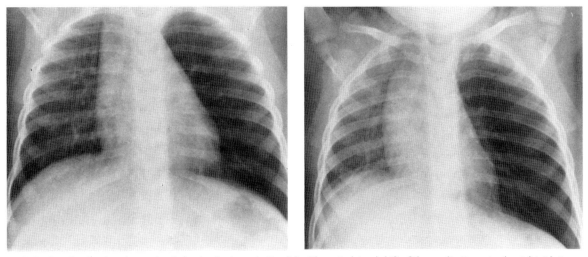

a

b

Fig. 5.**4 a, b**   Check-valve obstruction in foreign body aspiration (**a**) with contralateral shift of the mediastinum to the right side in expiration (**b**).

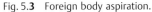 Computed Tomography

Helical CT will frequently allow direct visualization of the foreign body within the airway. Regional air trapping within the lung distal to the endobronchial body may be seen in cases of check-valve obstruction or atelectasis, and pneumonic consolidation may be present if the inhaled body leads to a high-grade obstruction.

Pneumoconiosis

■ Pathology and International Labor Office (ILO) Classification

The pneumoconioses are a group of lung diseases caused by inhalation of inorganic or organic dust of animal or plant origin. Typically, chronic environmental or domestic exposure leads to disease after a variable number of years. Minute dust particles up to a maximum diameter of 10 µm reach the alveoli during inspiration. There they are phagocytosed by macrophages and are deposited in the lung parenchyma. Larger particles are retained in the upper respiratory tract and are cleared by the mucociliary escalator.

In simple pneumoconiosis, the inhaled dust particles do not cause a reaction in the pulmonary parenchyma. *Foreign body reactions*, however, are frequent and result in eventual fibrosis. Dust particles may also bind with endogenous proteins; this complex then acts as an antigen and the *resulting allergic inflammatory response* may also progress to pulmonary fibrosis. Parenchymal fibrosis is characterized by cicatricial emphysema and a restrictive pattern on pulmonary function tests. An accompanying chronic bronchitis is frequent and results in a degree of obstructive ventilatory impairment. In addition, certain types of dust cause specific types of lung injury. For example, silicosis may be associated with tuberculous reactivation and asbestos exposure is associated with an increased risk of developing both bronchial carcinoma and mesothelioma.

Pneumoconioses are recognized as occupational diseases if a probable link between the occupation and the illness can be established. This "probability" is based on the history of exposure, abnormal pulmonary function tests, and appropriate findings on imaging studies. Lung biopsy is rarely necessary.

Goals of Diagnostic Imaging:
Detection of pneumoconiosis in "at-risk" individuals.
Evaluation of the extent and severity of change and particularly the presence of pulmonary fibrosis.
Detection of complications including silicotuberculosis and development of neoplasia.

The International Labor Office has established standardized criteria for the classification of pneumoconioses based on the categorization of pulmonary opacities on the posteroanterior (PA) chest radiograph (ILO 2000):
* *Shape and size of individual opacities*: Small round opacities are classified by size as p, q, or r. Small irregular opacities are classified as s, t, or u (fine, medium, or coarse). Opacities greater than 1 cm in diameter are categorized as A, B, or C on the basis of their combined diameters (Fig. 5.**5** and Table 5.**1**).

Table 5.**1** Pneumoconioses due to inorganic dusts (from Mathys 2001)

Syndrome	Source of antigen	Effects
Progressive pneumoconiosis due to silica-containing dusts, with relatively severe fibrosis:		
Talcosis	Chalk (magnesium, silicate), industrial lubricants, rubber products. Inhalation of pure talc, talc in association with silica (talcosiliosis), and talc in association with asbestos fibers (talcoasbestosis).	1. Changes similar to asbestosis but with sparing of the apices and costophrenic angles. 2. Confluence of nodules to give PMF-type appearance. 3. Hilar lymph node enlargement.
Kaolinosis (kaolin lung)	Aluminum silicate, porcelain, and ceramic industries.	Fibrosis due to the presence of quartz dust in kaolin.
Persistent pneumoconioses due to quartz-free dusts, with mild fibrosis:		
Anthracosis	Coal dust, coal mining, heaters.	No clinical effects or radiographic changes; black lungs seen at autopsy.
Siderosis	Iron oxide, arc welders, silver polishers, iron mining.	Inert deposits producing small opacities. Nodular opacification characteristically involving the midzones and reversible on cessation of exposure. Silicosiderosis: pulmonary fibrosis.
Bauxite lung	Aluminum manufacturing, smelting of aluminum ore to produce corundum.	Emphysema and pulmonary fibrosis.
Aluminum lung	Manufacture of explosives.	Fine reticular and focal opacities, spontaneous pneumothorax.
Berylliosis	Aircraft manufacturing.	Only 2% of exposed workers develop berylliosis; acute form manifest as alveolitis, chronic form is associated with generalized granulomatous disease similar to sarcoidosis.
Hard-metal lung disease	Tungsten, carbide, cobalt, titanium, vanadium, antimony, tin, steel tool manufacturing.	Spectrum of change from bronchitis and bronchiolitis through to subacute fibrosing alveolitis and giant cell interstitial pneumonia.

Section 4

Social security number [   ]

Name (first, last) [   ]

Date of radiograph

[ ][ ] . [ ][ ] . [ ][ ][ ][ ]

Day   Month   Year

Radiographic findings based on 2000 ILO Classification

Radiographic quality   ☐ +   ☐ ±   ☐ +/=   ☐ u   ☐ T   ☐ Lateral view available

Lung

Small opacities Profusion Rounded shape				Zones	
Size p q r ☐ ☐ ☐	☐ 0/- ☐ 1/0 ☐ 2/1 ☐ 3/2			☐ RU ☐ LU	
	☐ 0/0 ☐ 1/1 ☐ 2/2 ☐ 3/3			☐ RM ☐ LM	
	☐ 0/1 ☐ 1/2 ☐ 2/3 ☐ 3/+			☐ RL ☐ LL	

Irregular shape
Size s t u ☐ ☐ ☐

☐ 0/- ☐ 1/0 ☐ 2/1 ☐ 3/2   ☐ RU ☐ LU
☐ 0/0 ☐ 1/1 ☐ 2/2 ☐ 3/3   ☐ RM ☐ LM
☐ 0/1 ☐ 1/2 ☐ 2/3 ☐ 3/+   ☐ RL ☐ LL

Mixed shapes

☐ 0/- ☐ 1/0 ☐ 2/1 ☐ 3/2   ☐ RU ☐ LU
☐ 0/0 ☐ 1/1 ☐ 2/2 ☐ 3/3   ☐ RM ☐ LM
☐ 0/1 ☐ 1/2 ☐ 2/3 ☐ 3/+   ☐ RL ☐ LL

Large opacities   ☐ None   Size ☐ A   ☐ B   ☐ C
☐ RU ☐ LU
☐ RM ☐ LM
☐ RL ☐ LL

Symbols

☐   ☐ fr
☐ aa   ☐ hi
☐ at   ☐ ho
☐ ax   ☐ id
☐ bu   ☐ ih
☐ ca   ☐ kl
☐ cg   ☐ me
☐ cn   ☐ od
☐ co   ☐ pa
☐ cp   ☐ pb
☐ cv   ☐ pi
☐ di   ☐ px
☐ ef   ☐ ra
☐ em   ☐ rp
☐ es   ☐ tb

Pleura

Blunting of costophrenic angle   ☐ None   Side R ☐   L ☐

Pleural thickening
Diffuse
Lateral chest wall

Widening/thickness/<3 mm/en face widening/thickness/<3 mm/en face

R ☐ 1 ☐ a ☐ ☐ L ☐ 1 ☐ a ☐ ☐   ☐ RU ☐ LU
☐ None ☐ 2 ☐ b   ☐ 2 ☐ b   ☐ RM ☐ LM
☐ 3 ☐ c   ☐ 3 ☐ c   ☐ RL ☐ LL

Pleural thickening
Circumscribed
(plaque)

Widening/thickness/<3 mm/en face widening/thickness/<3 mm/en face

R ☐ 1 ☐ a ☐ ☐ L ☐ 1 ☐ a ☐ ☐   Site
☐ None ☐ 2 ☐ b   ☐ 2 ☐ b   Diaphragm R ☐ L ☐
☐ 3 ☐ c   ☐ 3 ☐ c   Chest wall ☐ ☐

Pleural calcification

☐ None   R ☐   L ☐

Diaphragm R ☐ L ☐
Chest wall ☐ ☐
Other ☐ ☐

Interpretation of occupational disease*)

☐ No evidence of notifiable disease

Definite evidence of notifiable disease)**

☐ Silicosis
☐ Silicotuberculosis
☐ Lung cancer in a patient with known quartz dust-associated lung disease

☐ Asbestosis
☐ Asbestos-induced pleural disease
☐ Asbestos-induced lung cancer

☐ Other abnormalities _____
☐ Asbestos-induced laryngeal cancer
☐ Pleural or peritoneal mesothelioma
☐ Disease caused by ionizing radiation

Cause of occupational disease, additional findings, recommendations and/or obligatory measures (please print)

_____

_____

_____

_____

_____

Physician stamp and signature

3683198456

*) Please check the appropriate box.
**) Please notify the insurance carrier and the insured.

Fig. 5.**5** Radiographic interpretation form based on the ILO Classification (see pp. 131–134 for coding and symbols).

- *Profusion of lesions in the pulmonary parenchyma* (number of small opacities per lung zone) is graded on a scale of 0–3 (Fig. 5.5).
- *Reactive pleural, pericardial, and hilar changes* are described and coded.

The ILO provides three guidelines for interpreting radiographic findings:
- Standard reference radiographs (e. g., Fig. 5.6). Classification aided by standard reference radiographs helps to minimize interobserver variability.
- Verbal definitions (see text pp. 131–134).
- Drawings and diagrams (Figs. 5.5–5.9). These materials are the least reliable and should be used only to reinforce verbal descriptions and letter codes.

Formal disability assessment by a specially trained and approved physician is based strictly on use of standard reference radiographs, computer-interpretable data sheets, and in some cases CT assessment. A simplified scheme based on overall impression of pulmonary involvement has been adopted for clinical use. The *predominant type of opacity* and the *predominant grade of profusion* are determined using the ILO verbal definitions. For example, grade qq 2/2 refers to numerous round opacities, 1.5–3 mm in diameter, scattered throughout both lungs but not obscuring pulmonary vascular markings; qt 2/2 refers to the additional presence of irregular opacities 1.5–3 mm in diameter. This simplified scheme by definition precludes a detailed account of all findings and, in particular, of regional variations in severity of change.

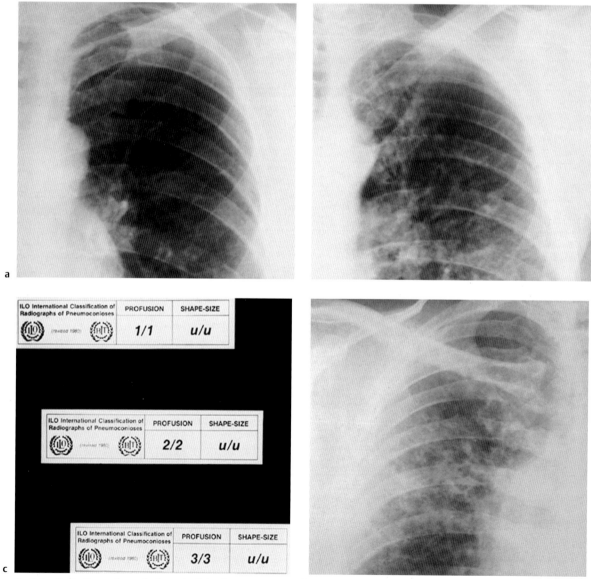

Fig. 5.**6**   Illustrative radiographs from the ILO reference series.

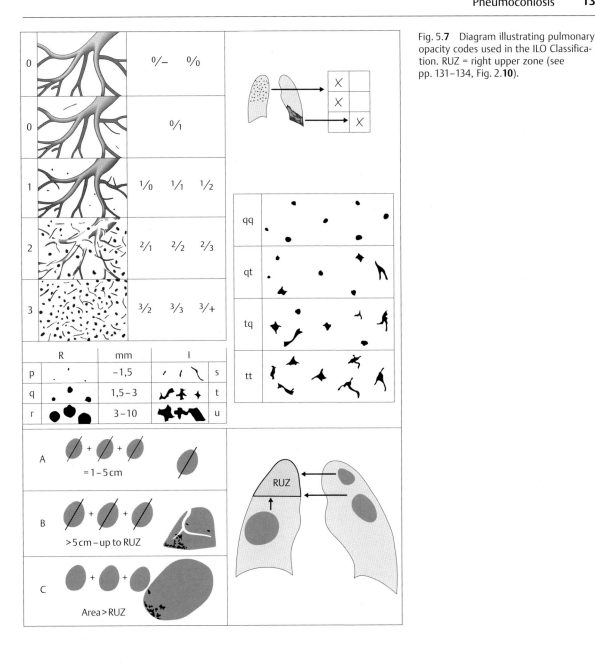

Fig. 5.**7** Diagram illustrating pulmonary opacity codes used in the ILO Classification. RUZ = right upper zone (see pp. 131–134, Fig. 2.**10**).

Interpretive criteria (from Hering 2003)

1 Radiograph quality:
- + Good;
- +/– Acceptable, with no technical defect likely to impair classification of the radiograph;
- +/– – Poor, with technical defects that limit evaluation of the lung or pleura;
- u Unreadable.

2 Small round opacities: well-defined nodular opacities that are classified according to the diameter of the predominant type of opacity.
- p smaller than 1.5 mm;
- q 1.5–3 mm in diameter;
- r 3–10 mm in diameter.

3 Small irregular opacities: linear, reticular, or reticulonodular opacities, which are classified according to their width.
- s smaller than 1.5 mm, fine, linear;
- t 1.5–3 mm, moderately coarse, still linear;
- u 3–10 mm, coarse.

4 Profusion and location: Profusion indicates the degree of parenchymal involvement relative to the standard reference radiographs. It is described in terms of the affected side and one or more affected lung zones, which are defined geometrically rather than anatomically. Profusion is classified on a four-point major category scale (from 0 to 3), with each major category divided into three parts, resulting in a 12-point scale:

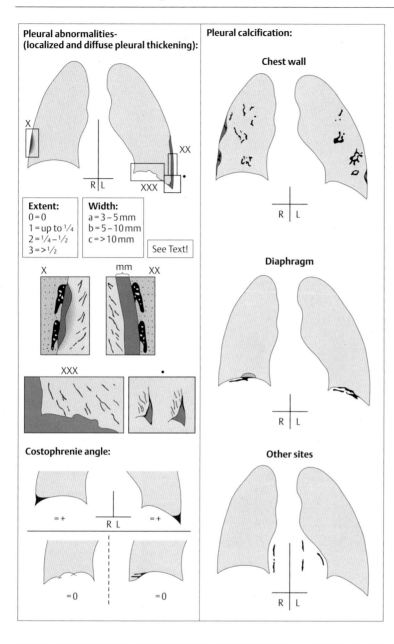

Fig. 5.**8** Review of pleural opacity codes used in the 1980 ILO Classification (see 6 below).

- 0   0/–   0/0   0/1
- 1   1/0   1/1   1/2
- 2   2/1   2/2   2/3
- 3   3/2   3/3   3/+

Examples: A radiograph that definitely fits category 2 when compared with ISO reference No. 2 is classified as 2/2. A study classified as 2/1 closely resembles the No. 2 reference radiograph but category 1 was also considered in classifying the radiograph. This scheme can be applied to the remaining categories in the same way.

Large opacities: This term is limited to opacities that are consistent with pneumoconiosis.

- A: This is a single opacity larger than 1 cm but no more than 5 cm in diameter or multiple opacities larger than 1 cm individually but that do not exceed a total combined diameter of 5 cm.
- B: One or more opacities larger than in category A but whose combined diameter does not exceed the equivalent of the right upper zone.
- C: One or more opacities larger than B and whose combined diameters exceed the equivalent area of the right upper zone.

6 Pleural thickening: Pleural thickening is classified as localized (plaque) or diffuse and both categories may coexist (Fig. 5.9). Each side is classified separately.

The pleural width or plaque thickness is measured from the inner margin of the chest wall to the sharp margin of the pleura/lung interface (a–c). Concomitant or exclusive "en-face" pleural thickening is recorded as being present (Y) or absent (N); its width cannot be measured.

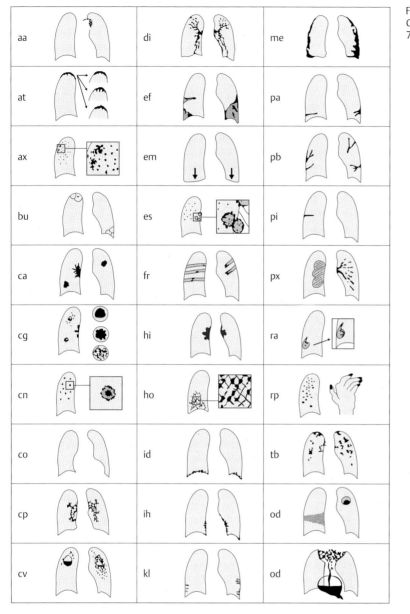

Fig. 5.**9** Coding symbols used in the ILO Classification (for key to symbols, see 7 below).

- a 3–5 mm
- b 5–10 mm
- c >10 mm

The maximum longitudinal extent of pleural thickening is based on the chest wall length for R and L from the lung apex to the costophrenic angle. This is determined individually for diffuse thickening or as the combined en-face or in-profile lengths of pleural plaques:

- 1 <1/4 the total length from the apex to the costophrenic angle on one side.
- 2 1/4 to 1/2 the total length from the apex to the costophrenic angle on one side.
- 3 >1/2 the total length from the apex to the costophrenic angle on one side.
- Diaphragmatic plaques with obliteration of the costophrenic angle are designated as being on

the right (R) or left (L) side and are reported as being present (Y) or absent (N).

The side and extent of pleural calcifications are reported separately for each side, and their location is categorized as chest wall, diaphragm, or "other" (mediastinal and pericardial pleura):

- 1 One or more calcifications with a total combined length <2 cm.
- 2 One or more calcifications with a total combined length of 2–10 cm.
- 3 One or more calcifications with a total combined length >10 cm.

7 Symbols: obligatory. Their expansions should be interpreted as if they were preceded by "suspected ..." or "findings consistent with ..."

- 0 None.
- aa Atherosclerotic aorta.

- at   Apical pleural thickening.
- ax   Coalescence of small opacities.
- bu   Bulla, additional information on emphysema.
- ca   Lung cancer.
- cg   Calcified granuloma.
- cn   Calcification in small pneumoconiotic opacities.
- co   Abnormality of cardiac size or shape.
- cp   Cor pulmonale or pulmonary hypertension.
- cv   Cavitation, liquefaction.
- di   Marked distortion of intrathoracic structures.
- ef   Free pleural effusion.
- em   Emphysema.
- es   Eggshell calcification of hilar and/or mediastinal lymph nodes.
- fr   Fractured rib(s).
- hi   Enlargement of hilar and/or mediastinal lymph nodes > 1.5–2 cm.
- ho   Honeycomb lung.
- id   Ill-defined diaphragmatic contour.
- ih   Ill-defined cardiac contour.
- kl   Kerley lines (indicate in cases with a suspected cardiac cause).
- me   Malignant mesothelioma of the pleura, pericardium, or peritoneum.
- od   Other significant disease.
- pa   Plate atelectasis.
- pb   Parenchymal bands.
- pi   Pleural thickening of an interlobar fissure (designate R/L side).
- px   Pneumothorax (also mark "ef" if effusion is also present).
- ra   Rounded atelectasis.
- rp   Rheumatoid pneumoconiosis.
- tba   Tuberculosis, active?
- tbu   Tuberculosis, inactive?

8 Comments: Comments may be added to this section to explain or describe findings in greater detail. The ILO Classification by definition is based on the PA chest radiograph. Information from other imaging modalities can and should be recorded in this section.

9 Conclusion: Finally, it is determined whether the coded changes are consistent with an occupational or environmental cause of pulmonary disease.

■ CT Classification

CT today plays an essential role in the diagnosis of pneumoconioses (Hering 2003). An international working group has issued guidelines for standardized classification of CT images (Fig. 5.10):

Interpretive criteria.
(1) Image quality:
Image quality is graded on a scale from 1 (good) to 4 (unreadable). The number of images may be limited in screening and/or follow-up examinations. If the study is limited to six reference slices, they should be acquired in the prone position: at the level of the carina,

which provides a reproducible reference point, and atequidistant levels above and below the carina using a 1–2 mm slice thickness and two window settings, such as C/W = 50/400 and C/W = –500/1500 to 2000.

(2) Smooth, well-circumscribed rounded opacities: Well-defined nodular opacities, which are coded according to the diameter of the predominant type: < 1.5 mm, also termed micronodular (P); 1.5–3 mm (Q); and 3–10 mm (R). The predominant size (P, Q, or R) is only indicated in the summation.

(3) Small, irregular, and/or linear opacities: Linear interlobular septal and intralobular nonseptal opacities or a focal centrilobular arrangement in the acinus. Subpleural curvilinear lines represent a specific distribution of intralobular structures. Parenchymal bands are residual scars longer than 2 cm that are located in the peripheral lung and generally are in contact with the pleura. If the images do not document contact with the pleura, the bands are classified as translobular.

(4) Other parenchymal abnormalities:
Inhomogeneous lung attenuation due to mosaic perfusion (MP) and ground-glass opacification (GGO). Honeycombing. Emphysema with a classification of type (e. g., acinar, panlobular, paraseptal, or cicatricial) may be entered under Additional Findings. Bullae are designated by the symbol BU.

(5) Large opacities:
Both pneumoconiotic and nonpneumoconiotic opacities larger than 1 cm in diameter are coded. Distinct areas of rounded atelectasis (RA) in contact with the pleura fall under the heading of visceral-type pleural thickening combined with the symbol RA.

(6) Pleural abnormalities:
Pleural changes may be parietal or visceral in type. Parietal change includes typical pleural plaques. There is no lower size limit; if pleural thickening is detectable by imaging, it should be coded. "Visceral" pleural change described as "diffuse pleural thickening," is frequently associated with subpleural fibrosis. When this is identified, then additional information should be given on small opacities and/or symbols should be added such as PB (parenchymal bands) or RA. Changes involving the mediastinal (M) and diaphragmatic (D) pleura may also be coded. W = wall, M = mediastinum, D = diaphragm.

(7) Symbols:
Symbols are an obligatory entry and should be interpreted as if they were preceded by "suspected …" or "findings consistent with …" Capital letters are used to distinguish them from the symbols in the ILO Classification.

(8) Additional findings:
Findings not covered in the interpretation form may be added as descriptive entries.

CT classification

Name, SSN		CT number, date				Quality	Position	
		Number of slices		Imaging technique	kV	1	Prone	
		Slice thickness		Single-slice spiral	mA	2	Supine	
		Window setting		Multislice Spiral	sec	3		
						4		

CT finding 2001

Is the radiograph negative? No   Yes

Symbols

0
AX
BE
BR
BU
CA
CG
CV
DI
DO
EF
ES
FP
FR
HI
ME
MP
OD
PB
RA
SC
TB
TD

Lung

Rounded opacities (sharply circumscribed)   No   Yes

	No	Yes	Most frequent size
P = < 1.5 mm			
Q = 1.5 - 3 mm			
R = > 3 - 10 mm			

Zones / Profusion

	R				L			
U	0	1	2	3	0	1	2	3
M	0	1	2	3	0	1	2	3
L	0	1	2	3	0	1	2	3

Total profusion

Irregular and/or linear opacities   No   Yes

	No	Yes	Most frequent type
Intralobular			
Interlobular			

Zones / Profusion

	R				L			
U	0	1	2	3	0	1	2	3
M	0	1	2	3	0	1	2	3
L	0	1	2	3	0	1	2	3

Total profusion

Nonhomogeneous opacity   No   Yes

Ground glass   Nein   Ja

	R				L			
U	0	1	2	3	0	1	2	3
M	0	1	2	3	0	1	2	3
L	0	1	2	3	0	1	2	3

Total profusion

Honeycombing   No   Yes

	R				L			
U	0	1	2	3	0	1	2	3
M	0	1	2	3	0	1	2	3
L	0	1	2	3	0	1	2	3

Total profusion

Emphysema   Nein   Ja

	R				L			
U	0	1	2	3	0	1	2	3
M	0	1	2	3	0	1	2	3
L	0	1	2	3	0	1	2	3

Total profusion

Large opacities   No   Yes

		R	L
A	U		
B	M		
C	L		

Most frequent parenchymal finding

RO	IR	GG	HC	EM	LO

Pleura

Pleural abnormalities   No   Yes

		No	Yes	Most frequent type
W	Parietal type			
	Visceral type			
M				
D				

	R	L
U		
M		
L		

Extent, thickness

	R				L			
	0	1	2	3	0	1	2	3
	0	a	b	c	0	a	b	c

Pleural calcifications   No   Yes

Site

W	M	D

Comments, summary

Date, signature

Date	Signature

Fig. 5.**10**   CT interpretation form based on the ILO Classification.

Pneumoconioses Due to Inorganic Dusts

Silicosis

Silicosis develops after prolonged exposure to quartz dust, usually over a period of 10–20 years. It primarily affects sandblasters, miners of quartz-rich stone, and workers in the polishing, ceramic, and porcelain industries. Pulmonary fibrosis develops as a result of both foreign body reaction and hypersensitivity-type allergic response. Changes may progress even when exposure has been discontinued.

■ Pathology

Inhaled dust particles reach the alveoli, are phagocytosed by macrophages, and transported to the interstitium. Here the phagocytosed particles act as a nidus for further aggregation of macrophages and fibroblasts, and a nodule of concentrically arranged collagen fibers develops. These silicotic nodules may coalesce and occupy an entire secondary lobule and appear radiographically as round opacities. Associated interlobular and intralobular septal fibrosis produces reticular shadowing and thickened intra- and interlobular septal lines on the chest radiograph. Finally, the nodules may coalesce to form large conglomerate fibrotic masses (progressive massive fibrosis).

Mixed-dust silicoses are much more common than pure silicosis. These pursue the same clinical course as the pathogenic agent is always silicon dioxide quartz dust but sometimes show more gradual progression. The total SiO_2 content of healthy lungs is less than 0.2 g; in silicosis it is increased by up to 100-fold. Quartz crystals are found on microscopic examination of histological specimens from silicotic nodules or from involved lymph nodes.

■ Clinical Features

Acute silicosis is rare and results from massive exposure to silica dust, usually in sandblasters. This disease is rapidly progressive and respiratory insufficiency develops within months. The radiology and histology of acute silicosis resemble pulmonary alveolar proteinosis. *Chronic silicosis* is much more common. Patients are usually asymptomatic when radiographic changes initially become visible. Fibrosis with cicatricial emphysema then develops gradually over a period of years and this is associated with increasing dyspnea progressing to cyanosis and eventual cor pulmonale. Pulmonary function tests show a mixed pattern with both obstructive and restrictive ventilatory impairment. Hy-

poxemia probably results from ventilation-perfusion mismatch.

Individuals exposed to quartz dust are at significantly higher risk for developing tuberculosis (silicotuberculosis). In men with silicosis, the relative risk has been estimated as 2.8 (Cowie 1994). The incidence of carcinoma also appears to be increased and there are cases in which bronchial carcinoma has been recognized as an occupational disease in German workers' compensation proceedings. Very rigorous criteria are applied in these cases including close proximity of the carcinoma to the fibrosis, profusion greater than category 1/1 or "large opacities."

■ Radiologic Findings

▢ Plain Chest Radiograph

Radiographic changes in silicosis may be classified into four types although mixed patterns are common (Fig. 5.**11**, 5.**12**):

- *Nodules*: Multiple, homogeneous, well-defined nodules 1–10 mm in diameter may produce a "snowstorm" appearance in the upper and mid zones. Nodular calcification occurs in 20% of cases (Fig. 5.**13 a**).
- *Diffuse fibrosis*: Fibrosis produces a generalized increase in linear and reticular markings. A honeycomb pattern may be seen in advanced cases (Fig. 5.**14**).
- *Lymph node enlargement showing an "eggshell" pattern of calcification*: There is hilar and mediastinal lymph node enlargement and these nodes show a peripheral, eggshell-like pattern of calcification in 5% of cases (Fig. 5.**15**). This appearance is very suggestive of silicosis although sarcoidosis occasionally may produce a similar appearance. Lymph node changes may precede the development of parenchymal involvement.
- *Progressive massive fibrosis (PMF)* is characterized by large, homogeneous opacities with radiating strands (pseudopodia) mainly involving the upper lobes. These conglomerate masses gradually shrink over a period of years and migrate towards the hilum (Figs. 5.**16**). Occasionally the centers of these masses may undergo autolytic degeneration but upper lobe cavitation may also indicate tuberculous reactivation.
- *Acute silicoproteinosis*: This very rare acute form of pneumoconiosis is only seen with massive exposure, usually in sandblasters. Radiographs show decreased pulmonary lucency consistent with ground-glass opacification and consolidation.

Computed Tomography

Thin-section CT images (collimation 1–3 mm) are helpful in classification of pulmonary parenchymal abnormality. CT features of silicosis include:

- *Diffuse pulmonary nodules* 2–5 mm in diameter in a perilymphatic (subpleural, paraseptal, and centrilobular) distribution. These sometimes may calcify (Fig. 5.**13 b**, Fig. 5.**17 a**).
- *Conglomerate masses in PMF*: irregular in outline and with fibrotic stranding radiating into the adjacent lung. These masses are frequently calcified and may undergo central degeneration with cavitation (Fig. 5.**18**).
- *Asymmetric nodules, consolidation, or cavitation* should raise the possibility of development of silicotuberculosis.

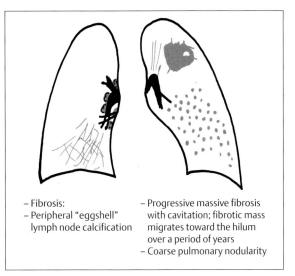

– Fibrosis:
– Peripheral "eggshell" lymph node calcification

– Progressive massive fibrosis with cavitation; fibrotic mass migrates toward the hilum over a period of years
– Coarse pulmonary nodularity

Fig. 5.**11** Silicosis.

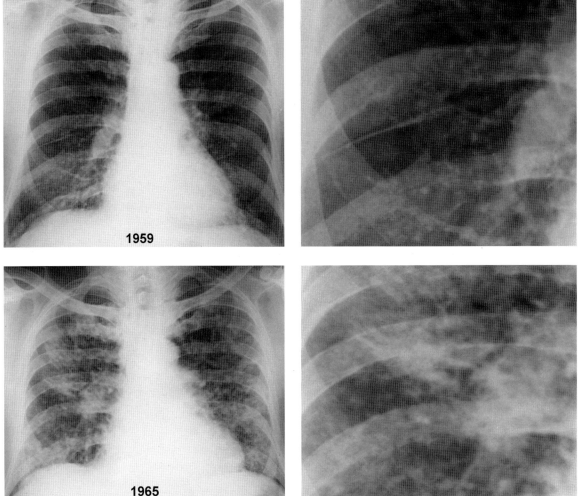

a   1959

c   1965

b

d

Fig. 5.**12 a–d** Progression of silicosis from small type q nodules in 1959 (**a**, **b**) to larger type r nodules (1965 **c**, **d**), and finally to diffuse fibrosis and conglomerate masses (1968 **e**, **f**) with apical emphysema. The 60-year-old coal worker was retired due to ill health in 1959 due to exertional dyspnea. His symptoms progressed slowly over years.   Fig. 5.**12 e, f** ▷

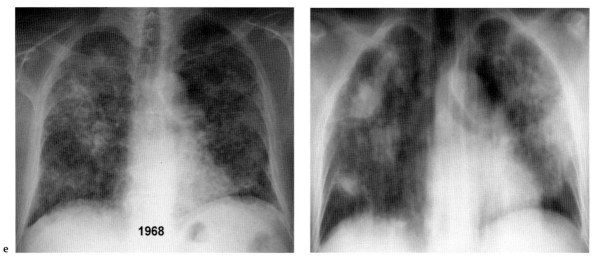

1968

e

f

Fig. 5.**12 e, f**

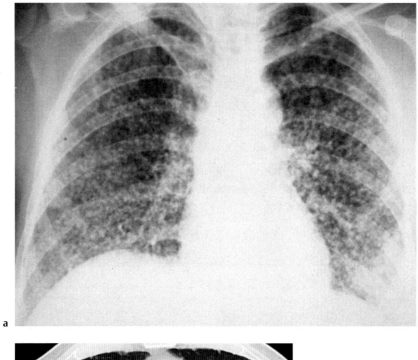

a

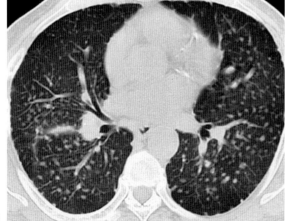

b

Fig. 5.**13 a, b**   Silicosis: Chest radiograph (**a**) and CT (**b**) show pulmonary nodularity.

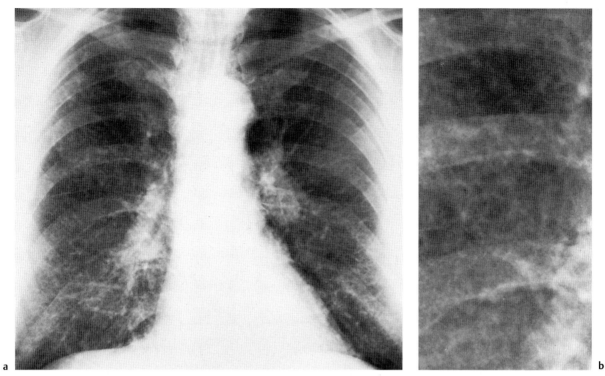

a   b

Fig. 5.**14 a, b**   Silicosis (t 3/3) with pulmonary fibrosis. Radiographs show reticulolinear interstitial shadowing.

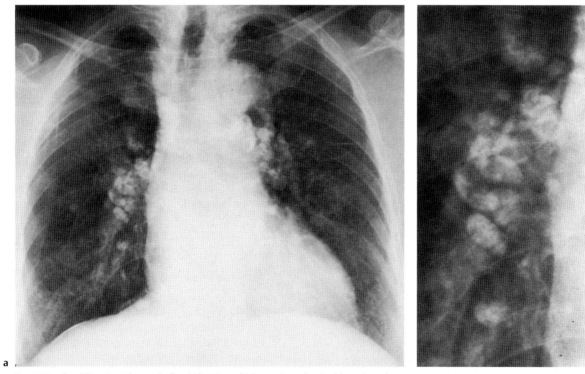

a   b

Fig. 5.**15 a, b**   Silicosis with eggshell calcification of hilar and mediastinal lymph nodes.

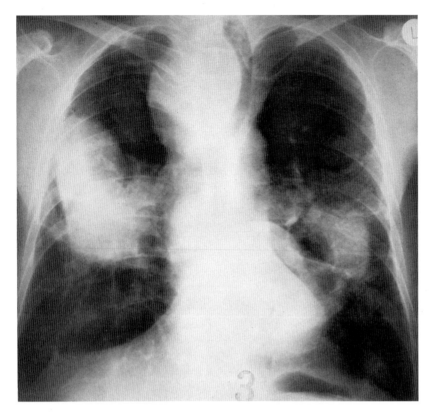

Fig. 5.**16** Silicosis (C, wd) with progressive massive fibrosis, confirmed histologically by biopsy of nodular masses. Incidental finding of right-sided thyroid goiter is also noted.

- *Hilar and mediastinal lymph node enlargement* which may show calcification (Fig. 5.**19**, Fig. 5.**17b**).
- *Acute silicoproteinosis*: CT findings include bilateral centrilobular nodules of ground-glass opacification, more diffuse patchy ground-glass opacification, and consolidation (Marchiori et al. 2001).

▦ Magnetic Resonance Imaging (MRI)

MRI may be useful in distinguishing between the conglomerate masses of progressive massive fibrosis and bronchial carcinoma. PMF-associated soft tissue masses tend to be hypointense on T2-weighted sequences whereas bronchial neoplasms generally show T2 hyperintensity (Matsumoto et al. 1998).

▦ PET

Lesions in PMF may show intense fluorodeoxyglucose (FDG) uptake and thus this may not be helpful in their differentiation from bronchial neoplasia (Chong et al. 2006).

Coal-Worker's Pneumoconiosis (CWP)

Coal-worker's pneumoconiosis results from exposure to "washed coal" which is almost free of silica. While histologically it differs from silicosis, imaging findings are similar with coal macules manifest as nodular opacities frequently centrilobular in distribution and sometimes less well defined than the nodules seen in silicosis. Complicated CWP is manifest as conglomerate masses (progressive massive fibrosis).

Asbestos-Induced Pleural Changes and Asbestosis

Asbestos is a magnesium silicate fiber used in the processing of insulation materials, textiles, paper, and plastic. Pulmonary parenchymal and pleural change usually becomes evident 10–20 years after initial exposure. The diagnosis is based on a history of exposure, the detection of asbestos fibers in the sputum, and typical radiologic findings. Lung biopsy for histological confirmation is very rarely performed.

Asbestos exposure is also associated with an increased risk of developing both bronchial carcinoma and

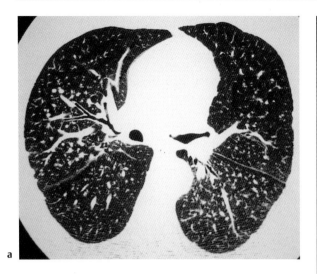

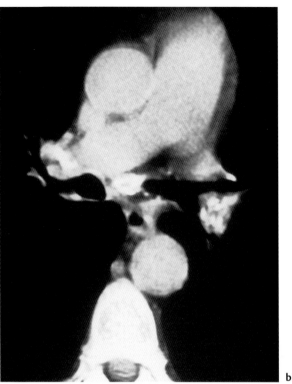

Fig. 5.**17 a, b**   Silicosis: CT shows pulmonary nodularity in a peri- ▷
lymphatic distribution (**a**). When study is viewed at mediastinal
window (**b**), there is bilateral hilar and mediastinal lymph node
enlargement which show eggshell calcification.

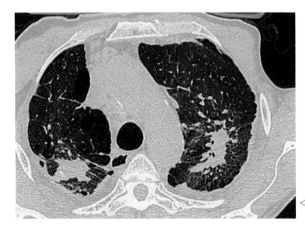

◁ Fig. 5.**18**   Silicotic masses of PMF in both upper zones with calcification and cicatricial emphysema.

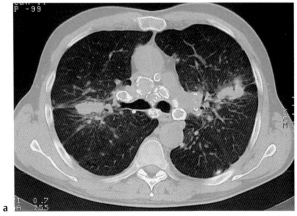

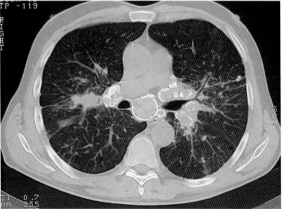

Fig. 5.**19 a, b**   Eggshell calcification of enlarged hilar and mediastinal lymph nodes in silicosis.

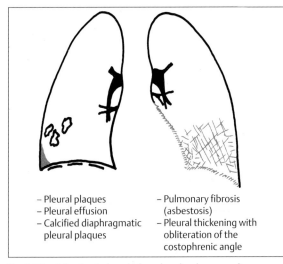

- Pleural plaques
- Pleural effusion
- Calcified diaphragmatic pleural plaques

- Pulmonary fibrosis (asbestosis)
- Pleural thickening with obliteration of the costophrenic angle

Fig. 5.**20** Asbestos-induced pleural and pulmonary disease.

malignant mesothelioma. These neoplasms also occur after a latent period of several years and are recognized as occupational diseases.

■ Pathology

Only asbestos fibers 20–150 μm in length can reach the lower respiratory tract and cause disease. On reaching the bronchioles and alveoli in the basal zones, fibers are phagocytosed and coated in a ferritin protein gel by macrophages (asbestos bodies).

Flat plaques of extrapleural fibrosis up to 10 cm in diameter form symmetrically on the diaphragmatic and costoparietal pleural surfaces. Plaques tend to spare the apices and costophrenic sulci. Calcification is frequent. Their pathogenesis is unclear but may result from mechanical irritation by asbestos fibers which perforate the visceral pleura.

Pulmonary fibrosis is initially peribronchiolar and then spreads along the peribronchovascular and septal connective tissue. Fibrosis is most marked in the lower zones with relative sparing of the apices. In contrast to silicosis, changes are diffuse and nodules are not seen. Fibrotic contraction leads to cicatricial emphysema with traction bronchiectasis and eventual honeycomb lung.

■ Clinical Features

Dyspnea and cyanosis may develop up to 20 years after initial exposure. Pulmonary function tests may show a mixed pattern of ventilatory impairment with both restrictive and obstructive features. Pulmonary diffusing capacity is reduced. Asbestos bodies sometimes may be detected in the sputum.

■ Radiologic Findings

▦ Chest Radiograph

Pleural involvement is frequently more conspicuous than the underlying pulmonary parenchymal change on the chest radiograph (Fig. 5.**20**).
- *Pleural plaques*: Plaques form on the parietal pleura and sites of predilection include the diaphragmatic pleura and the mid to lower anterolateral hemithorax. There tends to be preservation of the costophrenic sulcus. Calcification of pleural plaques is common occurring in 60–80% of cases (Fig. 5.**21**).
- *Recurrent pleural effusion*: This is a diagnosis of exclusion and may appear less than 10 years after initial exposure. It is unilateral in 90% of cases, and recurrent effusions may be associated with a smooth rind of pleural thickening. In a few cases, asbestos fibers may be detected in the pleural aspirate.
- *Diffuse pleural thickening*: Diffuse pleural thickening results from thickening and fibrosis of the visceral pleura with fusion to the parietal pleura often over a wide area (Solomon 1991). Its presence is less specific to asbestos exposure than pleural plaques as exudative effusions and hemothorax may also lead to diffuse pleural thickening and fibrosis.
- *Pulmonary fibrosis*: Reticular and linear shadowing is seen predominantly in the basal zones. Further progression leads to a honeycomb pattern with cicatricial emphysema and traction bronchiectasis. Nodules and massive fibrosis are usually an indicator of mixed dust exposure. In contrast to pure silicosis, however, this has a predilection for the lower zones when seen in association with asbestos exposure (Fig. 5.**22**).
- *The "shaggy-heart" sign*: Fibrosis of the mediastinal pleura adjacent to irregular pulmonary fibrosis in the paracardiac lung may produce an irregular cardiac contour called the shaggy-heart sign.
- *Ill-defined diaphragmatic contour*: Thickening of the diaphragmatic pleura together with contiguous pulmonary fibrosis obliterates the diaphragmatic border.

▦ Computed Tomography

High-resolution CT in both the supine and prone positions (Webb et al. 1992, Aberle 1988) or in the prone position (Friedman 1990) has been advocated for assessment of the lung bases. CT is superior to the chest radiograph in demonstration of early pleural and pulmonary changes and images acquired with the patient in the supine position may well be adequate for assessment.

CT features include:
- *Pleural plaques*: Parietal pleural plaques are sharply demarcated from the adjacent lung and are frequently calcified.
- *Diffuse pleural thickening* typically involves the posterolateral hemithorax inferiorly. CT helps in differen-

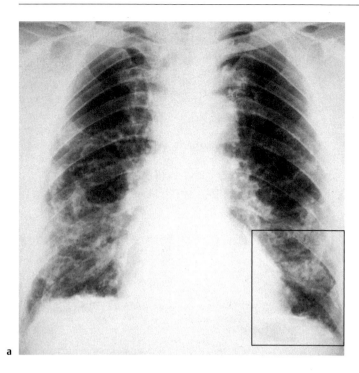

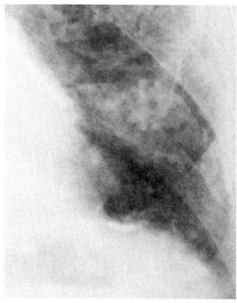

Fig. 5.**21 a, b** **a** Asbestosis and calcified pleural plaques, which particularly involve the diaphragmatic pleura. **b** Magnified view.

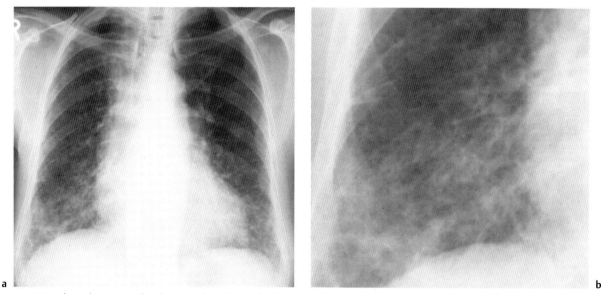

Fig. 5.**22 a, b** Asbestosis with asbestos-induced pleural plaques. Radiograph shows increased reticular markings and laterobasal pleural plaques. Asbestos fibers were found in significant numbers in the lung at postmortem.

tiation of diffuse pleural thickening from extrapleural fat deposition. However, extrapleural fat deposition is frequently seen in association with diffuse pleural thickening probably due to inward pleural retraction (Aberle and Balmes 1991).

- *Rounded atelectasis* appears as rounded juxtapleural opacities up to several centimeters in diameter. They

are seen subjacent to areas of pleural change, and a distinctive arching of vessels and bronchi is seen as they enter the area of infolded lung ("comet tail" sign, Figs 5.**23**, 5.**24 a, b**).

- *Asbestosis*: Dot-like opacities in the subpleural lung may be the earliest CT finding in patients with asbestosis (Webb et al. 1992). These represent centrilobu-

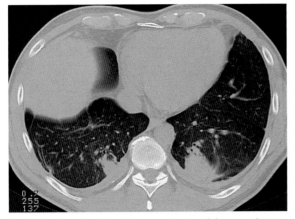

Fig. 5.**23**   Rounded atelectasis in a patient with known asbestos-induced benign pleural change. Note the comet-tail appearance of blood vessels entering the atelectatic lung.

lar peribronchiolar fibrosis (Akira et al. 1990). *Curvilinear subpleural lines* are beaded lines running parallel to and a few millimeters beneath the pleural surface (Fig. 5.25). They may represent confluent peribronchiolar fibrosis involving the subpleural terminal bronchioles but are not specific for asbestosis (Pilate et al. 1987). Later findings include irregular thickening of interlobular and intralobular septa progressing to a honeycomb pattern with traction bronchiectasis.

- *Parenchymal bands* may represent thickening of several marginating septa or fibrosis along the bronchovascular sheath (Akira et al. 1990).

Other Inorganic Pneumoconioses

See Table 5.**1**.

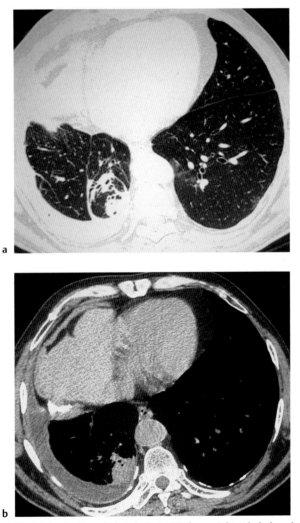

Fig. 5.**24 a, b**   Rounded atelectasis. CT shows right-sided pleural thickening and calcification (**a**) with associated infolded lung (**b**).

Extrinsic Allergic Alveolitis (EAA)/Hypersensitivity pneumonitis

■ Clinical Features

Organic dusts from plants and animals in isolation rarely cause pulmonary disease. Dust particles mixed with fungal antigens, however, may induce a hypersensitivity reaction in the lung. Animal proteins, particularly those of animal origin, also may cause disease. Dust particles 1–5 μm in diameter enter the gas exchange unit where they produce a granulomatous response centered on the bronchioles and surrounding alveoli.

The classic example of organic pneumoconiosis is *farmer's lung.* Its clinical and radiographic features resemble those of other known organic dust diseases (Table 5.2). An acute illness with symptoms of dry cough, dyspnea, fever, and malaise develops 4–12 hours after exposure to moist hay contaminated with thermophilic actinomycetes. These symptoms are usually of short duration, lasting for 12–24 hours, but recur with repeated exposure. The temporal association between exposure and symptoms suggests the diagnosis, which is confirmed by detection of serum precipitins against actinomycetes. Subacute illness is characterized by acute episodes of dyspnea superimposed on a progressive deterioration in lung function. The chronic form of EAA is associated with continuous low-grade exposure and irreversible pulmonary damage.

A number of recent studies have described the entity of **"hot-tub" lung** (Aksamit 2003, Cappelluti et al. 2003). This entity appears to be related to hot tub/spa use and affected individuals develop a hypersensitivity pneumonitis-type illness. Mycobacterium avium complex (MAC) organisms have been isolated from both patient specimens and the spa water with matching fingerprints by restricted fragment length polymorphism and electrophoresis. Hot-tub use appears to lead to high levels of infectious aerosols containing organisms found in the water. Whether this entity reflects an infective process or a true hypersensitivity pneumonitis is controversial, as some patients improve only after antimicrobial therapy while others improve on corticosteroid therapy and cessation of exposure.

■ Radiologic Findings

Chest Radiograph

In acute and subacute disease, a generalized haziness (sometimes described as ground-glass change) may be seen on the chest radiograph. Small pulmonary nodules (2–3 mm in diameter) are also a common finding. End-stage disease is characterized by upper lobe fibrosis with compensatory emphysema in the lower lobes.

Table 5.**2**   Extrinsic allergic alveolitis/hypersensitivity pneumonitis due to organic dusts (from Baum)

Syndrome	Source of antigen	Precipitins against
Farmer's lung	Moldy hay	Thermoactinomyces vulgaris
Bird fancier's lung	Bird droppings	Fecal proteins
Bagassosis	Bagasse (sugarcane fiber)	Fungal spores, Thermoactinomyces vulgaris
Mushroom worker's lung	Mushroom compost	Micropolyspora faeni and vulgaris
Cork worker's lung (suberosis)	Moldy cork	Cork dust
Wood dust lung (maple and poplar bark, sequoiosis)	Moldy sawdust	Cryptostroma corticale, C. graphium, C. altenaria
Cheese washer's lung	Moldy cheese dust	Penicillium casei
Malt worker's lung	Moldy barley	Aspergillus clavatus
Air conditioning alveolitis	Contaminated air humidifier	Molds
Cereal worker's lung	Infected cereal dust	Cereal beetle Sitophilus granarius

Numerous other diseases: hormone sniffer's lung (pituitrin in diabetes insipidus), coffee worker's lung, fishmeal worker's lung, detergent worker's lung, paprika splitter's lung.

High resolution CT

In early disease, patchy bilateral ground-glass opacification may be seen (Fig. 5.26 a). Centrilobular poorly defined nodules of ground-glass opacification are also a frequent finding. Air trapping indicative of a constrictive bronchiolitis may be seen on expiratory images (Small 1996, Figs. 5.26 b, 5.27 a, b).

Findings in hot-tub lung have been described and include centrilobular nodules, which may be well or poorly defined and which most commonly were symmetric in distribution, and areas of ground-glass opacification. Irregular linear opacities are occasionally seen (Hanak et al. 2005).

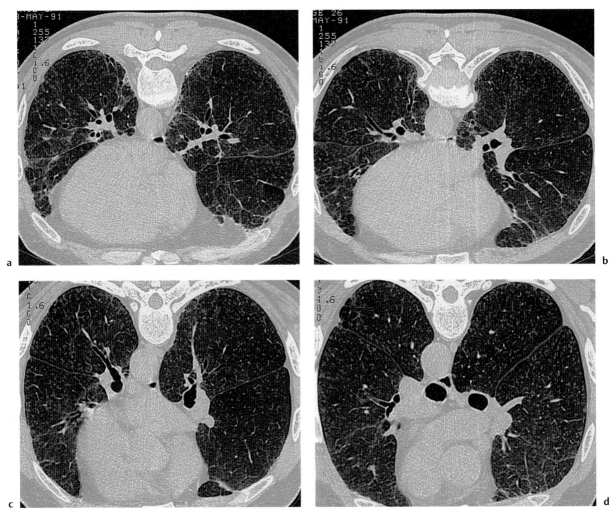

Fig. 5.**25 a–d**   Asbestosis: CT images were acquired with the patient prone. Note the subpleural curvilinear densities with reticular change, traction bronchiectasis, and fibrotic bands.

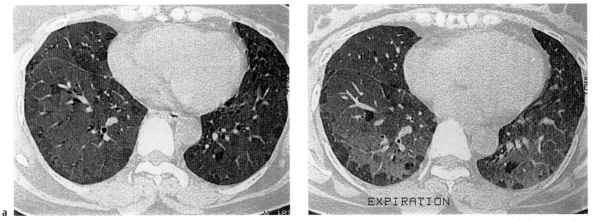

Fig. 5.**26 a, b**   Extrinsic allergic alveolitis/Hypersensitivity pneumonitis: CT in inspiration (**a**) shows extensive ground-glass opacification with areas of focal air trapping evident in expiration (**b**).

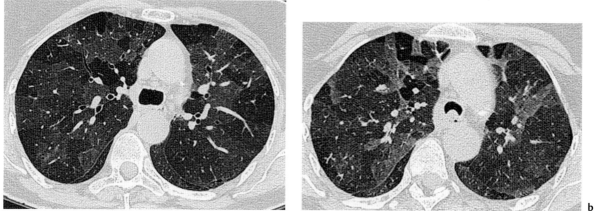

Fig. 5.**27 a, b**   Extrinsic allergic alveolitis/hypersensitivity pneumonitis: CT acquired in inspiration (**a**) shows a mosaic pattern of lung attenuation with evidence of extensive air trapping in expiration (**b**). Histology from VATS biopsy was consistent with EAA/HP.

Inhalation of Toxic Gases and Fumes

■ Clinical Features

Inhalation of noxious gases and vapors may precipitate an acute bronchitis, acute bronchiolitis, or pulmonary edema (Table 5.**3**). Solubility and permeability of the offending substances appear to determine whether damage is predominantly bronchial or alveolar. These injuries usually result from accidents in the chemical industry and changes are very often completely reversible. Environmental air pollution (smog) exacerbates preexisting bronchial disease although a causative association is often difficult to prove.

■ Radiologic Findings

The chest radiograph may show increased interstitial shadowing in acute bronchitis, pulmonary hypertransradiancy in constrictive bronchiolitis, or features of increased permeability pulmonary edema (Fig. 5.**28**).

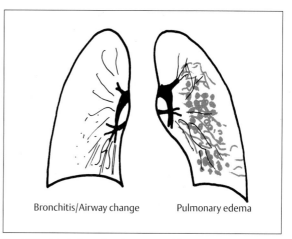

Bronchitis/Airway change   Pulmonary edema

Fig. 5.**28**   Inhalation of toxic gases and fumes.

Table 5.**3**   Pulmonary changes due to inhalation of toxic gases and fumes (from Baum and Mathys)

Substance	Source	Site of action
Oxygen	Respiration	Alveoli
Chlorine gas	Chemical and plastics industry	Bronchi > alveoli
Phosgene	Chemical and plastics industry	Alveoli > bronchi
Ammonia	Refrigerators, fertilizers	Bronchi > alveoli. Bronchiectasis with constrictive bronchiolitis. Pulmonary edema in severe cases.
Sulfur dioxide	Chemical industry, combustion of sulfur-containing oils	Bronchi > alveoli
Ozone	Bleach industry, electric arc welding	Bronchi > alveoli
Nitric oxide	Explosives, silos, automobile exhaust	Bronchi > alveoli
Toluylene isocyanate	Manufacture of polyurethane foam	Bronchi

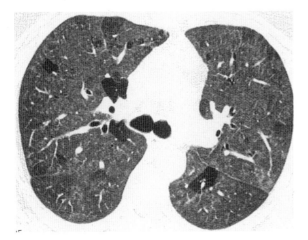

CT findings include features of bronchitis (see p. 116), bronchiectasis (see p. 117), constrictive bronchiolitis (see p. 123), and pulmonary edema (see p. 195) (Fig. 5.**29**).

Fig. 5.**29**   Chlorine gas poisoning. This patient developed dyspnea and cough 4 hours after an occupational accident. HRCT showed extensive ground-glass opacification with minor air trapping.

6 Tumors and Tumor-Like Lesions of the Lung

The Solitary Pulmonary Nodule (SPN)

A solitary pulmonary nodule is defined as a round or oval opacity less than 3 cm in diameter which is surrounded completely by pulmonary parenchyma and is not associated with lymph node enlargement, atelectasis, or pneumonia (Midthun et al. 1993).

Cytologic and/or histological evaluation is usually required to differentiate benign from malignant lesions. However, the following may also be helpful in evaluation of SPNs:

Lesion Size and Morphology

- *CT densitometry:* Central or laminated calcification is seen in granulomata while a "popcorn" pattern of calcification characteristically is seen in hamartomata. The presence of intralesional fat is also considered diagnostic of either a hamartoma or lipoma. Computed tomography (CT) also allows differentiation of lesions of soft tissue attenuation (called *solid* lesions) from those of ground-glass attenuation (called *nonsolid* lesions). Some nodules may comprise a combination of ground glass and soft tissue attenuation (called *partly solid* lesions). Henschke et al. evaluated the significance of nonsolid and partly solid lesions within the context of a lung cancer screening program in a high-risk population. They found an overall malignancy rate of 34% for partly solid/nonsolid lesions vs. 7% for solid lesions. The malignancy rate for partly solid lesions was 63% and for nonsolid lesions was 18%. Histologically, nonsolid and partly solid lesions were predominantly bronchioloalveolar carcinomas or adenocarcinomas with bronchioloalveolar features (Henschke et al. 2002). Aoki et al. correlated lesion attenuation with growth rate (tumor doubling time) and the Noguchi classification of peripheral lung adenocarcinoma (see Screening for Lung Cancer, p. 157). They found lesions of ground-glass attenuation showed slower growth (tumor doubling times of up to 24 months) and correlated with Noguchi types A and B lesions. Lesions of uniform soft tissue attenuation (solid lesions) show much more rapid growth (tumor doubling times of 3–4 months) and correlated histologically with the more aggressive Noguchi

types D to F. Partly solid lesions correlated with intermediate grade Noguchi lesions (Aoki et al. 2000).
- *Lesion measurement on serial studies.* No change in the size of a lesion over a period of 2 years has traditionally been accepted as being consistent with a benign lesion. This concept has been challenged by Yankelevitz and Henschke (1997) as substantial increases in the volume particularly of small nodules may be missed on serial radiographic assessment. CT assessment includes standard in plane measurements on axial CT images. There, however, may be a significant margin of error in the assessment of minor changes (i. e., less than 2 mm) in the diameter of smaller lesions. This is important as a 1 mm increase in the diameter of a 4 mm lesion equates to an increase in volume of approximately 100%. Volumetric analysis of interval growth has been shown to be much more accurate than in plane measurements in the assessment of indeterminate lesions (Yankelevitz and Henschke 2000). However, more recently Goodman and colleagues have reported a mean interscan variability of 13.1% in volumetric measurements using a semi-automated volumetric nodule sizing package (Goodman et al. 2006).

"Functional" Assessment

- *CT enhancement*: Image acquisition post intravenous injection of iodinated contrast medium may be of value in differentiating benign from malignant lesions. Helical volumetric CT images through the lesion may be acquired 1 and 2 minutes post administration of contrast medium. Swenson et al. have shown that enhancement of less than 15 Hounsfield units (HU) has a sensitivity of 98% for benign lesions greater than 5 mm in diameter. However, the specificity of this criterion was significantly lower at 58% as benign lesions may also show significant enhancement (Swenson et al. 2000).
- *Positron emission tomography (PET).* Malignant nodules are associated with an increased metabolic rate and hence increased fluorodeoxyglucose (FDG) uptake on PET evaluation. A number of studies have

shown sensitivities of 93–100% and specificities of 87–88% for all nodules (Gupta et al. 1996, Bury et al. 1996, Dewan et al. 1997). For lesions less than or equal to 15 mm in diameter, sensitivities of 80–83% and specificities of 95–100% have been reported (Dewan et al. 1997, Lowe et al. 1998). Benign inflammatory lesions may give false-positive results and some neoplasms such as bronchioloalveolar carcinoma and carcinoid tumors have low metabolic activity and may give false-negative results.

Miles et al. correlated CT enhancement measurements (standardized perfusion value [SPV]) of pulmonary nodules with their standardized uptake value (SUV) on PET and showed a positive correlation between the two values (Miles et al. 2001).

Evaluation of CT-Detected Small Pulmonary Nodules

In the past decade, detection of small pulmonary nodules has become routine on thin collimation helical volumetric CT. Data from multi-detector CT (MDCT) studies at 5 mm collimation indicate that approximately 50% of smokers over 50 years of age will have at least one visible nodule and another 10% will develop a new nodule over a 12-month period (Swenson et al. 2002). The clinical importance of these nodules appears to be very different from those detected on chest radiographs and the vast majority are benign (MacMahon et al. 2005).

Studies suggest that less than 1% of nodules which are less than 5 mm in diameter found in patients without a history of neoplasia will demonstrate malignant behavior (Henschke et al. 2004, Swenson et al. 2003, Henschke et al. 1999). Therefore, regular CT follow-up of these lesions may reflect poor use of resources, unnecessary patient anxiety, and impose a significant radiation dose particularly in young patients. On evaluation of Early Lung Cancer Action Project (ELCAP) data, Henschke et al. found no lung cancers in patients in whom the largest noncalcified nodule was less than 5 mm in diameter on initial CT. Therefore, there appears to be little point in short-term interval follow-up for nodules less than 5 mm even in high risk patients.

Bearing in mind these considerations, the Fleischner Society has recently issued the following recommendations for nodules detected incidentally at nonscreening CT in persons aged 35 years or older (MacMahon et al. 2005):

- Lesions ≤4 mm:
  - in a low-risk patient: no follow-up required;
  - in a high-risk patient: follow-up CT at 12 months and;
  - if unchanged, no further follow-up needed.
- Lesions >4–6 mm:
  - in a low-risk patient: follow-up CT at 12 months and if unchanged, no further follow-up required;
  - in a high-risk patient: initial follow-up CT at 6–12 months, then at 18–24 months if unchanged.
- Lesions >6–8 mm:
  - in a low-risk patient, initial CT follow-up at 6–12 months, then at 18–24 months if no change;
  - in a high-risk patient, initial CT follow-up at 3–6 months, then at 9–12 and 24 months if no change.
- Lesions >8 mms:
  - in both low- and high-risk patients: follow-up CT at 3, 9, and 24 months. CT enhancement, PET assessment, and/or biopsy.

Longer follow-up intervals may be appropriate for nonsolid and partly solid lesions given their slower growth rates and longer tumor doubling times.

Benign Tumors of the Lung

Benign tumors account for just 2% of pulmonary neoplasms. They may grow slowly or remain unchanged for several years (Table 6.1).

Clinical manifestations and radiographic findings are determined by their location (Fig. 6.1).

- *Central endobronchial lesions* present with cough, hemoptysis, distal pneumonic consolidation, wheezing, and dyspnea. *The chest radiograph* may occasionally show these endobronchial lesions as filling defects within the air-filled lobar and segmental bronchi (Fig. 6.2). In some instances, branching linear opacities representing mucoceles distal to the obstructing lesion may be seen.
- *Helical volumetric CT* through the central airways will confirm these findings and will show the degree of extrabronchial extension of these lesions. Histological confirmation from bronchoscopic biopsy with subsequent surgical resection of these tumors is usually feasible.
- *Peripheral parenchymal tumors* are frequently asymptomatic and these solitary pulmonary nodules are often an incidental finding on chest radiographs.

Table 6.**1**   WHO Classification of lung tumors (modified from Scholman et al. 1991)

	Benign	Malignant
I. Epithelial tumors	• Papillomas • Adenomas • (Dysplasias) • (Carcinoma in situ)	• Squamous cell carcinoma • Small cell carcinoma • Adenocarcinoma • Large cell carcinoma • Adenosquamous carcinoma • Carcinoid tumor • Bronchial gland carcinoma • Others
II. Non-epithelial (soft-tissue) tumors	• Lipoma • Fibroma • Neurofibroma • Lymphangioma • Hemangioma • Leiomyoma • Granular cell tumor • Chondroma	• Fibrosarcoma • Neurofibrosarcoma • Hemangiosarcoma • Leiomyosarcoma • Malignant hemangiopericytoma
III. Mesothelial tumors	(Benign) mesothelioma	Malignant mesothelioma
IV. Miscellaneous tumors	• Clear cell tumor • Paraganglioma • (Chemodectoma) • Teratoma	• Carcinosarcoma • Pulmonary blastoma • Malignant melanoma • Malignant lymphoma • Others
V. Metastases		
VI. Un-classified tumors		
VII. Tumor-like lesions	• Hamartomas • Lymphoproliferative processes • "Tumorlets" • Eosinophilic granuloma • "Sclerosing hemangioma" • Inflammatory pseudotumor • Others	

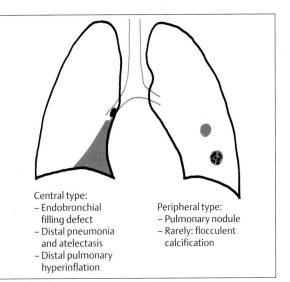

Central type:
– Endobronchial filling defect
– Distal pneumonia and atelectasis
– Distal pulmonary hyperinflation

Peripheral type:
– Pulmonary nodule
– Rarely: flocculent calcification

Fig. 6.**1**   Benign tumors.

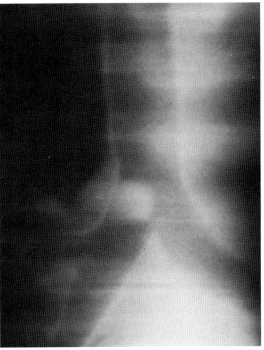

Fig. 6.**2**   Fibroma appears as a round filling defect within the tracheobronchial air column.

Pulmonary Hamartoma

Hamartomata account for 55% of benign and approximately 8% of all pulmonary neoplasms. These tumors contain cartilage, connective tissue, fat, and muscle. Approximately 80% are peripheral pulmonary nodules while the remainder are central endobronchial lesions.

Endobronchial lesions typically contain more fat than peripheral lesions (Gaerte et al. 2002) but frequently are inflamed and may be indistinguishable from bronchial carcinoma at bronchoscopy (Ahn et al. 1994, Fig. 6.**3 a**, **b**).

■ Radiologic Findings

The chest radiograph typically shows a well-circumscribed, homogeneous nodule which usually is less than 4 cm in diameter. Flocculent or popcorn calcification is

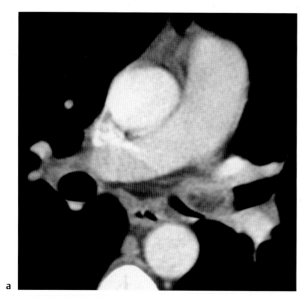

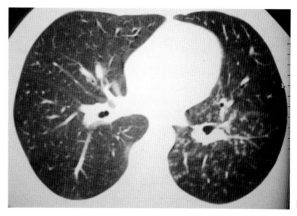

Fig. 6.**3a, b**   Endobronchial hamartoma. CT shows low density lesion possibly containing some foci of fat density with the left main bronchus (**a**). There are features of a cellular bronchiolitis within the left lower lobe distal to this lesion (**b**). Histology of resected specimen was consistent with a hamartoma.

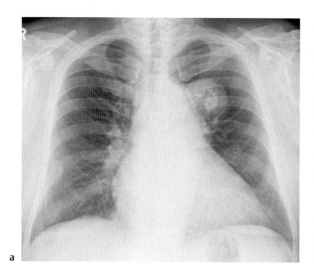

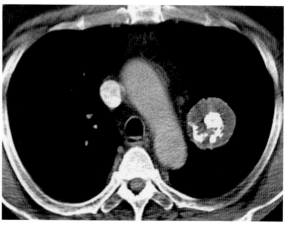

Fig. 6.**4a, b**   Pulmonary hamartoma appears as a well-defined round lesion and contains foci of calcification.

visible in up to 15% of cases (Figs. 6.**4**, 6.**5**). The presence of intralesional fat is also considered diagnostic.

Computed Tomography

Because of the superior contrast resolution of CT, fat and calcium within hamartomata are identified more easily. The prevalence of fat at CT has been reported to be from 5 to 50% (Erasmus et al. 2000). Fat is found in up to 50% of lesions and may be localized or generalized within the lesion (Siegelman et al. 1986, Erasmus et al. 2000, Fig. 6.**6a–c**).

Carcinoid, Mucoepidermoid, and Adenoid Cystic Carcinoma

The term "bronchial adenoma" in the past has been used to describe a group of lesions that included carcinoid tumor, mucoepidermoid carcinoma, and adenoid cystic carcinoma. The 1977 histologic classification considers carcinoid to be a separate entity while cylindroma or adenoid cystic carcinoma is classified with carcinoma of the tracheal wall glands (Tables 6.**1**, 6.**2**).

Bronchial carcinoid encompasses a spectrum of histology ranging from slow growing, locally infiltrative tumors to metastasizing lesions. Carcinoids may be typical (Kulchitsky cell carcinoma [KCC] type 1) or atypical (KCC type 2); the latter has cellular and clinical features

Table 6.**2**   TNM classification of bronchial carcinoma (UICC: TNM Atlas, 2nd ed. Berlin: Springer 1990)

TX	Positive cytology
T1	≤3 cm in greatest dimension
T2	>3 cm in greatest dimension, or extension to the hilar region, or invasion of visceral pleura, or a tumor that has caused partial atelectasis
T3	Extension to the chest wall, diaphragm, mediastinal pleura, or pericardium, etc., or a tumor that has caused complete atelectasis
T4	Invasion of the mediastinum, heart, great vessels, trachea, esophagus, etc., or the presence of malignant pleural effusion
N1	Metastasis to peribronchial or ipsilateral hilar lymph nodes
N2	Metastasis to ipsilateral mediastinal lymph nodes
N3	Metastasis to contralateral mediastinal lymph nodes, scalene lymph nodes, or supraclavicular lymph nodes

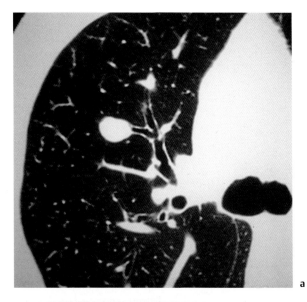

a

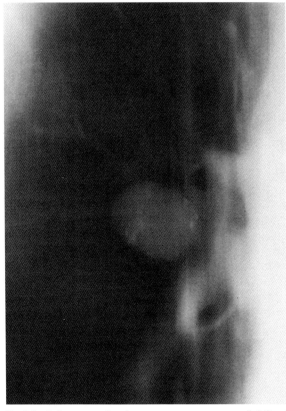

Fig. 6.**5**   Pulmonary chondroma appears as a well-defined nodule with flocculent calcification.

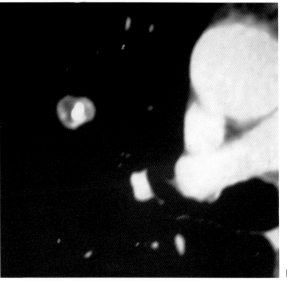

b

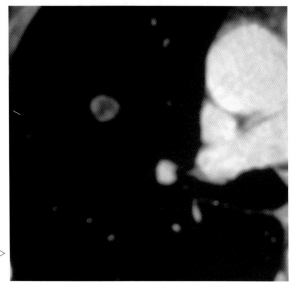

Fig. 6.**6 a–c**   Peripheral lung hamartoma. CT shows right upper ▷ lobe lesion with smooth contour (**a**), central nidus of calcification and surrounding rim of fat attenuation(**b** and **c**)

c

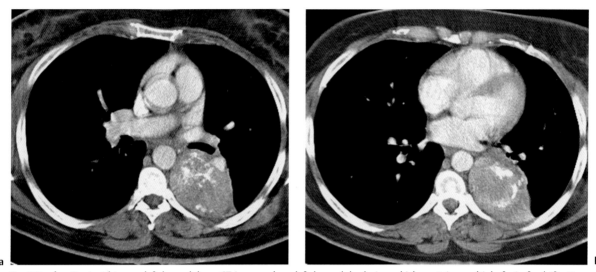

Fig. 6.**7a, b**   Carcinoid tumor left lower lobe – CT images show left lower lobe lesion which contains multiple foci of calcification. There is distal left lower lobe atelectasis. Histology of resected specimen was consistent with a typical carcinoid.

intermediate between those of typical carcinoid and small cell carcinoma (KCC type 3). Approximately 15 % of typical and 50 % of atypical carcinoids ultimately will metastasize (Armstrong et al. 1995).

Lesions distal to the level of the segmental bronchi are defined as peripheral carcinoids. Typical carcinoids characteristically are centrally located vascular tumors and may present with hemoptysis. Conversely, atypical carcinoids tend to have a peripheral location and presentation with hemoptysis is unusual.

■ Radiologic Findings

Most bronchial carcinoids are found within the major bronchi. The chest radiograph may be normal in 10 % of cases and then the diagnosis is established at bronchoscopy or following surgical resection of tumors initially detected at CT (Armstrong et al. 1995).

In those cases with an abnormal chest radiograph, the tumor may be visible as a well-defined hilar or perihilar mass. Partial or complete bronchial obstruction leads to distal atelectasis or pneumonic consolidation. Occasionally, collateral air drift maintains distal aeration even in the presence of total airway obstruction.

Tumors in segmental bronchi may cause obstruction with mucus retention in the distal airway; branching bronchoceles then may be the dominant radiographic finding. Ten to twenty percent of carcinoids present as peripheral pulmonary nodules or masses.

CT characteristically shows a spherical or ovoid nodule with a well-defined lobulated contour. Calcification is not often visible on the plain radiograph but is seen on CT in up to 30 % of lesions. It is seen more commonly in central than in peripheral lesions and may be diffuse or punctate in type (Chong et al. 2006, Fig. 6.**7a, b**).

Langerhans Cell Histiocytosis (LCH)

Langerhans cell histiocytosis comprises three disorders that show histologic similarities. These are:
1. Letterer–Siwe disease, a fulminant multisystem histiocytosis of young children.
2. Hand–Schuller–Christian disease, a chronic histiocytic disorder.
3. Eosinophilic granuloma of bone.

Isolated pulmonary involvement was first reported in 1951. Pulmonary Langerhans cell histiocytosis (PLCH) is today seen predominantly in young adults and has a smoking prevalence of 80–100 %. A much less common association with neoplasia including bronchial carcinoma and Hodgkin's lymphoma has been described.

The etiology of this condition remains poorly understood but it has been suggested that it may reflect an uncontrolled immune response to an unknown exogenous antigen in which Langerhans cells may serve as accessory cells in the activation of T lymphocytes.

Pathologically, multifocal peribronchiolar collections of Langerhans cells together with macrophages, lymphocytes, plasma cells, and eosinophils are seen. These cellular infiltrates are then replaced in a centripetal fashion by a fibroblastic proliferation which results in the classic stellate lesions. Over time, the cellular infiltrate disappears leaving behind fibrotic scars that are surrounded by enlarged and distorted air spaces. Temporal heterogeneity is commonly seen both within the pathologic specimen and within individual lesions (Abbott et al. 2004).

Patients may present clinically with a nonproductive cough and dyspnea. Less commonly, presentation may be with systemic symptoms of malaise and weight loss.

Pneumothorax occurs in up to 25% of cases over the course of the disease (Basset et al. 1978, Tazi et al. 2000) and may account for initial presentation.

Up to 25% of cases of PLCH may be asymptomatic and in these cases, the diagnosis may be due to incidentally discovered radiologic abnormalities.

■ Radiologic Findings

▦ Chest Radiograph

Radiographs during the early granulomatous stage may show multiple small nodules (1–10 mm in diameter). These are bilateral and symmetrical in distribution and show a predilection for the upper to mid zones (Figs. 6.**8**, 6.**9**). They give way to a coarse reticular pattern, honeycomb shadowing, and cystic change as the disease progresses. The presence of extensive cystic change may mimic bullous emphysema on the chest radiograph (Fig. 6.**10 a**).

▦ Computed Tomography

High-resolution CT (HRCT) in early-stage disease shows peribronchial or peribronchiolar nodularity with an upper to midzone predominance and with relative spar-

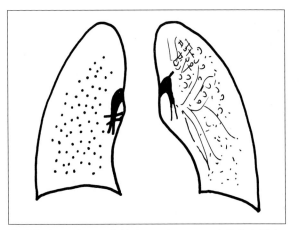

Fig. 6.**8** Langerhans cell histiocytosis presents initially with interstitial nodularity and may progress to cystic change and fibrosis.

ing of the lung bases. A combination of nodules and cystic lesions has been described as the commonest pattern (Brauner et al. 1989, Fig. 6.**11**) and the probable progression of change on CT has been postulated to be from nodules through to cavitary nodules, thick-walled cysts, then thin-walled cysts, and finally confluent cysts. Given this progression of change, it has been suggested that

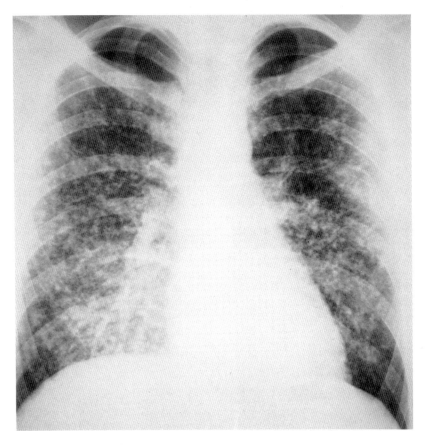

Fig. 6.**9** Langerhans cell histiocytosis—early-stage disease with extensive pulmonary nodularity.

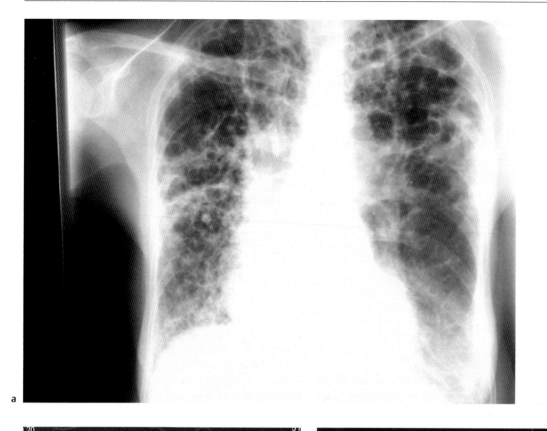

a

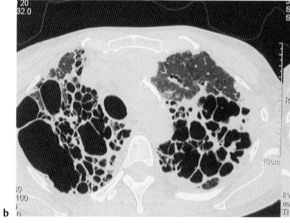

b

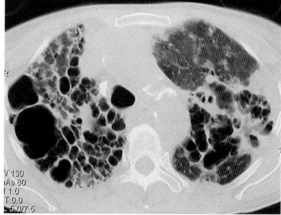

c

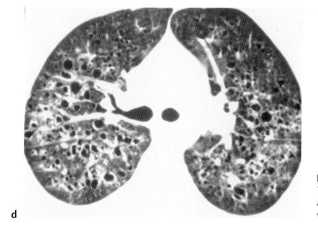

d

Fig. 6.**10 a–d** Advanced stage Langerhans cell histiocytosis. There is extensive pulmonary "cyst" formation with fibrosis most advanced in the upper zones with moderate midzone change and with relative sparing of the lung bases.

HRCT may be useful in evaluating the histopathologic activity of PLCH (Soler et al. 2000). Cystic lesions are frequently round or ovoid in shape but may exhibit rather bizarre configurations with bilobed, branching, and cloverleaf shapes (Fig. 6.**10b–d**).

The differential diagnosis is from lymphangiomyomatosis but this affects females and shows diffuse pulmonary involvement. Cystic change in pneumocystis pneumonia (see p. 87) may occasionally be indistinguishable from cystic change in PLCH (Webb et al. 2001).

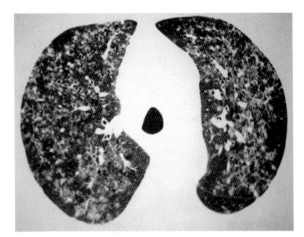

Fig. 6.**11** Pulmonary Langerhans cell histiocytosis. Histologically proven pulmonary Langerhans cell histiocytosis with areas of poorly defined nodular opacification and early cyst formation.

Bronchial Carcinoma

Bronchial carcinoma arises from the bronchial epithelium, grows by local expansion, and infiltrates local lymphatic channels and vessels to give rise to local and regional lymph node and distant metastases, respectively.

Its incidence in industrialized countries has increased 10-fold since 1930 (Müller 1983) and in Germany bronchial carcinoma is now second only to gastrointestinal malignancy as the most common organ tumor. Since the mid 1980s, the incidence appears to have plateaued in males but continues to rise in females. In the U.S. in 1988, the incidence of bronchial carcinoma surpassed that of breast carcinoma for the first time (Bragg 1994). It is estimated that approximately 85% of lung cancer may be attributable to cigarette smoking. The "rule of 20" states that in individuals who smoke 20 cigarettes per day for 20 years, the risk of bronchogenic carcinoma is increased 20-fold (Wynder et al. 1977).

Bronchial carcinoma is a particularly aggressive neoplasm with a high mortality. The reported 5-year survival rate in Germany in 1976 was only 2% (Heilmann and Doppelfeld 1976), and it remains a major cause of cancer deaths (27%) in both men and women over the age of 35 in the industrialized world. Current overall survival remains poor with a 10-year survival of just 7% in the U.S. National Cancer Database report (Fry et al. 1999). The early diagnosis and treatment of resectable nonsmall cell tumors offers some chance of cure with 5-year survival rates of 62–82% (Fry et al. 1999, Mountain 1997).

Screening for Lung Cancer

Large prospective studies on radiographic screening have been conducted in the U.S. (Fontana 1977). The Mayo Foundation reported very favorable results in 10 000 subjects: In the screened group who underwent sputum analysis and chest radiography at 4-month intervals, 62% of detected carcinomas were still operable and the calculated 5-year survival rate was 45%. This compares with resectable tumors in 28% of the control group and a 5-year survival rate of just 19%. This study found chest radiographs were rewarding much more frequently than sputum cytology.

Most other trial screening programs using chest radiographs and sputum cytology have failed to demonstrate improved survival in the screened group and they have emphasized the difficulties in detection of early lung cancer on plain radiographs (Bragg 1994).

A number of studies on CT screening for lung cancer have reported in the past decade:

Henschke and colleagues reported the results of the Early Lung Cancer Action Project in 1999 (Henschke et al. 1999). This two-center study enrolled 1000 patients more than 60 years of age with a smoking history of greater than 10 pack-years. Initial screening CT was performed at 10 mm collimation. The initial prevalence screen showed 1–6 noncalcified nodules in 233 (23%) of participants. In 27 (2.7%) of all participants, lung cancer was detected (cancer prevalence rate of 2.7%) and 23 (84%) of these neoplasms represented stage 1 disease. The initial incidence screen showed 26 new nodules, 10 of which were malignant and nine of which were primary bronchial carcinoma giving a cancer incidence rate of 0.9%.

More recently, Swenson et al. have reported the results of a 5-year prospective study on evaluation of a cohort at high risk of lung cancer with low-dose helical CT (Swenson et al. 2005). They enrolled 1520 individuals more than 50 years of age with a smoking history greater than 20 pack-years and residing within a so-called "histoplasmosis belt." After five annual examinations, 3356 uncalcified lung nodules had been detected in 1118 (74%) of participants. Sixty-eight cancers had been detected in 66 participants. Thirty-one of these were prevalence cancers of which 42% were adenocarcinomas, 19% were adenocarcinomas with bronchioloalveolar characteristics, and 13% were bronchioloalveolar carcinoma. There were 35 nonsmall cell incidence cancers, 17% of which were adenocarcinomas and 29% were squamous cell carcinomas. Sixty-one percent of incidence cancers were stage 1 disease.

These studies suggest that screening CT allows detection of early-stage lung cancer but the detection rate of benign nodules is high and it remains uncertain if early-stage detection represents a true stage shift or over diagnosis.

The U.S. National Lung Screening Trial by the U.S. National Cancer Institute is a randomized controlled trial which aims to determine if there is a disease-specific mortality benefit (Hillman and Schnall 2003). Until this study is completed, it has been suggested that CT screening should only be performed in the setting of a clinical trial (Earnest et al. 2003, Stanley 2001).

Goals of Diagnostic Imaging.
Early diagnosis of bronchial carcinoma. In everyday practice, most primary lung cancers are detected initially on the chest radiograph.

Staging of carcinoma: Some preliminary information may be derived from the *chest radiograph*. Tumor size, atelectasis, the presence of a pleural effusion. Mediastinal and hilar changes may be visible (Bragg 1994).

CT of the thorax and upper abdomen is then performed for further evaluation. *Magnetic resonance imaging* (MRI) is useful in demonstrating neurovascular involvement in Pancoast (superior sulcus) tumor and in assessment of extrathoracic spread in selected instances (see Fig. 6.**13**).

PET-CT is useful in determining the presence and extent of regional lymph node and distant metastatic spread and now is routinely employed in cases of nonsmall cell lung carcinoma (NSCLC) being considered for surgical resection.

Identification of predisposing factors other than tobacco smoking such as asbestos exposure.

Detection of concomitant disease such as emphysema or congestive heart failure which may preclude or increase the risk of surgical resection.

■ Pathology

Classification of bronchial carcinoma by location may have important implications for surgical management:
- *Central bronchial carcinoma* (75–80%) has its origin in the lobar, segmental, or subsegmental bronchi. These tumors grow into the bronchial lumen along the peribronchial lymphatics and through to the interstitium.

- *Peripheral bronchial carcinoma* (15–30%) originates in the mucosa of the smaller bronchi and initially the tumor may form a solitary pulmonary nodule. *Peripheral bronchial carcinoma arising in the subpleural parenchyma* may involve the pleura at an early stage. Bronchial carcinoma arising at the lung apex (Pancoast or superior sulcus tumor) may infiltrate the brachial plexus and the sympathetic trunk to produce the typical syndromes of pain in the upper limb (Pancoast syndrome) and the Horner's triad, respectively.

- *Diffuse, infiltrating, pneumonic forms of lung cancer* almost always are bronchioalveolar in type. In 1977, they accounted for just 2.8% of primary lung cancer. Their relative incidence has increased considerably in the past three decades and now they may account for up to 15% of primary lung cancer (Armstrong et al. 1995, Vincent et al. 1977, Auerbach and Garfinkel 1991).

Tumor spread may initially be via the lymphatics to the hilar, mediastinal, and supraclavicular lymph nodes. Hematogenous spread may also occur with metastatic seeding to the brain, adrenals, liver, and bones.

Bronchial carcinoma is classified histologically according to World Health Organization guidelines (Table 6.**2**).

The most common histologic types are (Fig. 6.**12**):
- *Small cell carcinoma* has the most irrefutable association with cigarette/tobacco smoking. It is predominantly a central tumor (90%) but growth is mainly along anatomic tissue planes. Small cell carcinoma tends to metastasize early; systemic spread is present in two-thirds of cases at presentation. Small cell carcinoma is classified as limited or extensive. Surgical resection plays no role in its management with chemotherapy ± radiotherapy forming the basis of treatment.

The following histologic types collectively are called nonsmall cell lung carcinoma and in early-stage disease (stage I and II ± stage IIIa), surgery offers the best chance of cure. The International Staging System developed by the Task Force on Lung Cancer of the American Joint Committee on Cancer (AJCC) was introduced in 1986 (Mountain 1986, Stitik 1990). The TNM (Tumor, Nodes, Metastasis) classification defines the primary tumor (T), the presence of nodal disease (N), and of distant metastases (M) (Tables 6.**2**, 6.**3**). This TNM classification is used to define the stage of disease (Fig. 6.**13**, Table 6.**4**).
- *Squamous cell carcinoma* is most commonly a central tumor developing at the level of the lobar, segmental, or subsegmental bronchi in 66% of cases. These tumors frequently are lobulated and have a tendency to cavitate. Squamous cell carcinoma arises peripherally in one-third of cases.
- *Adenocarcinoma* is the third most common histologic type in Germany. In the United States, its incidence is increasing, and it may now be the most common cell type in females and in nonsmokers. Adenocarcinoma

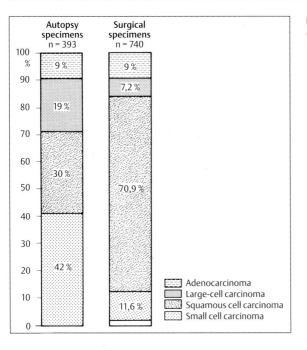

Fig. 6.**12** Bar graphs indicate the histologic types of bronchial carcinoma found at autopsy (Münster Institute of Pathology, 1965–1975) and at surgical resection (from Hinson et al.).

Table 6.**3** TNM clinical classification of bronchial carcinoma

T: Primary tumor

TX   Primary tumor cannot be assessed, or tumor proven by the presence of malignant cells in sputum or bronchial washings but not visualized by imaging or bronchoscopy

T0   No evidence of primary tumor

Tis   Carcinoma in situ

T1   Tumor ≤ 3 cm in greatest dimension, surrounded by lung or visceral pleura, without bronchoscopic evidence of invasion more proximal than the lobar bronchus (i. e., not in the main bronchus)[1]

T2   Tumor with any of the following features of size or extent:
- > 3 cm in greatest dimension
- Involves main bronchus, ≥ 2 cm distal to the carina
- Invades the visceral pleura
- Associated with atelectasis or obstructive pneumonitis that extends to the hilum but does not involve the entire lung

T3   Tumor of any size that directly invades any of the following: chest wall (including superior sulcus tumors), diaphragm, mediastinal pleura, parietal pericardium; or tumor in the main bronchus < 2 cm distal to the carina[1], but without involvement of the carina itself; or tumor associated with atelectasis or obstructive pneumonitis of the entire lung

T4   Tumor of any size that invades any of the following: mediastinum, heart, great vessels, trachea, esophagus, vertebral body, or carina; or satellite tumor nodules within the lobe containing the primary tumor; or presence of malignant pleural effusion[2]

N: Regional lymph nodes

NX   Regional lymph nodes cannot be assessed

N0   No regional lymph node metastasis

N1   Metastasis of ipsilateral peribronchial and/or ipsilateral hilar lymph nodes, and intrapulmonary nodes involved by direct extension of the primary tumor

N2   Metastasis to ipsilateral mediastinal and/or subcarinal lymph node(s)

N3   Metastasis to contralateral mediastinal, contralateral hilar, ipsilateral or contralateral scalene, or supraclavicular lymph node(s)

M: Distant metastasis

MX   Presence of distant metastasis cannot be assessed

M0   No distant metastasis

M1   Distant metastasis present

[1] Rare superficial tumors of any size with invasive components limited to the bronchial wall that extend proximal to the main bronchus are also classified as T1.

[2] Most pleural effusions in lung cancer are caused by the tumor. But there are a few patients in whom serial cytologic examinations of the pleural effusion are negative and the effusion is not bloody or exudative. When these findings and the clinical evaluation exclude a tumor-related effusion, the effusion should not be scored as a malignant effusion for staging purposes, and the tumor should be classified as T1, T2, or T3.

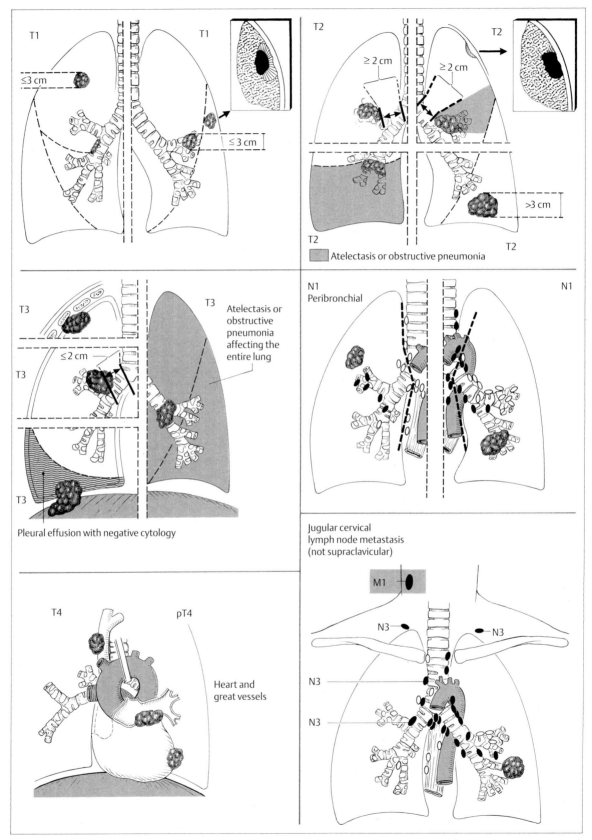

Fig. 6.**13** TNM classification of bronchial carcinoma (UICC: TNM Atlas. Berlin: Springer 1990).

is a peripheral tumor in 75% of cases with a predilection for the upper lobes. Initially, it was thought that adenocarcinoma had a predilection for regions of parenchymal fibrosis (*scar* carcinomas). More recently, this concept has been challenged and it has been suggested that some peripheral adenocarcinomas may induce a desmoplastic reaction to the tumor and form central fibrosis (Aoki et al. 2000). The histologic subtype of adenocarcinoma, bronchioloalveolar carcinoma grows mainly within the alveoli respecting interstitial boundaries. Bronchioalveolar carcinoma may be unifocal or multifocal and when multifocal may produce alveolar cell carcinosis. Immunohistochemical expression of **thyroid transcription factor 1 (TTF1)** has been shown to be a highly specific marker for primary lung adenocarcinoma (Reis-Filho et al. 2000). TTF1 has also been shown to be positive more frequently in peripheral than in central primary lung adenocarcinoma (Stenhouse et al. 2004). This therefore may be helpful in distinguishing a peripheral primary lung adenocarcinoma from a solitary pulmonary metastasis.

- Noguchi Classification: The Noguchi classification of adenocarcinoma was published in 1995. Noguchi types A/B showed a "replacement" growth pattern, no lymph node metastases and was associated with an excellent prognosis. Type C comprised the lepidic growth pattern of types A/B but in addition showed foci of fibroblastic proliferation. Types D–F represented "nonreplacement" forms of adenocarcinoma and had a less favorable prognosis (Noguchi et al. 1995).
- Large cell carcinoma tends to be a diagnosis of exclusion. Microscopically, these large cells with prominent nucleoli lack features of squamous, adeno, or small cell differentiation.

Table 6.**4** Staging of bronchial carcinoma

Occult carcinoma	TX	N0	M0
Stage 0	Tis	N0	M0
Stage IA	T1	N0	M0
Stage IB	T2	N0	M0
Stage IIA	T1	N1	M0
Stage IIB	T2	N1	M0
	T3	N0	M0
Stage IIIA	T1, T2	N2	M0
	T3	N1, N2	M0
Stage IIIB	Any T	N3	M0
	T4	Any N	M0
Stage IV	Any T	Any N	M1

■ Clinical Features

Patients are frequently asymptomatic until the disease has reached an advanced stage. Respiratory manifestations include cough with recurrent episodes of pneumonia and hemoptysis. Systemic features of neoplasia including lethargy, cachexia, anorexia, elevated erythrocyte sedimentation rate (ESR), and anemia indicate advanced disease. Local invasion of extrapulmonary structures may lead to venous obstruction (superior vena cava), dysphagia (esophagus), hoarseness (recurrent laryngeal nerve), Horner syndrome (sympathetic trunk), and arm pain (brachial plexus).

Distant metastases especially to the brain and skeleton may also be the initial manifestation of bronchial carcinoma.

■ Radiologic Findings

■ Chest Radiograph (Fig. 6.14):

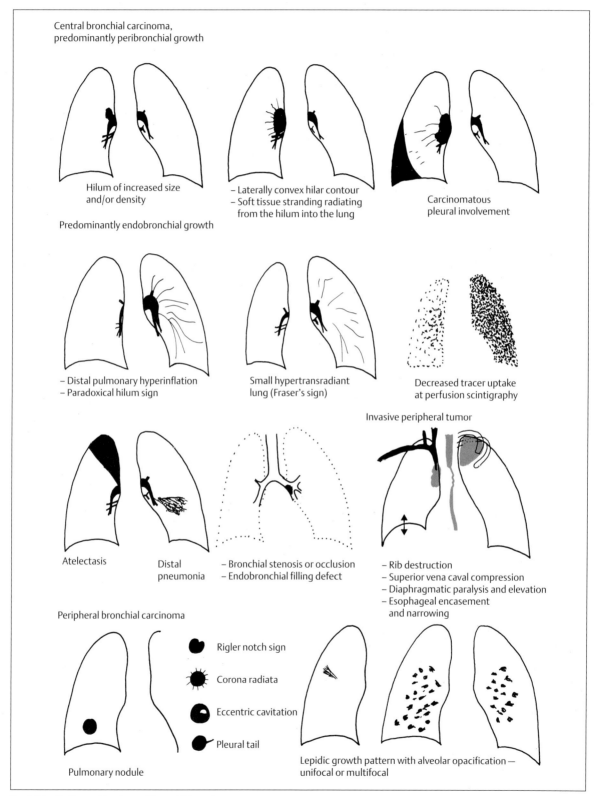

Fig. 6.**14** Radiographic signs of bronchial carcinoma.

Bronchial Stenosis/Occlusion

Most central bronchial carcinomas exhibit either endoluminal or transmural growth and bronchial stenosis/occlusion with associated distal parenchymal changes are a common finding. Occasionally, bronchial stenosis is directly visible on the chest radiograph. Much more frequently, the following indirect signs suggest the presence of a central obstructing lesion:

- *Partial or complete atelectasis* is a common finding in bronchial carcinoma. Segments, lobes, or occasionally an entire lung no longer are aerated (Fig. 6.**15**, and see Fig. 6.**24**). There may be associated displacement of the adjacent interlobar fissure, mediastinum, or hemidiaphragm.
- *Distal pneumonia* presents as lobar or segmental consolidation which may resolve partially with antibiotic therapy. In patients with appropriate risk factors and recurrent or persistent pneumonia, further evaluation with CT and/or bronchoscopy to exclude a central endobronchial tumor is merited.
- *Distal hyperinflation* is unusual and is seen in less than 2% of cases (Fraser and Paré 1983). Partial bronchial occlusion creates a check-valve obstruction with inspiratory expansion and expiratory air trapping. Hyperinflated lung is seen radiographically as a region of hypertransradiancy and there may be associated displacement of neighboring structures. Mediastinal shift to the contralateral side and an enlarged contralateral hilum are additional features. This hilar enlargement, which may also result from decreased perfusion on the side of the carcinoma, is the "paradoxical hilum" sign. Unilateral hyperinflation is sometimes more obvious on expiratory views
- *Reflex oligemia.* Partial obstruction causes ventilatory impairment even when the volume of the affected lung is normal or increased. Hypoxic vasoconstriction (the Euler Liljestrand reflex) then results in reduced perfusion. This is manifest radiographically as a decrease in vessel caliber. Oligemia may also result from encasement and compression of the pulmonary artery. Vessel attenuation in the affected lung then results in hypertransradiancy.
- *Hilar mass.* Growth of some central bronchial carcinomas is predominantly peribronchial in the initial stages (see Fig. 6.**19**). The chest radiograph in these cases may show a hilar mass. Initially the hilum is altered in contour and enlarged, then the mass may obliterate the lateral hilar concavity and finally normal

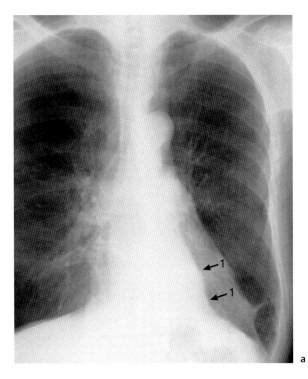

a

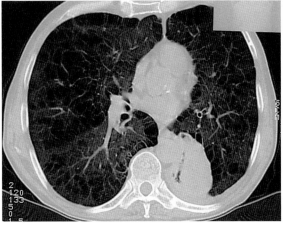

b

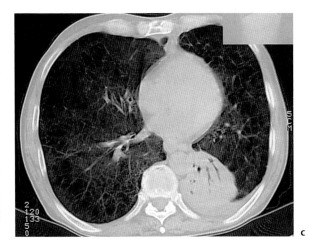

Fig. 6.**15** Left lower lobe atelectasis in a patient with bronchoscopically confirmed carcinoma. Note the triangular opacity projected behind the heart and inability to visualize the left lower lobar artery on the chest radiograph (**a**). CT images (**b, c**) show the atelectatic LLL with visible air bronchograms and a small left pleural effusion. Changes are superimposed on a background of advanced centrilobular emphysema.

c

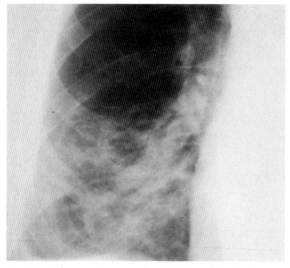

Fig. 6.**16** Adenocarcinoma of the right lower lobe displaying a lepidic type growth pattern with radiographic evidence of pulmonary consolidation. Histology confirmed alveolar infiltration by carcinoma cells.

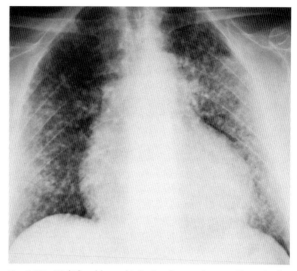

Fig. 6.**17** Multifocal bronchioloalveolar carcinoma. There is also cardiac enlargement due to the presence of a malignant pericardial effusion.

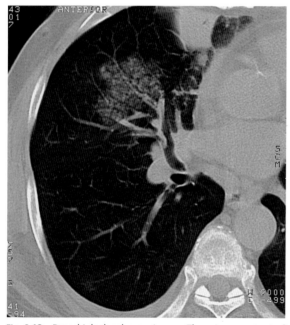

Fig. 6.**18** Bronchioloalveolar carcinoma. There is a segment of peripheral consolidation in the subpleural lung anteriorly with an area of "alveolar" type opacification also seen in the right middle lobe.

nodules greater than 1 cm may be missed due to superimposition of normal structures. While a specific diagnosis is not possible from radiologic findings, the following features suggest a diagnosis of bronchial carcinoma:

- Larger lesions are more likely to be malignant.
- Ill-defined margins are present in 85 % of malignant tumors (Müller and Fraser 2001).
- The corona radiata corresponds to radial striated markings at the interface with lung parenchyma; these represent centrifugal tumor spread along the lymphatics.
- Notching of the contour, which represents the vascular hilum of the tumor and is termed the "Rigler notch" sign.
- A cavitating lesion is typical of either primary bronchial squamous cell carcinoma or a metastatic deposit from a squamous cell carcinoma of uterine cervix or skin.

Pneumonic Form of Carcinoma

This pattern of disease appears as an ill-defined, patchy, or homogeneous consolidation in a segmental or nonsegmental distribution. An air alveologram and air bronchogram may be seen (Figs. 6.**16**–6.**18**). Initially, this appearance simulates an infective consolidation but lack of radiologic and/or clinical response to antibiotic therapy should lead to biopsy and diagnosis. Histologically, the majority of these tumors are bronchioloalveolar carcinomas or adenocarcinoma with bronchioloalveolar characteristics.

Mediastinal Lymph Node Enlargement

Bulky paratracheal, tracheobronchial, and aortopulmonary lymph nodes lead to widening of the mediastinum while large volume subcarinal lymph node enlargement

hilar structures may become completely obscured. Linear stranding extending into the perihilar lung may represent lymphatic infiltration with desmoplastic reaction.

Peripheral Pulmonary Nodule

The size threshold for detection of small lesions on the chest radiograph is 7 to 9 mm (Armstrong et al. 1995), but may cause splaying of the carina. Mediastinal widening may be the first radiographic sign of lung cancer particularly in small cell carcinoma (Table 6.**5**).

Intrathoracic Spread of Bronchial Carcinoma
The following radiographic features suggest locally infiltrative carcinoma (Fig. 6.**19**):
- Upper lobe tumor with local chest wall invasion (Fig. 6.**20**).
- Diaphragmatic paralysis secondary to *phrenic nerve involvement*. The inspiratory view shows elevation of the ipsilateral hemidiaphragm and paradoxical motion is evident at fluoroscopy.
- *Esophageal involvement*: Dilatation proximal to a stenotic segment may occasionally be visible on the chest radiograph. A contrast swallow will demonstrate the level and degree of obstruction.
- *Ipsilateral pleural effusion* may signify malignant pleural involvement and this is confirmed by cytology of pleural aspirate plus or minus percutaneous pleural biopsy. Occasionally, lymphatic obstruction by a central bronchial carcinoma results in a pleural effusion and in these cases resolution is expected as the tumor responds to therapy. Pleural effusion is present in approximately 15% of cases at presentation and is found in over 50% of patients at some stage during the course of their illness.

Hematogenous Spread of Bronchial Carcinoma
Osteolytic bone lesions and pathologic fractures may signify hematogenous spread of disease.

Computed Tomography

Helical MDCT is today the standard imaging modality for further evaluation of suspected bronchial carcinoma. It confirms the presence of tumor and allows initial imaging staging of disease.

Thin collimation helical volumetric CT through the thorax in the systemic arterial phase and through the upper abdomen in the portal venous phase of enhancement is routinely acquired.

These allow assessment of:
1. The primary tumor including its size and to some degree, the extent of local invasion (Figs. 6.**21**, 6.**22**). Image acquisition through the thorax accurately identifies airway involvement and may serve as a road map for the bronchoscopist (Figs. 6.**23**, 6.**24b**, **c**).
2. The presence and volume of hilar and mediastinal lymph node enlargement (Fig. 6.**25a**, **b**). Lymph nodes greater than 10 mm in short axis are considered to be abnormal while lymph nodes that are less than this value are determined to be free of disease. However, the sensitivity and specificity of CT using these size criteria has been shown to be moderate (Fig. 6.**26**). Metastatic involvement has been reported in up to 21% of "normal" nodes (Arita et al. 1995) and up to 40% of enlarged nodes have been

Table 6.**5** Radiographic signs related to tumor histology (from Müller and Fraser: *Diseases of the Chest*. Philadelphia: Saunders 2001)

Occult carcinoma	Squamous cell carcinoma	Small cell carcinoma	Adeno-carcinoma	Large cell carcinoma
Hilar mass	40%	78%	18%	32%
Peripheral mass	27%	29%	71%	59%
Large mass (>4 cm)	(18%)	(26%)	(8%)	(41%)
Apical Mass	(3%)	(2%)	(1%)	(4%)
Multiple masses	(0%)	(1%)	(2.4%)	(2%)
Atelectasis	36%	17%	10%	13%
Pneumonia	15%	22%	15%	23%
Cavitation	7%	0%	2%	4%
Mediastinal lymph nodes	1%	13%	2%	10%

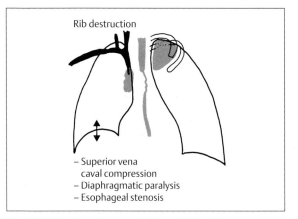

Fig. 6.**19** Intrathoracic spread of bronchial carcinoma.

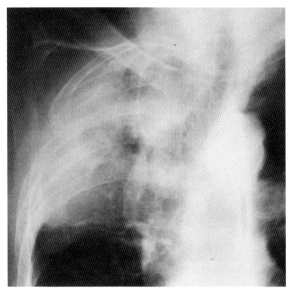

Fig. 6.**20** Pancoast tumor. Squamous cell carcinoma in the right upper lobe with associated destruction of the third to fifth ribs.

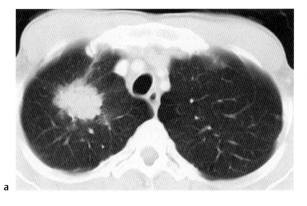

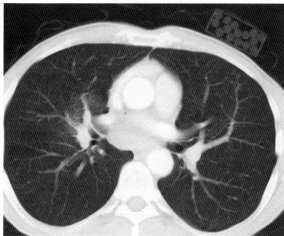

Fig. 6.**21 a, b**   Right upper lobe bronchial carcinoma in a heavy smoker (who was reluctant to part with his cigarettes even during CT!).

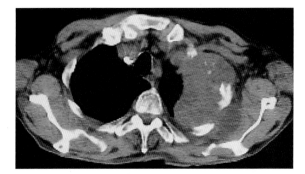

Fig. 6.**22**   Left upper lobe tumor with rib destruction and infiltration of subscapularis muscle.

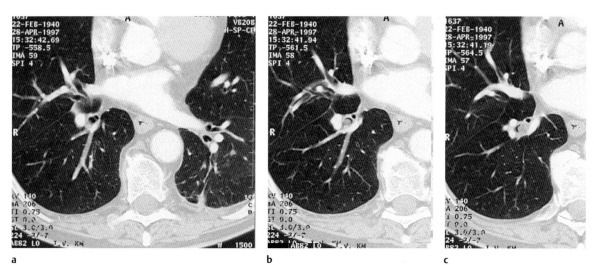

Fig. 6.**23 a–c**   Endobronchial tumor. CT demonstrates soft tissue lesion that is partially obstructing the right lower lobe bronchus as it branches into segmental bronchi. Confirmed at bronchoscopy.

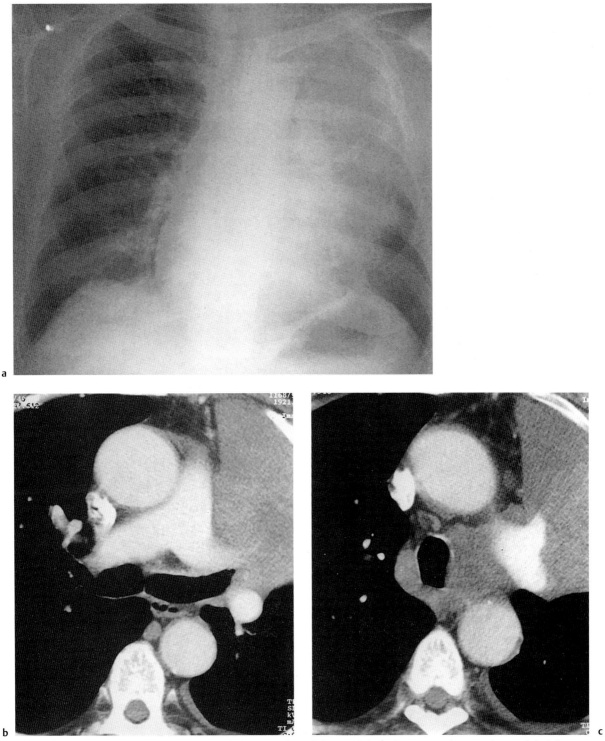

Fig. 6.**24 a–c**   CT: Bronchial carcinoma. Chest radiograph (**a**) shows left upper lobe atelectasis. CT shows occlusion of the left upper lobe bronchus (**b**) and tumor infiltration of the mediastinum (**c**).

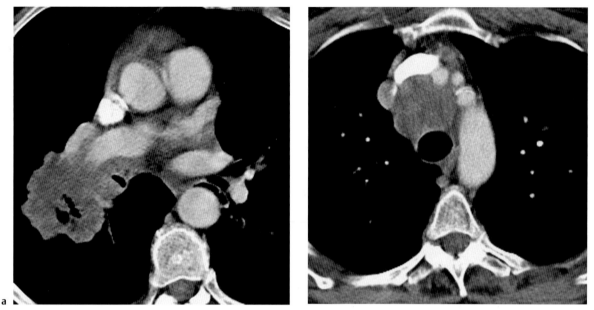

Fig. 6.**25 a, b**   Bronchial carcinoma with mediastinal lymph node metastases. CT (**a**) shows cavitating right hilar/lower lobe mass with confluent pretracheal lymph node mass (**b**).

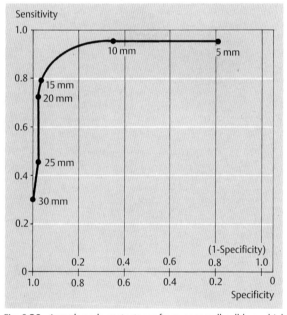

Fig. 6.**26**   Lymph node metastases from nonsmall-cell bronchial carcinoma: sensitivity and specificity of CT detection versus the transverse diameter of the lymph nodes. When a lymph node diameter of 10 mm is used as the value for lymph node involvement, the specificity is 70 % and the sensitivity is 95 %. When this is increased to 15 mm, the specificity rises to 95 % while the sensitivity falls to 80 %.

shown to be disease free at sampling during bronchoscopy or mediastinoscopy (Arita et al. 1996).

3. Compression and invasion of mediastinal vascular structures may be identified. Gross mediastinal invasion can be identified accurately by CT (Figs. 6.**27**–6.**31**). However, neither CT nor MRI allows accurate differentiation between direct invasion and simple contact between the tumor and the mediastinum (Rendina et al. 1987, Martini et al. 1985, Glazer et al. 1989). In fact, Glazer et al. found that when contact of the tumor with the mediastinum was less than or equal to 3 cm, the arc of contact with the aorta was less than 90 degrees and/or the fat plane with the mediastinum was preserved, the tumor was resectable in 97 % of cases.

4. Thin collimation images may be reconstructed on a high-resolution algorithm at lung windows and allow for assessment of the presence of both pulmonary metastases and lymphangitis carcinomatosa.

5. Hepatic and adrenal involvement may be identified on images through the upper abdomen.

6. Reformatted images in the coronal and sagittal planes when viewed at bone windows (WW = 2500, WW = 500) may demonstrate lytic skeletal metastases.

Fig. 6.**28 a, b**   Bronchial carcinoma with superior vena caval ▷ encasement. CT shows right upper lobe mass which is occluding the right upper lobe bronchus (**a**). There is mediastinal invasion with tumor encasement and extrinsic compression of the superior vena cava (**b**).

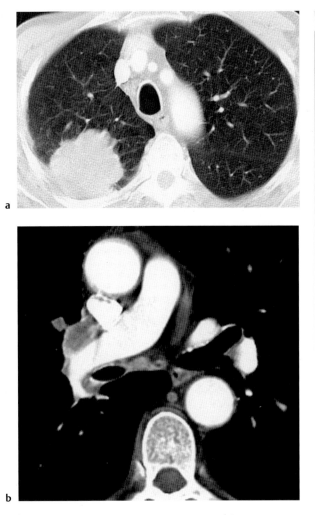

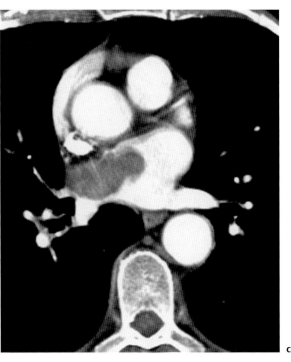

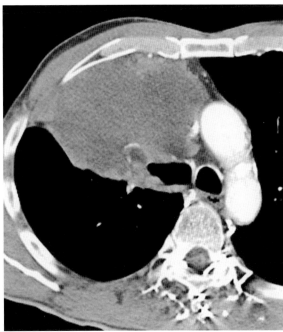

Fig. 6.**27 a–c** Bronchial carcinoma with pulmonary venous thrombosis. CT shows right upper lobe tumor (**a**). There is occlusion of the right superior pulmonary vein by probable tumor thrombus (**b**) and this extends proximally into the left atrium(**c**).

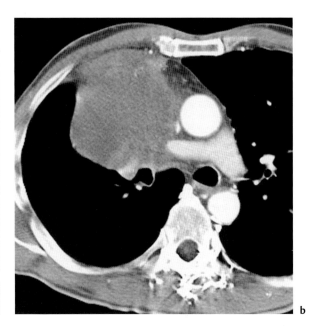

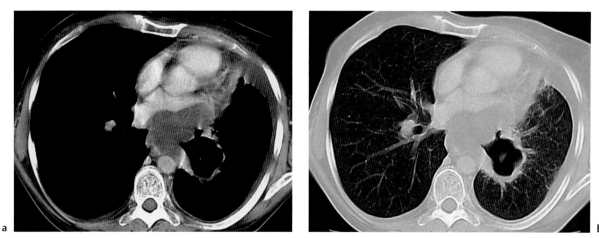

Fig. 6.**29 a, b**   Squamous cell carcinoma with cavitation and direct left atrial invasion.

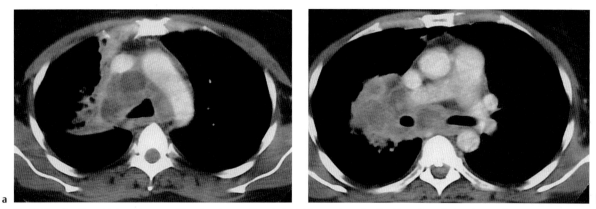

Fig. 6.**30 a, b**   Bronchial carcinoma with extensive confluent right hilar and mediastinal lymph node involvement.

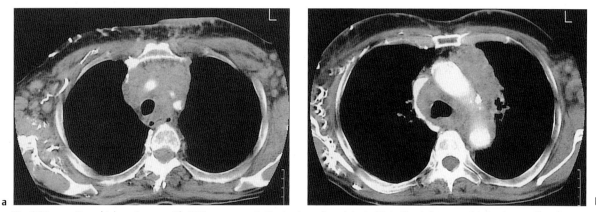

Fig. 6.**31 a–c**   Bronchial carcinoma with SVC encasement. Contrast medium injected into the right antecubital vein opacifies the azygos vein via chest-wall collateral veins and then opacifies the SVC inferior to the level of tumor encasement.

Fig. 6.**31 c**   ▷

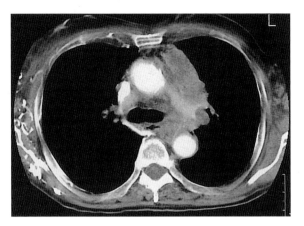

Fig. 6.**31c**

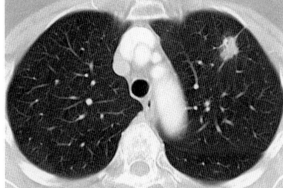

a

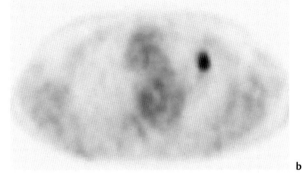

b

▣ Sonography

Ultrasound may be useful in determining the optimal site for pleural aspiration and percutaneous biopsy particularly in the presence of phrenic nerve paralysis and an elevated hemidiaphragm.

▣ Radionuclide Bone Scintigraphy

Patients with systemic features of malignancy, patients with bone pain, and those with plain radiographic evidence of osteolysis may be evaluated with radionuclide bone scintigraphy to assess the extent and distribution of skeletal involvement.

▣ Positron Emission Tomography-Computed Tomography (PET-CT)

The past decade has seen PET-CT being incorporated into the diagnostic pathway in the imaging staging of patients with nonsmall cell lung carcinoma (Fig. 6.**32**).

Evaluation of nodal stage: As described above, CT has been shown to have substantial limitations in determination of local/regional lymph node involvement in bronchial carcinoma. PET shows increased sensitivity and specificity in determination of nodal stage. Dwamena et al. (1999) performed a meta-analytic comparison of FDG-PET and CT for mediastinal staging incorporating a number of studies performed in the 1990s. They reported a sensitivity of 79% and a specificity of 91% for PET and a sensitivity of 60% and a specificity of 77% for CT. More recently, Shim et al. have compared the accuracy of PET-CT and CT alone in preoperative staging of NSCLC. For depiction of malignant nodes the sensitivity, specificity, and accuracy of CT were 70, 69, and 69% and for integrated PET-CT, the corresponding values were 85, 84, and 84% (Shim et al. 2005 b).

Combined N and M staging: Marom et al. compared PET with "conventional" imaging staging in 100 patients

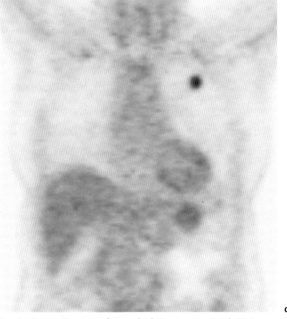

c

Fig. 6.**32 a–c** Staging of Bronchial Carcinoma. Axial CT image (**a**) shows T1/T2 tumor in left upper lobe. Axial (**b**) and coronal (**c**) images from staging PET study show increased FDG uptake in primary tumor but no evidence of hilar or mediastinal lymph node or distant metastatic spread consistent with stage 1 disease.

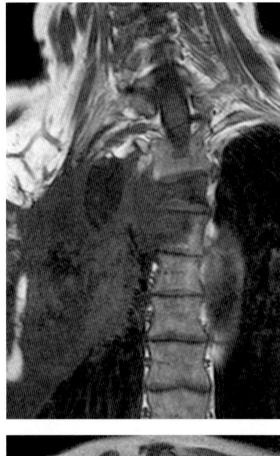

a

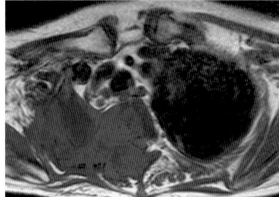

b

with newly diagnosed bronchogenic carcinoma. Conventional imaging staging comprised thoracic CT, radionuclide bone scintigraphy, and CT/MRI brain. They showed an overall accuracy in staging of 83% for PET and of 65% for conventional imaging. Nine percent of patients had metastases at PET not demonstrated on conventional imaging whereas 10% suspected of metastatic spread at conventional imaging were shown correctly by PET to have no metastases (Marom et al. 1999).

FDG PET has also been evaluated in the assessment of patients who had completed treatment for NSCLC. Patients with a positive PET study had a median survival of 12 months whereas in patients with a negative study, 85% were still alive at a median follow-up of 34 months (Patz et al. 2000).

Magnetic Resonance Imaging

Magnetic resonance imaging plays a complementary role to CT in selected instances.

Superior sulcus tumors: Magnetic resonance remains the modality of choice for imaging superior sulcus tumors. Extent of tumor invasion and neurovascular involvement may be demonstrated (Fig. 6.33a, b), and the intrinsic contrast between the low intensity of the tumor and the high intensity of fat on T1-weighted sequences is valuable.

The role of MRI in assessment of chest wall invasion at other sites remains more equivocal (Musset et al. 1986, Webb et al. 1991).

CNS involvement: Up to 40% of patients with adenocarcinoma and mediastinal node involvement will have CNS metastases, and magnetic resonance brain imaging may be appropriate in this group.

Fig. 6.**33a, b**   MRI shows large right upper lobe tumor which is involving the lower cords of the brachial plexus (**a**). There is also invasion and destruction of the upper thoracic vertebrae with spinal cord compression (**b**).

Pulmonary Metastases

Pulmonary metastases occur in 20 to 30% of all malignancies (Weiss et al. 1973) and usually result from hematogenous spread of tumor cells. Less commonly, they result from lymphatic spread; this occurs most frequently with gastric, pancreatic, and breast carcinoma. Endobronchial spread is unusual but sometimes may be found in head and neck malignancies as well as in renal and breast carcinoma (Fig. 6.34). Pulmonary metastases may be classified according to their growth pattern (Fig. 6.**35**):

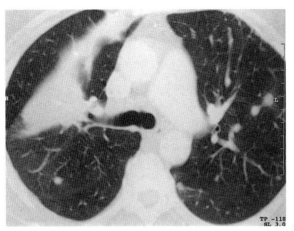
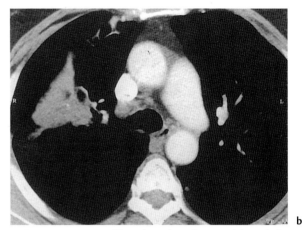

a

b

Fig. 6.**34 a, b** Metastatic breast carcinoma: pulmonary and endobronchial metastases. Helical CT images show bilateral nodular pulmonary metastases (**a**). There is also occlusion of the anterior and posterior segmental bronchi to the right upper lobe with distal lung atelectasis (**a**, **b**). Biopsies acquired at bronchoscopy showed metastatic breast carcinoma.

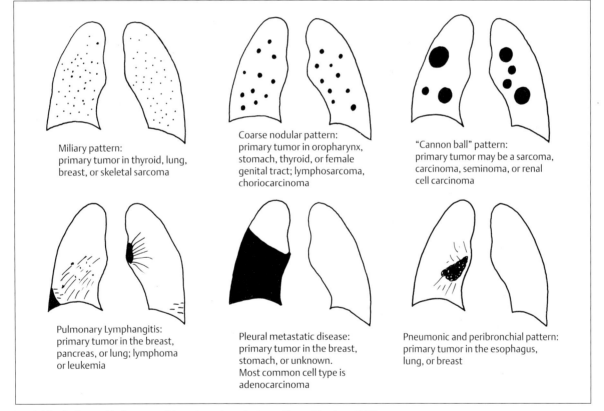

Miliary pattern:
primary tumor in thyroid, lung,
breast, or skeletal sarcoma

Coarse nodular pattern:
primary tumor in oropharynx,
stomach, thyroid, or female
genital tract; lymphosarcoma,
choriocarcinoma

"Cannon ball" pattern:
primary tumor may be a sarcoma,
carcinoma, seminoma, or renal
cell carcinoma

Pulmonary Lymphangitis:
primary tumor in the breast,
pancreas, or lung; lymphoma
or leukemia

Pleural metastatic disease:
primary tumor in the breast,
stomach, or unknown.
Most common cell type is
adenocarcinoma

Pneumonic and peribronchial pattern:
primary tumor in the esophagus,
lung, or breast

Fig. 6.**35** Radiographic features of intrathoracic metastases (from Meschan 1981).

- *Discrete pulmonary nodules* show a spherical expansile type of growth. Metastatic deposits range from fine miliary nodules to mass lesions several centimeters in diameter. Multiple nodules of uniform size scattered throughout both lungs suggest simultaneous growth. Some correlation may exist between the primary tumor and the pattern of metastases.
- *Pulmonary lymphangitis carcinomatosa* (PLC) is characterized by permeation of the lymphatics of the pulmonary interstitium by tumor cells.

- *Pleural carcinomatosis* may cause massive pleural effusion with or without neoplastic pleural thickening.
- *Endobronchial spread.*

■ Pathology

Different tumor types metastasize with varying frequency (Table 6.**6**). Tumor cells are filtered by pulmonary capillaries and lymphatics, proliferate and develop into expansively growing spherical masses. Permeation of the capillary wall with growth into the lymphatics, small airways and alveoli may occur. Histologically, metastases show good correlation with the cell type of the primary tumor, e. g., ossification is seen in metastases from osteogenic sarcoma.

Quint et al. evaluated the frequency of single lung metastasis, bronchogenic carcinoma, and benign lesions in patients with a solitary pulmonary nodule and a known extrapulmonary neoplasm. In patients with carcinomas of the head and neck, bladder, breast, cervix, bile ducts, esophagus, ovary, prostate, and stomach, a SPN was more likely to represent a primary bronchogenic carcinoma than a metastatic deposit whereas in patients with melanoma, sarcoma, and testicular carcinoma, a SPN was more likely to reflect a metastatic deposit (Quint et al. 2000).

Perihilar metastases are supplied by the bronchial arterial system while peripheral lung lesions are supplied by the pulmonary circulation. In pulmonary lymphangitis carcinomatosa, strands of neoplastic cells grow in the subpleural, septal, and peribronchovascular interstitium. There is an associated desmoplastic reaction which leads to decreased pulmonary compliance.

■ Clinical Features

Pulmonary metastases may be asymptomatic or when profuse may cause dyspnea. Pulmonary lymphangitis carcinomatosa may be associated with cough and marked dyspnea. Pleural carcinomatosis frequently yields a serosanguinous blood-stained effusion containing tumor cells.

■ Radiographic Findings

▨ Plain Chest Radiograph

- *Nodular metastases.* These homogeneous nodules are usually smooth with well-defined margins (Figs. 6.**36**–6.**38**). Cavitation is unusual (4%) and occurs predominantly in squamous cell metastases. Calcification and ossification are found in metastases from chondro- and osteosarcoma, respectively.
- *Pulmonary lymphangitis carcinomatosa* is characterized by reticulolinear markings including Kerley A and B lines. Associated loss of volume may result in a small hemithorax. Pleural effusion is present in 50% of cases. In metastatic breast carcinoma, pleural and pulmonary changes are ipsilateral to the breast primary in two-thirds of cases, presumably resulting from contiguous extension (Janower and Blennerhassett 1971, Lange and Minck 1983).
- *Pleural carcinomatosis*: Radiographic findings include pleural effusion with or without neoplastic pleural thickening. Pleural carcinomatosis is especially common in breast, bronchogenic, and gastrointestinal adenocarcinoma.
- *Endobronchial metastases* lead to distal atelectasis.

▨ Radionuclide Scintigraphy

Thyroid scintigraphy: Metastases from well-differentiated thyroid carcinoma may concentrate radioactive iodine as does the primary tumor (Fig. 6.**40**).

▨ Computed Tomography

Discrete pulmonary nodules: CT is superior to the chest radiograph in demonstrating small pulmonary nodules. These tend to have well-defined smooth contours and be more numerous in the mid to lower zones in keeping with hematogenous spread. Metastases from a squamous cell primary lesion may show cavitation and meta-

Table 6.**6** Incidence of pulmonary metastasis associated with various primary tumors (after Dähnert 2002)

Primary tumors accounting for __% of pulmonary metastases	
Breast	22
Kidney	11
Heat and neck tumors	10
Colorectal carcinoma	9
Uterus	6
Pancreas	5
Ovary	5
Prostate	4
Stomach	4
Frequency with which primary tumors metastasize to the lung	
Kidney	75
Osteosarcoma	75
Choriocarcinoma	75
Thyroid gland	65
Melanoma	60
Breast	55
Prostate	40
Head and neck tumors	30
Esophagus	20

static deposits from osteo- and chondrosarcoma typically show ossification and chondroid-type calcification,
respectively.

Pulmonary lymphangitis carcinomatosa: Thin colli-
mation/high-resolution CT is optimal for demonstration of PLC. Findings include smooth or beaded thick-

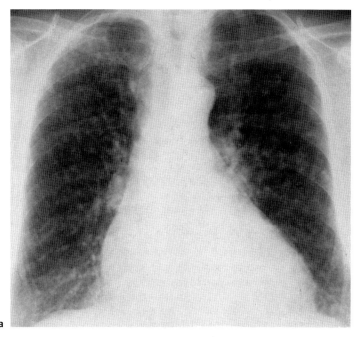

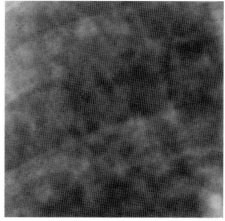

Fig. 6.**36 a, b**   Pulmonary metastases appear as
multiple small nodules in a patient with known
gastric carcinoma.

Fig. 6.**37**   "Cannon ball" pattern of
pulmonary metastases from a
testicular teratocarcinoma.

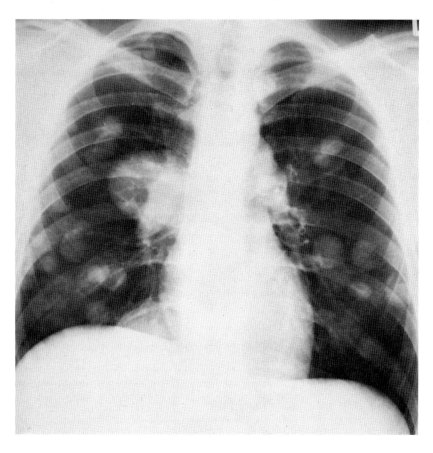

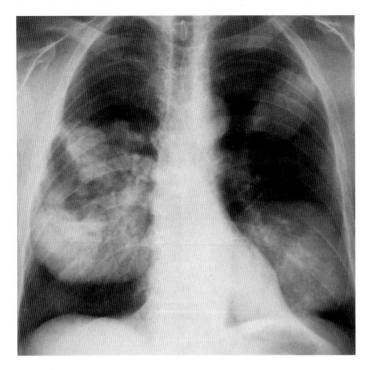

Fig. 6.**38** Very large pulmonary metastases from a tibial fibrosarcoma.

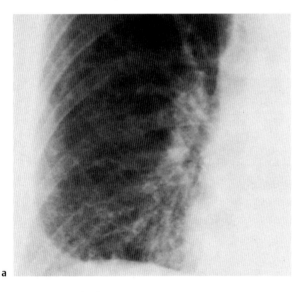

a

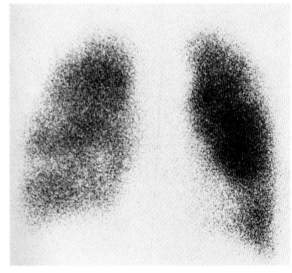

b

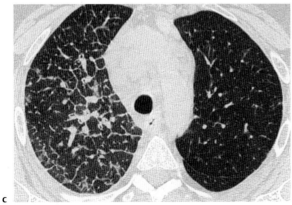

c

Fig. 6.**39 a–c** Pulmonary lymphangitis carcinomatosa (PLC): Increased reticular markings are seen in the mid and lower zones with an associated pleural effusion (**a**). Radionuclide scintigraphy shows some decrease in right pulmonary perfusion (**b**). HRCT (**c**) shows extensive interlobular septal and centrilobular thickening consistent with PLC. There is also significant mediastinal lymph node enlargement. Patient had presented clinically with severe dyspnea.

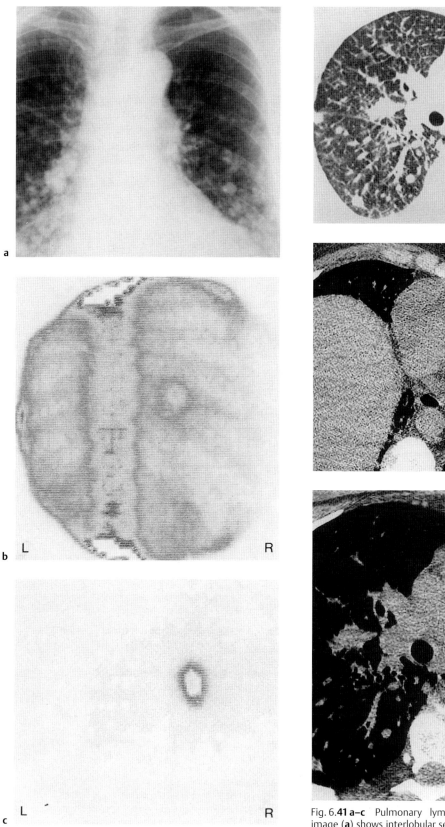

Fig. 6.**40 a–c**   Pulmonary nodules in a patient with known follicular thyroid carcinoma. Thyroid scintigraphy (^{99m}Tc-MOP and ^{131}I) show a solitary iodine-concentrating lesion in the parenchyma of the left lung.

Fig. 6.**41 a–c**   Pulmonary lymphangitis carcinomatosa: HRCT image (**a**) shows interlobular septal and centrilobular thickening, features consistent with PLC. Multiple discrete nodular metastases are also present. Images viewed at mediastinal windows show evidence of a pericardial effusion (**b**) and subcarinal lymph node enlargement (**c**). Final diagnosis was "metastatic adenocarcinoma with unknown primary."

ening of the peribronchovascular and centrilobular interstitium and of the interlobular septa (Fig. 6.**39** and Fig. 6.**41**).

Lymphoma

Lymphoma represents a neoplastic proliferation of lymphoid tissue and accounts for approximately 2% of all malignancies. Hodgkin disease (HD) shows a peak incidence in childhood and in the 2nd and 3rd decades while non-Hodgkin lymphoma (NHL) is most common in the 5th to 7th decades. Intrathoracic involvement is common with mediastinal adenopathy being found in 67 to 84% of patients with HD at initial presentation. Extranodal disease in the pulmonary parenchyma is less common. Diagnosis and histological classification are usually based on node biopsy, but occasionally lung biopsy may yield the diagnosis.

> **Goals of Diagnostic Imaging:**
> Initial staging of lymphoma.
>
> Monitoring radiological response to therapy, imaging complications of treatment, and detecting evidence of relapse.

■ Pathology

HD is characterized by lymphocyte proliferation and the presence of Reed–Sternberg cells. The Kiel classification is used in NHL, and further characterization is based on specific immunologic markers (Table 6.**7**).

■ Clinical Features

Patients may present with cervical, axillary, or inguinal lymph node enlargement or with systemic manifestations such as fever, lethargy, weight loss, and night sweats. Occasionally, massive mediastinal lymph node enlargement may lead to respiratory symptoms of cough, dyspnea, and retrosternal pain.

■ Radiologic Findings

▦ Plain Chest Radiograph

- *Mediastinal and hilar lymph node enlargement*: Paratracheal lymph node enlargement causes widening of the superior mediastinum (Figs. 6.**42**, 6.**43 a**). On the lateral view, the superior retrosternal space may be narrowed or obliterated by enlarged pretracheal

Endobronchial metastases: Helical volumetric CT through the central airways may show bronchial occlusion and distal atelectasis/consolidation (see Fig. 6.**34**).

Table 6.**7** Classification of Hodgkin and non-Hodgkin lymphomas

Ann Arbor staging classification of Hodgkin and non-Hodgkin lymphoma	
Stage I	Involvement of a single lymph node region
Stage I e	Involvement of a single extralymphatic organ or site (e. g., pulmonary nodule)
Stage II	Involvement of two or more lymph node regions on the same side of the diaphragm
Stage II e	Localized involvement of an extralymphatic organ or site and of one or more lymph node regions on the same side of the diaphragm (e. g., including perihilar parenchymal invasion with ipsilateral lymphadenopathy and unilateral pleural effusion with hilar lymphadenopathy)
Stage III	Involvement of lymph node regions on both sides of the diaphragm
Stage III e	Stage III, accompanied by localized involvement of an extralymphatic organ or site
Stage IV	Diffuse involvement of one or more extralymphatic organs or tissues (e. g., including multifocal lung involvement, bilateral effusion)

Histologic classification of Hodgkin disease (Rye classification)
1. Lymphocyte predominant (paragranuloma), incidence 15%
2. Nodular sclerosing, incidence 40%
3. Mixed cell, incidence 30%
4. Lymphocyte depleted (Hodgkin sarcoma), incidence 15%

WHO classification of non-Hodgkin lymphoma
(I) Low-grade lymphomas (low risk)
- B-cell lymphoma:
  Lymphocytic lymphoma, CLL
  Immunocytic lymphoma (Waldenström disease)
  Hairy cell leukemia
  Marginal zone lymphoma
  Extranodal MALT B-cell lymphoma
  Follicle center lymphoma
  Mycosis fungoides, Sézary syndrome

(II) Aggressive lymphomas (intermediate risk)
- B-cell origin:
  Plasmacytoma
  Mantle cell lymphoma
  Follicle center lymphoma
  Diffuse large-cell B-cell lymphoma
  Thymic B-large cell lymphoma
  High-grade B-cell lymphoma
- T-cell origin:
  Peripheral T-cell lymphoma
  Angioimmunoblastic lymphoma
  Angiocentric lymphoma
  Anaplastic T-cell lymphoma

(III) Very aggressive lymphomas (high risk)
- B-cell origin:
  Burkitt lymphoma
  Plasma cell leukemia
- T-cell origin:
  Adult T-cell lymphoma

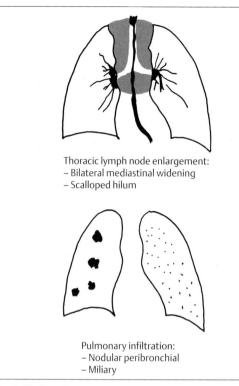

Thoracic lymph node enlargement:
– Bilateral mediastinal widening
– Scalloped hilum

Pulmonary infiltration:
– Nodular peribronchial
– Miliary

Fig. 6.**42**   Lymphoma.

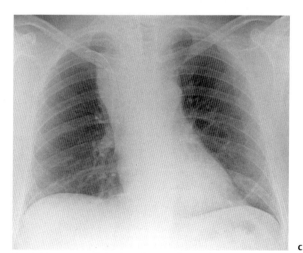

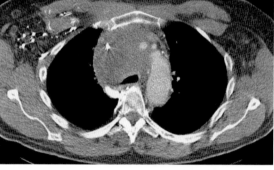

lymph nodes. Hilar lymph node enlargement frequently is bilateral and symmetrical with lobulated lateral contours.

- *Pulmonary parenchymal involvement* in HD is usually associated with mediastinal lymph node enlargement (Kaplan et al. 1987); in NHL, it may be found in the absence of mediastinal change. Direct extension from the hilum into the adjacent lung is most common and results in nodular shadowing around patent bronchi in the perihilar lung, giving visible air bronchograms. Pulmonary involvement may also be manifest as multiple nodules, which may have a peribronchial distribution or very occasionally may cavitate.

▓ Computed Tomography

CT forms an integral part of initial staging of lymphoma. It allows accurate assessment of the size and extent of mediastinal and hilar lymph node enlargement (Figs. 6.**43 b**, 6.**44**, 6.**45 a**). All node groups except for the paracardiac and posterior mediastinal nodes are more frequently involved by HD than by NHL. Involvement by contiguity is typically found in HD but may be absent in NHL.

Fig. 6.**43**   Non-Hodgkin lymphoma: Chest radiograph (**a**) shows mediastinal widening. Thoracic CT (**b**) shows extensive confluent lymph node enlargement in the superior mediastinum with SVC compression and with intravenous contrast medium within right chest wall collateral vessels and within the azygos vein. Patient had clinical signs of SVC obstruction. Chest radiograph (**c**) one week later shows of a stent within the SVC.

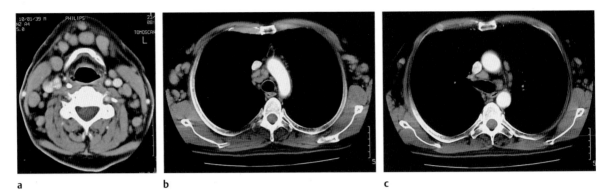

Fig. 6.**44 a–c**   Hodgkin disease. CT demonstrates cervical, axillary, and mediastinal lymph node enlargement.

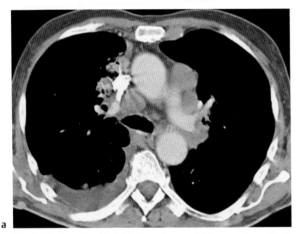
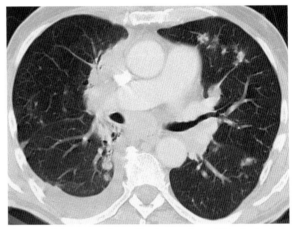

Fig. 6.**45 a, b**   Non-Hodgkin Lymphoma: CT image at mediastinal windows (**a**) shows precarinal, aortopulmonary, and left hilar lymph node enlargement. CT image viewed at lung windows (**b**) shows nodular areas of opacification confirmed histologically to reflect pulmonary parenchymal involvement.

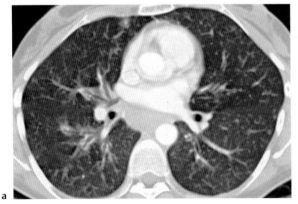
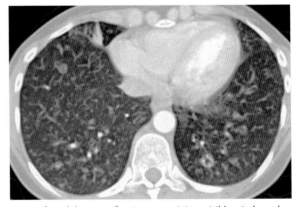

Fig. 6.**46 a, b**   Pulmonary involvement in recurrent low-grade follicular lymphoma. CT shows peribronchial infiltration and posterior mediastinal lymph node enlargement (**a**) There are also areas of nodular opacification containing visible air bronchograms (**b**).

Lymphoma involving the lung by direct extension from the hilum may be seen as soft-tissue nodules surrounding patent bronchi. Discrete pulmonary nodules frequently have ill-defined borders (Figs. 6.**45 b**, 6.**46 a**, **b**).

Primary Pulmonary Lymphoma

Three distinct entities are now covered by the definition of primary pulmonary clonal lymphoid proliferation (primary pulmonary lymphoma). These comprise:
1. Low-grade pulmonary B-cell lymphoma.
2. High-grade pulmonary B-cell lymphoma.
3. Inclusion of lymphomatoid granulomatosis (LG) remains controversial.

Low grade B-cell lymphoma arises from mucosa-associated lymphoid tissue (MALT) and is the most frequent form of primary pulmonary lymphoma **(MALT lymphoma)**. It tends to be indolent, has an excellent prognosis, and treatment is controversial (Cadranel et al. 2002).

The CT findings in MALT lymphoma have been described. These included nodular and linear areas of increased attenuation and areas of consolidation. All of these changes had their epicenter on the airway which appeared dilated, and they correlated histologically with lymphomatous infiltration in a peribronchovascular distribution (Wislez et al. 1999, Fig. 6.**47**).

High grade B-cell lymphoma usually occurs in patients with underlying immunodeficiency and its prognosis tends to be poor.

AIDS-Related Lymphoma

See p. 98.

Lymphomatoid Granulomatosis

Inclusion of lymphomatoid granulomatosis is controversial and debate continues as to whether this reflects a vasculitis or a neoplastic entity. Lee et al. have described CT features in LG that include a peribronchovascular distribution of nodules, coarse irregular opacities, thin-walled cysts, and large masses (Lee et al. 2000).

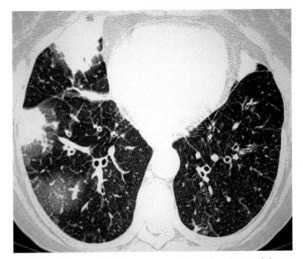

Fig. 6.**47** Baltoma. CT shows areas of peripheral consolidation with visible air bronchograms.

Treated Lymphoma

CT is routinely used to assess response to therapy and for regular follow-up of patients in remission. It is also appropriate for imaging complications of lymphoma therapy.

For radiation-induced complications, see p. 107.

For complications of chemotherapy, see drug-induced lung disease, p. 108.

Indirect complications of therapy are frequently secondary to bone marrow suppression and steroid therapy. Thrombocytopenia may give rise to hemorrhagic complications including diffuse pulmonary hemorrhage. Neutropenia and lymphopenia result in increased susceptibility to infection. Bacterial pneumonia may develop but these individuals are also at risk of developing opportunistic infections.

▪ Radionuclide Scintigraphy

Gallium citrate (^{67}Ga) has been advocated for diagnosis and staging of both HD and NHL, but caution is required in image interpretation as ^{67}Ga is not particularly tumor specific.

▪ FDG PET/PET-CT

The role of PET/PET-CT in lymphoma has been evaluated and PET may play an important role in evaluation and management of lymphoma (Kazama et al. 2005). Residual abnormality at CT after completion of chemotherapy is not uncommon. This may reflect either residual disease or necrotic/fibrotic tissue.

Schaefer et al. retrospectively compared coregistered FDG PET-CT to contrast-enhanced CT in staging and re-staging of both Hodgkin disease and high-grade non-Hodgkin lymphoma. For lymph node involvement, PET-CT had a sensitivity and specificity of 94 and 100% vs. values of 88 and 86% for CT. For organ involvement, PET-CT had a sensitivity and specificy of 88 and 100% respectively vs. values of 50 and 90% for CT (Schaefer et al. 2004).

Reinhardt et al. evaluated the role of FDG-PET in predicting progression-free survival of patients with HD and NHL after completion of therapy. They found that FDG-PET allowed stratification of patients into those at low ($<$20%) and those at high ($>$80%) risk of recurrence (Reinhardt et al. 2005).

These and other studies show FDG-PET to be more accurate than CT in assessing residual disease and in identifying patients who require more intense therapy. However, post-treatment PET may not identify minimal residual disease and as it is not tumor-specific, it sometimes may be positive in benign conditions so clinical and imaging correlation is appropriate.

7 Pulmonary Hypertension and Edema

Pulmonary Hypertension

Pulmonary arterial hypertension is defined as a mean pulmonary artery pressure of greater than 25 mmHg at rest or greater than 30 mmHg during exercise with increased pulmonary vascular resistance (Burke et al. 1991). Pulmonary artery pressures greater than 70 mmHg are consistent with severe hypertension.

Ohm's Law (P_{pa}–P_{pv} = $R \times I$) indicates that chronic elevation of pulmonary arterial pressure (P_{pa}) may result from increased blood flow (I), increased resistance (R), or an increase in pulmonary venous pressure (P_{pv}). Pulmonary hypertension may therefore be due to (Table 7.1):

* *Increased pulmonary vascular resistance (precapillary pulmonary hypertension)* in longstanding cardiac left-to-right shunt, chronic thromboembolic disease, pulmonary parenchymal diseases including chronic obstructive pulmonary disease (COPD) and diffuse interstitial pulmonary fibrosis, vasospasm secondary to alveolar hypoventilation, and may be idiopathic in primary pulmonary hypertension (PPH). 60–70% of the pulmonary vascular bed must be occluded before there is an appreciable increase in pressure.
* *Increased pulmonary venous pressure* (postcapillary pulmonary hypertension) is usually secondary to elevated left atrial pressure and may be seen in left ventricular failure, mitral valve stenosis, longstanding left atrial myxoma, or may be idiopathic in pulmonary veno-occlusive disease (PVOD) (Table. 7.1).

Goals of Diagnostic Imaging:

Identify imaging features of pulmonary hypertension. Further evaluation with echocardiography, computed tomography (CT), magnetic resonance imaging (MRI), and right heart catheterization with pulmonary angiography may then be appropriate.

Determine if it reflects pre- or postcapillary hypertension.

Determine if there is an underlying cause or if it is idiopathic (i.e., primary pulmonary hypertension or pulmonary veno-occlusive disease).

Table 7.1 Classification of pulmonary hypertension

Precapillary Causes
* Chronic thrombo-embolic disease (CTEPH), fat and parasitic pulmonary emboli.
* Secondary to a longstanding left-to-right cardiac/vascular shunt.
* Pulmonary parenchymal disease: COPD, Diffuse interstitial pulmonary fibrosis.
* Vasospasm due to alveolar hypoventilation (muscular dystrophy, poliomyelitis, Pickwickian syndrome, Ondine curse syndrome).
* Idiopathic: primary pulmonary hypertension (PPH)

Postcapillary Causes
* Left ventricular failure.
* Mitral valve disease, Left atrial myxoma.
* Idiopathic: Pulmonary veno-occlusive disease (PVOD).

■ Pathology

Changes seen in all forms of precapillary pulmonary hypertension include intimal cellular proliferation and medial smooth muscle hypertrophy. These changes are characteristically seen in the muscular arteries. In addition, plexiform lesions and necrotizing arteritis are seen in primary pulmonary hypertension and in pulmonary hypertension secondary to a cardiac shunt. A plexiform lesion is defined as a focal disruption in the internal elastic lamina of a muscular artery by a "glomeruloid" plexus of endothelial channels which proceed to ramify into alveolar septal capillaries.

Postcapillary hypertension is characterized by venous medial hypertrophy and intimal proliferation with marked prominence of the venous internal elastic lamina (Frazier et al. 2000).

■ Clinical Features

All forms of pulmonary hypertension are associated with progressive dyspnea, which in advanced disease may be severe and associated with cyanosis. Clinical manifestations of right heart failure include peripheral edema, elevated jugular venous pressure, hepatomegaly, and ascites.

Precapillary Pulmonary Hypertension

Primary Pulmonary Hypertension

PPH is relatively rare. Its existence as a separate entity has on occasion been queried by those who suggest that it may result from clinically latent microemboli (Shinnick et al. 1974 a, b). Nevertheless, the following appear to justify its recognition: It shows a familial incidence and primarily affects young to middle-aged adults with a 3–5:1 female to male ratio. Acetylcholine infusion has been shown to reduce the pulmonary arterial pressure (Fishman and Pietra 1980). In the 1960s, clusters of cases were reported in Germany, Austria, and Switzerland; this was subsequently attributed to use of the appetite suppressant Menocil (Fig. 7.1). Evidence suggests that endothelial injury to small pulmonary arteries and arterioles with resulting vasoconstriction may act as an inciting mechanism for PPH (Frazier et al. 2000).

Clinical features include dyspnea, chest pain, syncope, cyanosis, and right ventricular (RV) failure. Electrocardiographic (ECG) changes in advanced disease are those of cor pulmonale.

■ Radiologic Findings

The pulmonary circulation is a low-pressure system. This results in part from the high compliance of the pulmonary vessels. An increase in pressure is associated with a radiologically appreciable increase in vessel caliber (Fig. 7.2).

The frontal chest radiograph shows central pulmonary artery dilatation. Apparent prominence of the pulmonary segment of the left heart contour results from vascular dilatation and from a degree of cardiac rotation associated with right ventricular hypertrophy. Chronically elevated pulmonary arterial pressure leads to right ventricular overload. Initial adaptation is with ventricular muscular hypertrophy, but eventually the right ventricle becomes dilated and right ventricular failure supervenes.

On the lateral view, right ventricular dilatation may be associated with narrowing or obliteration of the retrosternal space. Pulmonary vascularity is variable.

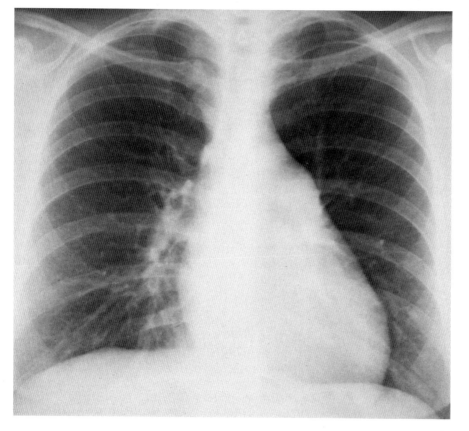

Fig. 7.1 Primary pulmonary hypertension in a patient who had used appetite suppressants.

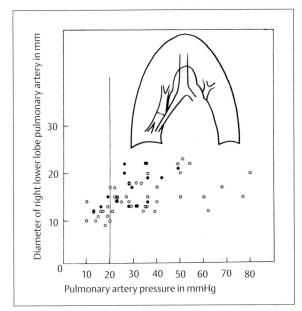

Fig. 7.**2** Correlation of pulmonary arterial pressure with the diameter of the right lower lobe pulmonary artery (from Meschan: *Analyse der Röntgenbilder*, vol. II. Stuttgart: Enke; 1981).

Computed Tomography

CT demonstrates central pulmonary artery dilatation (Figs. 7.**3 a**, 7.**4 a**). The diameter of the main pulmonary artery is measured at the level of the bifurcation perpendicular to the long axis of the vessel (Naidich et al. 1999). A diameter of > 29 mm demonstrates a sensitivity of 87 % and specificity of 89 % for prediction of pulmonary hypertension.

When a main pulmonary artery diameter of > 29 mm is associated with an elevated segmental arterial/bronchial ratio (i. e., > 1) in three of four lobes, the specificity for pulmonary hypertension increases to 100 % (Fig. 7.**3 b**) (Tan et al. 1998).

A main pulmonary artery to ascending aortic diameter ratio of > 1 also has a strong correlation with pulmonary hypertension (PH) particularly in patients who are less than 50 years of age (Ng et al. 1999).

There may be dilatation of right heart chambers and paradoxical bowing of the interventricular septum towards the left ventricle may be seen in severe PH (Fig. 7.**3 c**, and see Fig. 7.**17 b**).

High-resolution images through the lungs in severe pulmonary hypertension sometimes show small centrilobular nodules that may reflect the presence of cholesterol granulomata (Nolan et al. 1999, Fig. 7.**4b**, **c**).

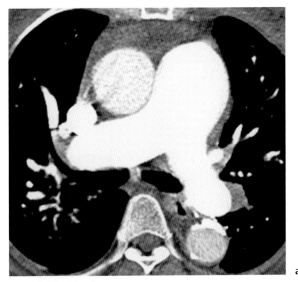

a

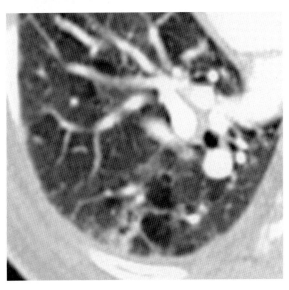

b

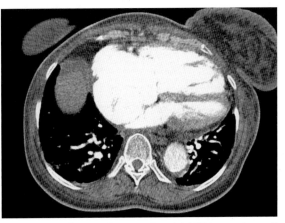

c

Fig. 7.**3 a–c** Pulmonary hypertension: Axial CT image shows dilatation of the main pulmonary artery (**a**). Arterial-bronchial diameter ratio is increased in the right lower lobe (**b**). There is marked dilatation of the right heart chambers (**c**). Subcutaneous edema and ascites are consistent with right ventricular decompensation (cor pulmonale).

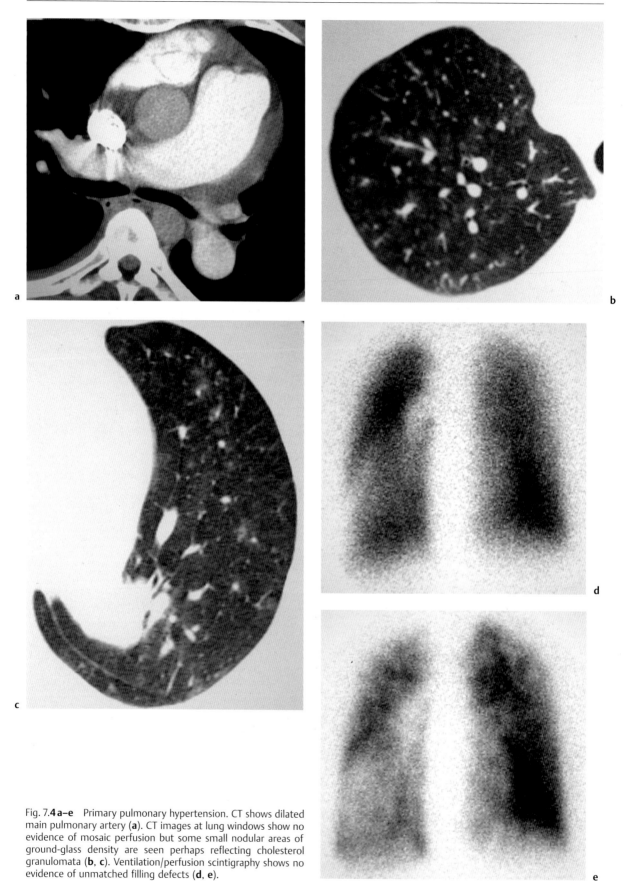

Fig. 7.**4 a–e**   Primary pulmonary hypertension. CT shows dilated main pulmonary artery (**a**). CT images at lung windows show no evidence of mosaic perfusion but some small nodular areas of ground-glass density are seen perhaps reflecting cholesterol granulomata (**b**, **c**). Ventilation/perfusion scintigraphy shows no evidence of unmatched filling defects (**d**, **e**).

Magnetic Resonance Imaging

MRI shows features of pulmonary hypertension including central pulmonary artery dilatation, right heart chamber dilatation, and paradoxical bowing of the interventricular septum. Abnormal intravascular signal related to slow flow within pulmonary arteries may be seen on ECG-gated spin echo sequences.

Velocity-encoded gradient echo sequences provide a two-dimensional velocity map of a cross-sectional area of a vessel and allow calculation of aortic and pulmonary artery flow as well as flow volumes to the right and left lungs.

The role of combined magnetic resonance (MR) perfusion and magnetic resonance angiography (MRA) has recently been evaluated by Nikolaou et al. who report a sensitivity of 90% for this technique in differentiating patients with PPH from those with chronic thromboembolic disease (Nikolaou et al. 2005).

Ventilation–Perfusion Scintigraphy (VQS)

Ventilation–perfusion scintigraphy is characteristically normal or of low probability in PPH (Fig. 7.**4d**, **e**).

Pulmonary Angiography/Right Heart Catheterization

Right heart catheterization reveals elevated pulmonary vascular resistance with normal capillary wedge and left atrial pressures. Pulmonary angiography shows dilated central vessels and a diffuse pattern of abruptly tapering and pruned subsegmental vessels (Frazier et al. 2000).

Acute Pulmonary Embolism (PE) and Chronic Thromboembolic Pulmonary Hypertension (CTEPH)

■ Pathology

Pulmonary thromboembolism may be found in up to 65% of autopsies, making it the most common pathologic finding in hospitalized patients. However, pulmonary emboli remain clinically silent in up to 80% of cases. An embolus within a pulmonary artery results in either a reduction or a cessation in distal perfusion. Collateral flow from the bronchial arterial system is usually sufficient to maintain lung viability.

Pulmonary infarction develops in 10 to 15% of cases usually when there is associated pulmonary venous hypertension. It results from local hypoxia leading to capillary damage, exudation, hemorrhage, and coagulation necrosis. Macroscopic examination of the hemorrhagic infarct shows a firm, airless, livid dark-red segment of lung. Pulmonary infarcts are revascularized gradually from the periphery. Subsequent organization of smaller infarcts leads to complete resolution or contracted scar formation. Pulmonary infarcts very occasionally may become infected leading to abscess formation.

■ Clinical Features

Clinical diagnosis of acute pulmonary embolism may be difficult as the classic triad of sudden onset of chest pain, dyspnea, and hemoptysis is present in only a minority of cases. Hypoxia may be found on arterial blood gas analysis. Studies have reported both a high sensitivity and negative predictive value of D-dimer assay in investigation of acute PE in ambulant patients (Hogg et al. 2006, Hlavac et al. 2005). This test is less reliable in immobile hospitalized and pregnant patients.

It is estimated that 1–5% of patients with acute PE progress to CTEPH (Frazier et al. 2000). The incidence of CTEPH is higher in females and lupus anticoagulant and anticardiolipin antibody may be positive.

■ Radiologic Findings

Chest Radiograph

The chest radiograph in acute PE may be normal or findings may be nonspecific, even in severely symptomatic patients (Fig. 7.**5**).

The posterobasal segments are sites of predilection for pulmonary thromboembolism because of the relatively high proportion of pulmonary blood flow which they receive. Conversely, only 10% of emboli involve the upper lobes.

Features of acute pulmonary embolism without infarction include:
- *Local oligemia* (the Westermark sign) with regional hyperlucency. This finding, in isolation on a single chest radiograph is unreliable. However, its occurrence as a new finding when previous radiographs have been normal may be significant (Fig. 7.**6**).
- *Areas of discoid atelectasis*. These probably result from surfactant deficiency in the involved lung. On the chest radiograph, discoid or plate atelectasis is seen as intrapulmonary linear opacities 1–3 mm in thickness and up to several centimeters in length. These may extend to the pleura.
- *Elevation of the hemidiaphragm*: This may result from reflex splinting due to pleuritic pain but may also be secondary to surfactant deficiency with a resultant reduction in pulmonary compliance.
- *Pleural effusion*, which may yield serosanguinous fluid.

Radiographic features of acute PE with infarction include:
- *Wedge-shaped or oval opacities* (the Hampton hump; Hampton and Castleman 1940). This opacity typically

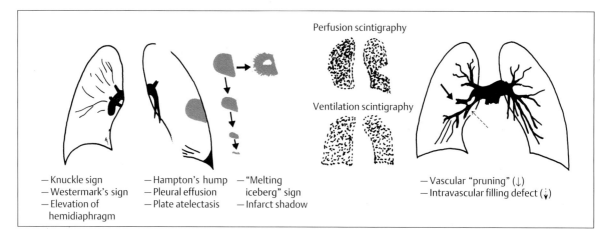

Fig. 7.**5** Pulmonary embolism and infarction.

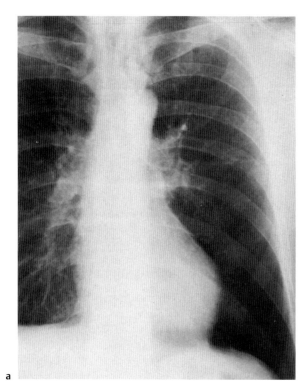

a

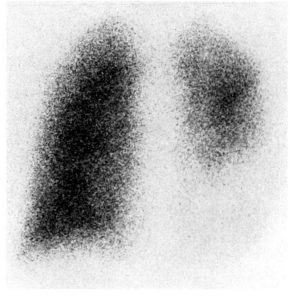

b

Fig. 7.**6 a, b** Pulmonary embolism. Frontal chest radiograph shows attenuated vascular markings in the left lower zone (Westermark's sign) correlating with large perfusion defect at scintigraphy.

appears 24 hours after the embolic event and usually measures 3–5 cm in diameter. The base of the wedge-shaped infarct abuts the visceral pleura while the rounded apex points towards the hilum. Resolution of the opacity in 4–7 days suggests simple alveolar edema and hemorrhage. An opacity that regresses gradually over a period of 3–5 weeks indicates parenchymal necrosis. Characteristically, these opacities shrink from the periphery and remain homogeneous (*melting iceberg*). This differs from the pattern in pneumonic consolidation which usually resolves from the center towards the periphery.

- Infarcts that become infected may show a transient increase in size and may cavitate. Superinfection also delays resolution (Fig. 7.**7**).
- *Pleural effusion* that is usually hemorrhagic on aspiration.
- Features of *pulmonary hypertension in CTEPH* may be indistinguishable from radiographic findings in PH due to other causes (see p. 183).

Radionuclide Scintigraphy

A normal ventilation/perfusion study excludes acute pulmonary embolism in up to 95% of cases (PIOPED study). However, only approximately 25% of patients fall into this category. Pulmonary emboli causing vascular occlusion may produce wedge-shaped perfusion defects.

Pulmonary infarcts produce scintigraphic defects that are larger than the corresponding opacities on the chest radiograph, but definite differentiation from pneumonic consolidation is not possible.

An unmatched perfusion defect with a normal ventilation study is consistent with pulmonary embolism. This is in contrast to the typical findings of matched perfusion and ventilation defects in emphysema. Multiple unmatched perfusion defects at scintigraphy are seen when multiple acute pulmonary emboli are present (high probability study Fig. 7.**8a–d**) and also are frequently seen in CTEPH (Fig. 7.**9b**, **c**).

Computed Tomography

Contrast-enhanced helical and electron-beam CT allow direct visualization of pulmonary emboli. In the 1990s, a number of studies reported sensitivities for single-row helical CT of greater than 90% for detection of emboli in the central (main, lobar, and segmental) vessels with specificities comparable to those for pulmonary angiography (Goodman et al. 1995, Remy-Jardin 1992). CT pulmonary angiography (CTPA) using this technology was shown to be less sensitive for detection of thromboemboli confined to subsegmental vessels (Goodman et al. 1995).

Four-, 16-, and now 64-slice multi-detector row CT (MDCT) scanners are in widespread clinical use today. Their improved spatial resolution together with their subsecond gantry rotation times show improved detection of emboli within subsegmental vessels. The PIOPED II study is currently evaluating the accuracy of MDCT in this setting and should yield important information (Patel and Kazerooni 2005).

Emboli appear as filling defects within contrast-enhanced vessels (Fig. 7.**10**). In cases of pulmonary infarction, peripheral wedge-shaped areas of pulmonary opacification may be seen (Fig. 7.**11**).

In CTEPH, CT may directly visualize *endothelialized thromboemboli* which tend to lie asymmetrically within the vessel lumen (Figs. 7.**9a**, 7.**12a**, **b**, 7.**13a**). *Vascular occlusions, changes in vessel caliber, and mural irregularity* may also be seen (Schwickert et al. 1993). Heinrich et al. evaluated the role of preoperative helical CTPA in predicting surgical outcomes of post pulmonary thromboendarterectomy. They found that the absence of central thrombi at CTPA was a significant risk factor for inadequate hemodynamic improvement postsurgery (Heinrich et al. 2005).

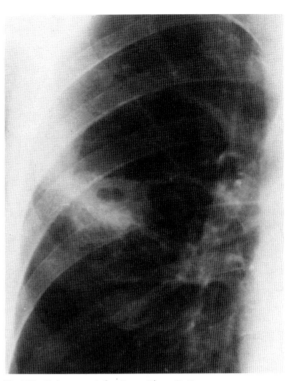

Fig. 7.**7** Pulmonary infarction with cavitation.

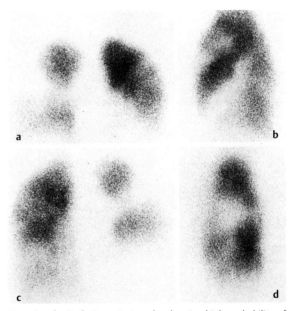

Fig. 7.**8a–d** Perfusion scintigraphy showing high probability of pulmonary embolism with multiple perfusion defects seen bilaterally. **a** Prone, **b** LLD, **c** supine, and **d** RLD.

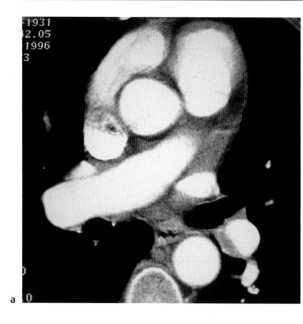

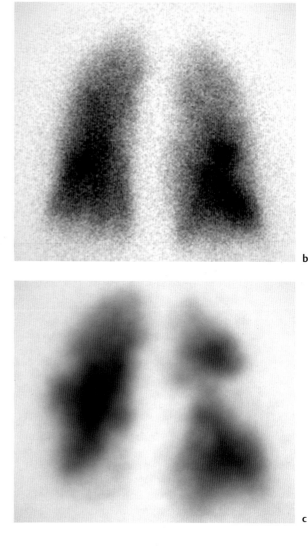

Fig. **7.9 a–c** Chronic thromboembolic disease. CT shows endothelialized thrombus within the left inferior pulmonary artery (**a**). Ventilation-perfusion scintigraphy shows multiple unmatched perfusion defects consistent with a high probability for pulmonary embolism (**b**, **c**).

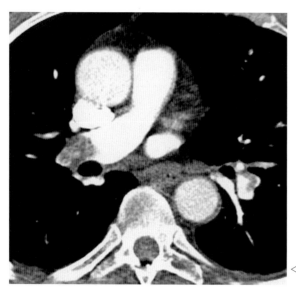

◁ Fig. **7.10** Acute pulmonary embolism. CT shows bilateral filling defects within the central pulmonary arteries.

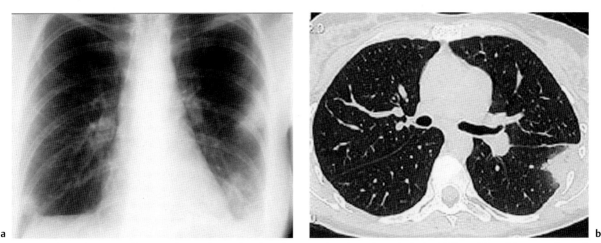

a

b

Fig. 7.**11 a, b** Pulmonary infarction. Chest radiograph and CT show a wedge-shaped opacity in the left lower lobe with concomitant effusion in a patient with a history of pelvic and lower extremity venous thrombosis.

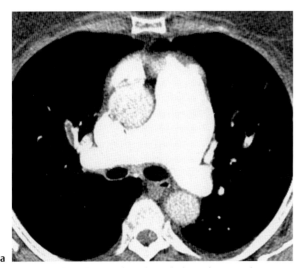

a

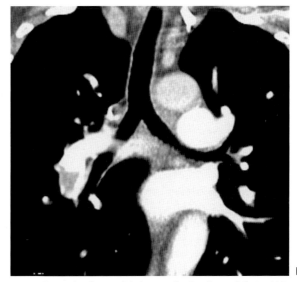

b

Fig. **7.12 a, b** Chronic thromboembolic pulmonary hypertension (CTEPH): Axial CT image (**a**) shows dilatation of the central pulmonary arteries and a filling defect within the right upper lobe

artery. Coronal reformat (**b**) shows a further large defect within the interlobar artery.

Dilated systemic collateral vessels and most commonly dilated bronchial arteries may be seen. Remy-Jardin et al. reported this finding to be more common in patients with CTEPH (73%) than in those with primary pulmonary hypertension (14%) (Remy-Jardin et al. 2005).

Features of PH including increased diameter of the main pulmonary artery, elevated arterial-bronchial ratio, and increased pulmonary artery–ascending aortic ratio may be seen. CT features of cor pulmonale include right heart dilatation, peripheral edema, pleural effusions, and ascites (see Fig. 7.3 c).

At lung windows, CT may show a *mosaic pattern of attenuation* as a sign of inhomogeneous lung perfusion (Figs. 7.13 b, 7.14 a). This pattern has been shown to be more common in PH secondary to vascular disease than in cases due to cardiac or lung disease (Sherrick et al. 1997).

Pulmonary Angiography

Pulmonary angiography has largely been replaced by CTPA in the diagnosis of acute pulmonary embolism. Typical angiographic features include intraluminal filling defects with abrupt cutoff of the contrast column. Equivocal signs include (1) regions of absent or delayed perfusion and (2) increased tortuosity of subsegmental arteries (Fig. 7.**15**).

Pulmonary angiography in CTEPH shows nonhomogeneous distribution of pulmonary vessels with abrupt

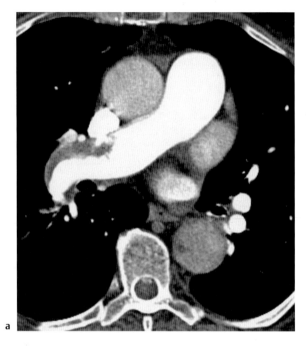

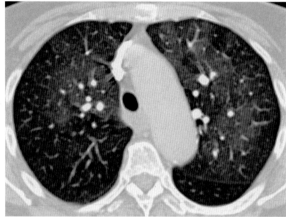

a

b

Fig. **7.13 a, b**   CTEPH: CT image at mediastinal windows shows endothelialized thrombus within the distal right main and inferior pulmonary artery (**a**). CT at lung windows shows mosaic perfusion (**b**).

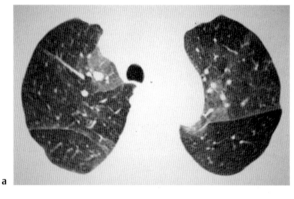

a

Fig. 7.**14 a–c**   CTEPH: High-resolution CT shows inhomogeneous lung attenuation consistent with mosaic perfusion (**a**). Pulmonary angiography (**b**, **c**) shows vascular occlusions, rapid "cutoffs," and stenoses.

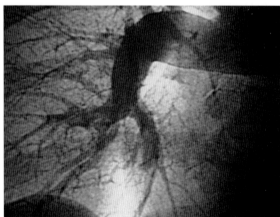

b

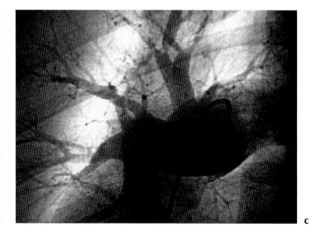

c

vascular cut-offs, stenotic and absent arterial segments, and intravascular webs and bands (Fig. 7.**14 b**, **c**)

Cardiac Defects with a Left-to-Right Shunt

■ Clinical Features

In the normal individual, equal volumes of blood flow through both the pulmonary and systemic circulation. When a congenital left-to-right shunt is present, pulmonary blood flow will increase 3- to 6-fold relative to the systemic circulation. When an atrial or ventricular septal defect (VSD), patent ductus arteriosus (PDA), or aortopulmonary window is present, blood is shunted from the left heart through the defect into the right heart or pulmonary artery and is recirculated through the lung. An effective left-to-right shunt is also present with anomalous pulmonary venous drainage to the vena cava or right heart.

Because of the compliance of the pulmonary vessels, pulmonary arterial pressure is initially normal in the presence of increased flow. Pulmonary arterial hypertension eventually develops in untreated cases and is secondary to sclerosis of pulmonary arterioles in response to increased flow, leading to increased pulmonary vascular resistance. Pathologic changes in the pulmonary vessels may be classified by the Heath and Edwards's system. Grades I and II are characterized by medial hypertrophy, intimal proliferation, and "muscularization" of the pulmonary arterioles; these changes reflect potentially reversible disease. By contrast, grades IV to VI are characterized by plexiform lesions, aneurysmal muscular arteries, and sites of necrotizing arteritis that reflect severe irreversible disease (Katzenstein et al. 1997, Frazier et al. 2000).

Increased pulmonary vascular resistance, in turn leads to right ventricular hypertrophy, and when right ventricular pressure eventually exceeds that of the left ventricle, the shunt reverses (Eisenmenger reaction). The age at which shunt reversal occurs depends in part on initial shunt volume. Presenting symptoms include exertional dyspnea and palpitations. Characteristic auscultatory findings include systolic (VSD) or continuous (PDA) murmurs. The electrocardiogram may show features of right ventricular hypertrophy and strain.

■ Radiologic Findings

Chest Radiograph

There is cardiomegaly of RV configuration. The central pulmonary vessels are dilated and often tortuous (Fig. 7.**16**). Initially there is associated pulmonary ple-

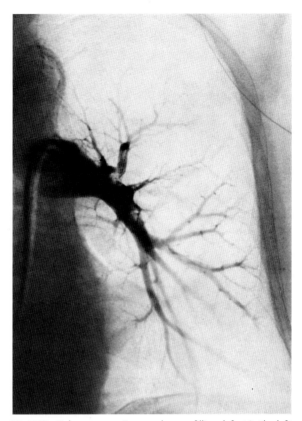

Fig. 7.**15** Pulmonary angiogram shows a filling defect in the left upper lobar artery and poststenotic vascular attenuation; findings consistent with a pulmonary embolus.

thora but with shunt reversal, pulmonary oligemia develops. The so-called "hilar dance" sign seen in the past when fluoroscopy was performed routinely in these cases represents the vigorous pulsations of the central pulmonary arteries. This phenomenon was best appreciated in the right lower lobe artery. In patent ductus arteriosus, pulsations are less conspicuous as flow through the shunt continues throughout the cycle.

Echocardiography determines the level of the shunt and provides estimation of both its volume and pulmonary arterial pressure.

Computed Tomography

CT may show features of pulmonary hypertension, right heart dilatation ± cor pulmonale (Fig. 7.**17 a**, **b**). Linear calcification may be evident within the central pulmonary arteries. In cases of patent ductus arteriosis, mural calcification and dilatation of the ductus may be seen (Virmani et al. 1987).

Magnetic Resonance Imaging

MRI shows features of pulmonary hypertension and the site and size of the intracardiac shunt may be seen.

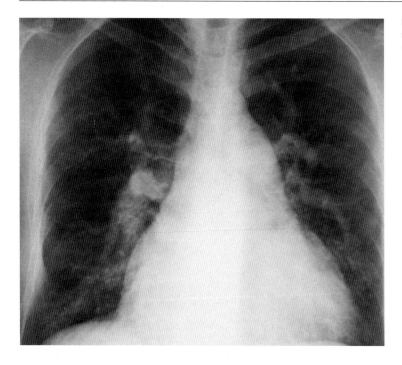

Fig. 7.**16**   Atrial septal defect with a left-to-right shunt characterized by central pulmonary artery dilatation.

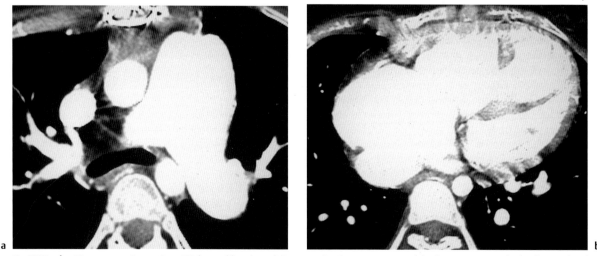

a   b

Fig. 7.**17 a, b**   Eisenmenger's reaction: CT shows dilatation of the central pulmonary arteries (**a**). There is very marked right atrial and ventricular dilatation with paradoxical bowing of the interventricular septum toward the left atrium (**b**).

■ Cardiac Catheterization

Cardiac catheterization is performed in some cases if surgical correction is still feasible before development of Eisenmenger's reaction, particularly in older patients with suspected concomitant ischemic heart disease. Right heart catheterization will reveal increased oxygen saturation in the right heart chambers and will also document the level and size of the shunt.

Pulmonary Hypertension Due to Alveolar Hypoventilation

Pulmonary hypoventilation results in a reflex hypoxic vasoconstriction of the pulmonary arterioles. A persistent reduction in ventilation results in gradual development of pulmonary hypertension. This may be due to the following:

Ondine's Curse Syndrome

This refers to a congenital or postencephalitic hyposensitivity of the respiratory center to CO_2. These patients intermittently "forget" to breathe, and diaphragmatic pacing is occasionally beneficial.

Pickwickian Syndrome

This syndrome, also known as obstructive sleep apnea, is associated with inspiratory pharyngeal collapse and produces snoring and upper airway obstruction, particularly in obese patients. This in turn leads to hypoxic vasoconstriction. There may be secondary loss of hypercapnic responsiveness in the respiratory center. This phenomenon may also result from inspiratory muscle weakness due to poliomyelitis, muscular dystrophy, amyotrophic lateral sclerosis, etc.

Chronic Hypercapnia Syndrome

Chronic alveolar hypoxia and hypercapnia resulting from perfusion ventilation mismatch due to bullous emphysema and chest wall deformity may induce a refractory state in the respiratory center leading to further hypoventilation.

Postcapillary Pulmonary Hypertension

Pulmonary Veno-Occlusive Disease

Pulmonary veno-occlusive disease is a rare cause of pulmonary hypertension. It may be difficult but it is important to distinguish it from PPH as the vasodilator therapy used to treat PPH may be fatal in PVOD. The histologic changes in PVOD include intravascular webs, recanalized thrombosis, and intimal fibrosis within the pulmonary veins. Proliferative lesions referred to as capillary "hemangiomatosis" may also be present or this may reflect a distinct variant. In addition to the changes seen in precapillary hypertension, the capillary wedge pressure is elevated in PVOD.

Imaging studies suggest the diagnosis when changes of pulmonary hypertension are seen in association with features of interstitial edema in the presence of a normal left atrium (Frazier et al. 2000). Reston et al. studied CT findings in PVOD. They found that the presence of ground-glass opacities particularly in a centrilobular distribution, subpleural septal thickening, and lymph node enlargement were more common in PVOD (Reston et al. 2004). The same group studied CT features which predict epoprostenol therapy failure and found similar CT features including the presence of ground-glass opacities, septal thickening, and pleural effusion (Reston et al. 2002, Fig. 7.**18**).

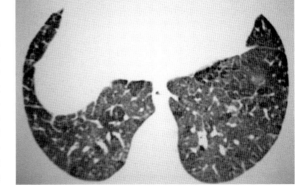

Fig. 7.**18** Pulmonary veno-occlusive disease (PVOD): CT shows ground-glass opacification with some interlobular septal thickening.

Pulmonary Congestion and Edema

Pulmonary edema occurs when pulmonary venous return is impaired, primarily in left ventricular failure and mitral stenosis. The increased pulmonary venous pressure is transmitted to the pulmonary arteries as valves are absent in the pulmonary circulation. There is a marked increase in intravascular volume as pulmonary vessels are also very compliant. Later, an increase in capillary pressure leads to fluid transudation into the interstitium and alveolar airspaces. Acute pulmonary edema is reversible, but chronic edema results in a degree of interstitial fibrosis. Left ventricular impairment commonly results in pulmonary edema and therefore this is a common radiologic diagnosis. The radiologist's role includes recognition of pulmonary edema and identification of precipitating factors such as valvular heart disease. Frontal and lateral chest radiographs are usually adequate for imaging evaluation. Although radiographic signs of interstitial edema may precede clinical symptoms in up to 30% of cases, some of these features are relatively nonspecific and clinical correlation is helpful when making the diagnosis.

■ Pathology

At autopsy, acutely congested lungs are large, heavy, and engorged with blood. There is capillary dilatation, which may compress the alveoli.

Interstitial edema is most pronounced at the lung bases because of higher hydrostatic pressure in these zones. This unequal gravitational distribution of edema also leads to a redistribution in perfusion; this is also evident on the chest radiograph.

At least two factors account for flow redistribution to the upper zones. First, basal edema reduces compliance in the lower zones and the vessels cannot expand normally during inspiration. Second, reduced pulmonary elasticity leads to hypoventilation, hypoxic vasoconstriction (by the von Euler–Liljestrand reflex), and decreased perfusion to the lower zones (see Figs. 1.**36** and 1.**37**).

With further increases in left atrial and pulmonary venous pressures, alveolar edema develops. Initially, fluid-filled lobules are interspersed among normally aerated lung, producing a radiographic pattern of mottled opacification. As edema becomes more diffuse, homogenous opacification is seen.

In chronic pulmonary edema, fibroblasts produce collagen in the alveolar wall and interlobular septa. This increases the texture of the blood-engorged lung (red induration). Eventually, hemorrhage through the capillary walls and phagocytosis of red cells by macrophages results in "brown" induration.

■ Clinical Features

Clinical manifestations of congestive heart failure include cough productive of frothy blood-stained sputum, dyspnea, orthopnea, cyanosis, and peripheral edema. Auscultatory findings include moist rales or crackles.

■ Radiologic Findings

Plain Chest Radiograph

While florid pulmonary edema is easily recognized, interpretation of the chest radiograph in the initial stages remains more controversial with significant interobserver variation. Plain radiographic findings include:
- Pulmonary vascular dilatation due to raised pulmonary venous pressure
- Upper-zone redistribution of blood flow
- Interstitial edema
- Alveolar edema

The radiographic equivalents of these changes include (Fig. 7.**19**):
- *Dilated lobar and segmental vessels*: Given the variation in normal vessel caliber, dilatation is best evaluated on serial radiographs. Widening of the interlobar artery at the level of the bronchus intermedius

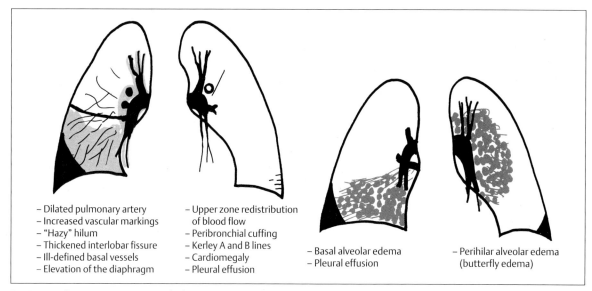

– Dilated pulmonary artery
– Increased vascular markings
– "Hazy" hilum
– Thickened interlobar fissure
– Ill-defined basal vessels
– Elevation of the diaphragm

– Upper zone redistribution of blood flow
– Peribronchial cuffing
– Kerley A and B lines
– Cardiomegaly
– Pleural effusion

– Basal alveolar edema
– Pleural effusion

– Perihilar alveolar edema (butterfly edema)

Fig. 7.**19** Pulmonary congestion and edema.

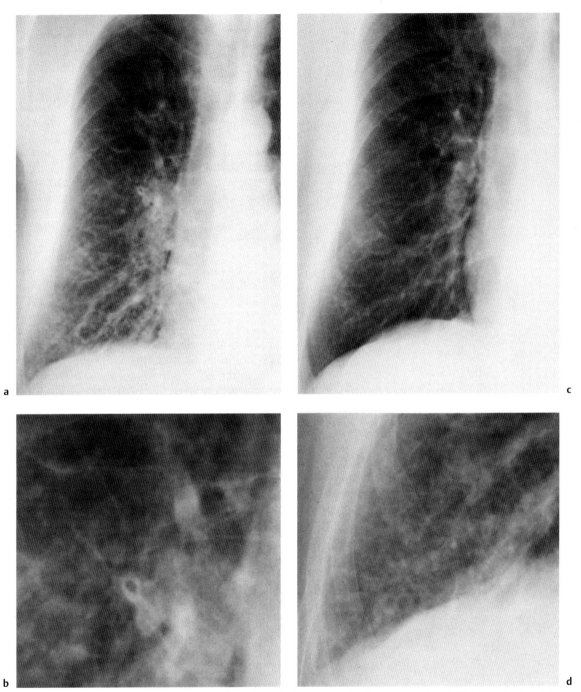

Fig. 7.**20 a–d**   Radiographic features of pulmonary edema include dilated central pulmonary vessels with ill-defined borders (**a**), peribronchial cuffing with Kerley A lines (**c**) and Kerley B lines (**d**). Changes resolved on anti-failure therapy (**b**).

to more than 18 mm is considered pathologic (Fig. 7.**20**).

- *Increased vascular markings*: Dilatation of small, previously indefinable vessels increases the number of radiologically visible vascular markings. Also, decreased pulmonary compliance results in reduced lung volume, which in turn leads to crowding of vascular markings.

- *Dilated perihilar vessels seen in cross section*: Dilated segmental and subsegmental arteries running parallel to the x-ray beam appear as round or oval opacities.

- *Upper-zone redistribution of blood flow*: In the normal individual standing upright, upper zone vessels are smaller in caliber than those to the lower zones, the apical-to-basal cross-sectional ratio being approximately 0.8. With flow redistribution to the upper

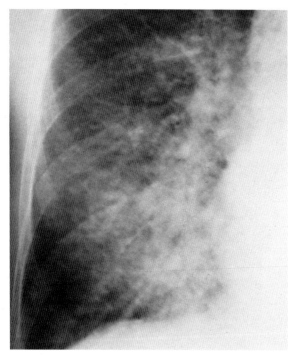

Fig. 7.**21**   Confluent acinar shadowing in pulmonary edema.

zones, this ratio may increase to values in the range from 1 to 3.

- *Hilar haze*: Peribronchovascular edema surrounding the hilar structures and extending into the lung parenchyma may partially obscure the hilar contours resulting in a "hilar haze."
- *Peribronchial cuffing*: The bronchial wall appears thickened as a result of mucosal and peribronchial interstitial edema. This is seen particularly in the ante-

rior segmental bronchi to the upper lobes which appear end on as thick-walled ring shadows (Fig. 7.**20**).

- *Fissural thickening*: Subpleural edema thickens the interlobar fissures, which become radiographically visible if tangential to the beam.
- *Septal lines* correspond to thickened, edematous interlobular septa. Kerley B lines are thin horizontal lines approximately 10 mm in length and are usually seen in the costophrenic angles. Kerley A lines are approximately 40 mm in length and radiate from the hila into the adjacent lung (Fig. 7.**20**).
- *Basal pulmonary edema*: Confluent airspace shadows approximately 5 mm in diameter in dependent lung represent fluid-filled acini (Fig. 7.**21**). Radiographically, these appearances may be difficult to distinguish from bronchopneumonia.
- *"Butterfly" distribution of pulmonary edema.* Pulmonary edema is perihilar/central in distribution in approximately 5% of cases (Fig. 7.**22 a**, **b**). This is the so-called butterfly or bat's wing pattern of edema. This results from the racemous branching pattern of the perihilar arteries which tends to raise capillary pressure. It is also assumed that the pumping action of respiratory excursions enhances pulmonary lymph flow; this effect is more pronounced in the lung periphery than in the perihilar zone.
- *Localized pulmonary edema*: In patients with preexisting lung conditions such as emphysema, edema accumulates in well-perfused lung. The underlying lung disease accounts for the atypical distribution of the edema.
- *Chronic pulmonary edema* may lead to some degree of interstitial fibrosis. Occasionally, multiple small granulomata in the lung parenchyma result from capillary hemorrhage and lead to miliary nodulation (hemosiderosis). These granulomata are most numer-

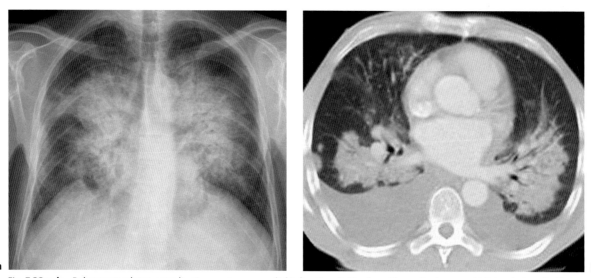

a   b

Fig. 7.**22 a**, **b**   Pulmonary edema complicating acute myocardial infarction. Butterfly pattern of edema and bilateral pleural effusion are seen.

ous in the lower zones and may show a degree of mineralization.

The following frequently are associated with pulmonary edema:

- *Cardiomegaly* usually represents left ventricular dilatation.
- *Pleural effusion*, which often is more pronounced on the right than on the left side (Fig. 7.**19**). This phenomenon has been attributed to the anatomical enlargement of the visceral pleural surface area by the middle lobe, resulting in greater transudation, and to the lymphatics in the right hemidiaphragm, which normally drain peritoneal fluid into the pleural cavity (Light 1983).
- *Elevation of the diaphragm*: This is attributable to the decrease in pulmonary compliance which results from interstitial edema.

Computed Tomography

CT features of interstitial edema include thickened interlobular septa with ground-glass opacification in a dependent or perihilar distribution. More confluent and denser opacification is seen with progression to alveolar edema (Fig. 7.**23**a, **b**). Pleural and pericardial effusions may also be present.

Echocardiography

Echocardiography assesses left ventricular function, allowing estimation of left ventricular ejection fraction and thus helping in differentiation of cardiac and noncardiogenic edema. It also allows detection of cardiac valve dysfunction and the presence of a pericardial effusion/pericardial tamponade.

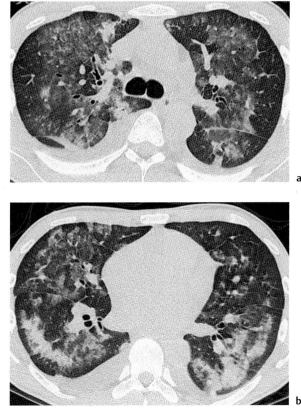

Fig. 7.**23**a, **b** Pulmonary edema: CT images show patchy ground-glass opacification, areas of confluent consolidation, and some interlobular septal thickening.

8 Thoracic Trauma

In this, the age of motorized transport, road traffic accidents (RTAs) frequently result in nonpenetrating chest injury. In Northern Europe, penetrating injuries from gunshot and stab wounds are less common. Thoracic injuries are important as they account for up to 50% of trauma deaths (Wiot 1975). Imaging is initially with chest radiographs proceeding in many cases to computed tomography (CT) and less commonly to aortography.

Multiple injuries are frequent but the following anatomic classification is helpful:
- Chest wall
- Pleural
- Pulmonary
- Mediastinal/vascular injury
- Diaphragmatic injuries

Chest Wall Injuries

Rib Fractures

■ Clinical Features

Isolated rib fractures occur at sites of limited impact. Wide impact injuries deform the chest wall over a large area and result in multiple rib fractures which most commonly occur posteriorly adjacent to the costotransverse

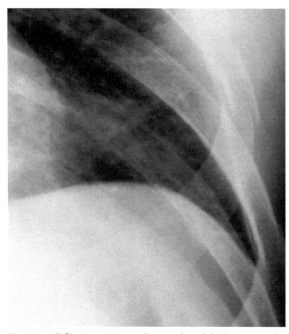

Fig. 8.1 Rib fractures. Minor adjacent pleural thickening may be due to a small hematoma.

articulations. There may be accompanying fractures through the lateral ribs (Fig. 8.1) and costal cartilages. When a large segment of the chest wall loses continuity with the remainder of the bony thorax, there are paradoxical respiratory excursions that may cause life-threatening ventilatory impairment (*flail chest*, Fig. 8.2).

Fractures through the 1st and 2nd or 11th and 12th ribs are unusual but they are frequently complicated by vascular (aortic, subclavian artery) and visceral (liver, spleen, kidneys) injury, respectively. *Arch aortography* will demonstrate aortic and subclavian artery transection and helical CT now plays an important role in patient selection for angiography. Upper abdominal visceral injury is best evaluated with contrast-enhanced CT of the abdomen.

Rib fractures may appear as radiolucent lines, step-like contour deformities, or overriding bone fragments on the chest radiograph (Fig. 8.3). Fractures of the costal cartilages are not visible on standard radiographs and are detected only when there is gross displacement (Fig. 8.4). While isolated rib fractures may not be significant, when they are present it is important to exclude associated pleural, vascular, and visceral injury and particularly pneumothorax.

Sternal Fractures

Sternal fractures result from severe direct trauma such as from a sudden forward thrust against the steering wheel of a car during rapid deceleration of the vehicle. They sometimes are visible on the chest radiograph but are imaged optimally with computed tomography. Kehdy et al. recently have described the utility of three-

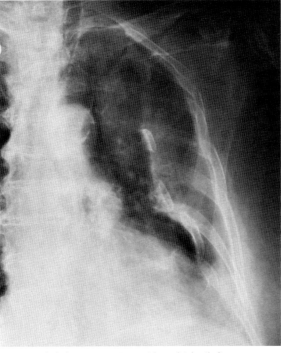

Fig. 8.**2**   Flail chest in a patient with multiple rib fractures.

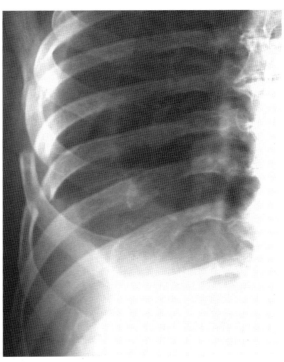

Fig. 8.**3**   Multiple rib fractures on the right side with hemothorax.

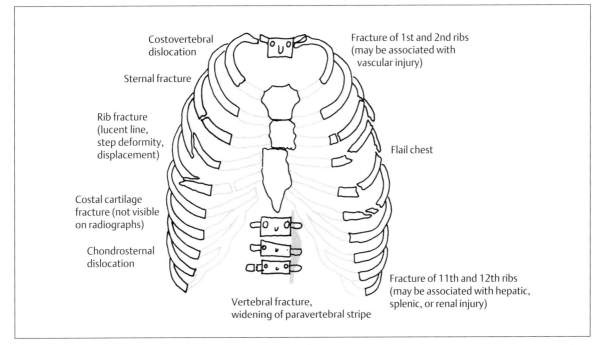

Fig. 8.**4**   Fractures and dislocations of the bony thorax.

dimensional CT reconstructions in diagnosis and evaluation of sternal fractures (Kehdy et al. 2006). There is frequently an associated pneumomediastinum, pneumothorax, or pulmonary contusion (see Fig. 8.**16**).

Vertebral Fractures

Thoracic vertebral body fractures usually result from hyperflexion injuries.

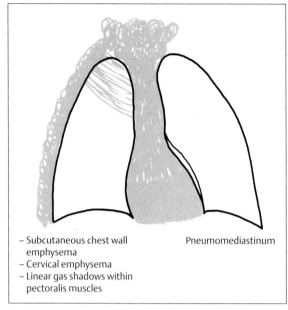

– Subcutaneous chest wall   Pneumomediastinum
  emphysema
– Cervical emphysema
– Linear gas shadows within
  pectoralis muscles

Fig. 8.5   Pneumomediastinum and chest-wall emphysema.

▓ Radiologic Findings

The lateral chest radiograph/lateral thoracic spine may show vertebral body wedging. There may be a step-like deformity of the anterior vertebral margin as the compressed spongiosa produces a line of sclerosis. The degree of vertebral body fragment retropulsion is important to assess. On the frontal radiograph, associated paravertebral soft-tissue hematoma may cause a convex lateral bulge of the paravertebral stripe.

CT of the thoracic spine with sagittal and coronal reformatted images will define accurately the extent of both bony and associated soft tissue injury. Magnetic resonance imaging (MRI) may be complementary to CT when there is clinical evidence of spinal cord or peripheral nerve root injury.

Subcutaneous Emphysema

Subcutaneous chest wall emphysema occurs when intrathoracic air leaks into the soft tissues. There is usually an associated pneumothorax or pneumomediastinum. A characteristic subcutaneous crackling sensation is noted on palpation.

▓ Radiologic Findings

The chest radiograph shows vesicular or linear gas shadows and there may be quite marked thickening of the subcutaneous tissues. Characteristically, air also spreads along the fibers of the pectoralis major muscle and produces fan-shaped linear lucencies overlying the upper thorax (Figs. 8.5, 8.6).

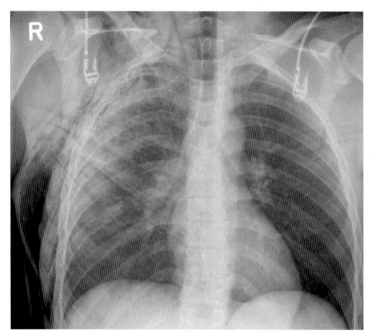

Fig. 8.6   Subcutaneous chest-wall and cervical emphysema. Linear gas shadows outline fibers of pectoralis major muscle.

Pleural Injuries

Pneumothorax

■ Pathology

Air entering the pleural space results in a pneumothorax. Leakage is most commonly from the lung. A pleurocutaneous fistula resulting from penetrating chest injury and a bronchopleural fistula will also produce pneumothoraces. Traumatic bronchopleural fistulas usually result from nonpenetrating compressive trauma with sudden elevation of intra-alveolar pressure; this leads to alveolar rupture and tearing of the visceral pleura. The negative intrapleural pressure then draws air into the pleural cavity. Sharp rib fragments may also injure the pleura and result in pneumothorax.

The elastic recoil of the lung may lead to closure of pleural tears through relaxation atelectasis. Occasionally, the visceral pleural flap may produce a check-valve obstruction with air entering the pleura during inspiration and air trapping within the pleura during expiration. This leads to a tension pneumothorax with mediastinal displacement and compression of major vessels and the contralateral lung. A tension pneumothorax constitutes a medical emergency.

The following are relatively unusual causes of a pneumothorax; they, however, have important implications for patient management:

• *Bronchial rupture.* The presence of pneumomediastinum, pneumothorax, and partial pulmonary atelectasis together with fractures of the 1st to 3rd ribs should raise suspicion of bronchial rupture. The diagnosis may be confirmed at bronchoscopy.

• *Esophageal rupture* is associated with hydropneumothorax and dysphagia. The diagnosis may be confirmed by upper gastrointestinal endoscopy or contrast swallow with water-soluble contrast medium.

■ Clinical Features

A small pneumothorax may be asymptomatic but if it occupies more than 25% of the hemithorax it may lead to significant pulmonary atelectasis with hypoxemia and dyspnea. The hemithorax is hyperresonant to percussion and on auscultation breathing sounds are diminished. Tension pneumothorax is associated with progressively increasing chest pain, dyspnea, and cyanosis.

■ Radiologic Findings

Chest Radiograph (Fig. 8.7)

When possible, an upright chest radiograph should be acquired. In severely traumatized patients, cross-table lateral or supine views only may be possible. On the frontal chest radiograph, the visceral pleura is separated from the chest wall and becomes visible as a laterally convex "pleural line" that parallels the chest wall (Fig. 8.8). Pulmonary vascular markings are absent lateral to this line. On both upright and decubitus views, intrapleural air is seen at the most superior point in the hemithorax except when loculation from adhesions is present. Tension pneumothorax is associated with complete pulmonary atelectasis. There is flattening of the ipsilateral hemidiaphragm, widening of intercostal spaces, and mediastinal shift to the contralateral side (Fig. 8.9).

In the supine position, air tends to collect anteriorly. Radiographic findings in anterior pneumothorax include increased clarity of the mediastinal contours and costophrenic angle on the affected side. These signs frequently are subtle and may not be detected in the patient with multiple trauma (Dee 1995d). A number of studies have shown that only 40 to 50% of pneumothoraces are detected on supine radiographs in

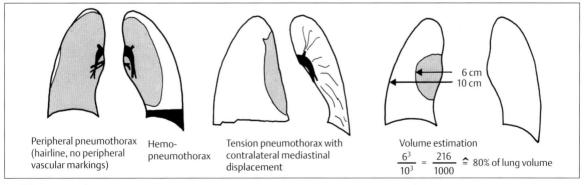

Peripheral pneumothorax (hairline, no peripheral vascular markings) — Hemopneumothorax — Tension pneumothorax with contralateral mediastinal displacement — Volume estimation $\frac{6^3}{10^3} = \frac{216}{1000} \hat{=} 80\%$ of lung volume

Fig. 8.**7** Pneumothorax.

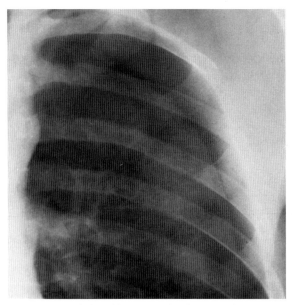

Fig. 8.**8**   Visceral pleural line in peripheral pneumothorax.

the clinical setting of acute trauma (Wall 1983, Tocino 1984).

Pleural aspiration is advocated by some sources if the volume of the pneumothorax exceeds 25% of the hemithorax, if serial radiographs show a progressive increase in intrapleural air or if the pneumothorax persists for more than 1 week (Light 1983). Tension pneumothorax is life-threatening and requires immediate aspiration.

■ Computed Tomography

Computed tomography is highly accurate in detection of pneumothoraces that may be missed on supine radiographs; sensitivities of up to 100% have been reported (Wall 1983, McGonigal 1990). The most superior images through the lung bases therefore should be reviewed at lung windows when CT abdomen is performed in patients with suspected intra-abdominal visceral trauma.

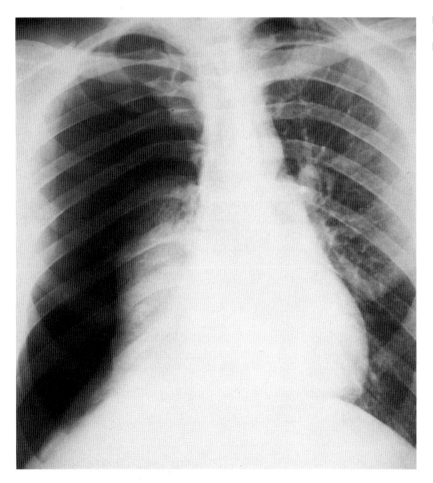

Fig. 8.**9**   Tension pneumothorax with contralateral mediastinal displacement.

Hemothorax

■ Clinical Features

Blood in the pleural cavity may be due to transection of pulmonary, mediastinal, or intercostal vessels. Large volumes of blood are unlikely to be secondary to pulmonary parenchymal injury as the expanding hemothorax tends to compress the lung and tamponade the hemorrhage. All except trivial hemothoraces should be evacuated to prevent development of fibrothorax. If the volume of the hematoma is more than 1500 mL or if drainage from the chest tube is more than 100 mL per hour, thoracotomy may be indicated (Light 1983).

■ Radiologic Findings

▨ Chest Radiograph

When the patient is in the upright position, appearances are those of a pleural collection/effusion. Blood accumulates in the lower hemithorax and obliterates the costophrenic angle forming a medially concave meniscus that is continuous laterally with the chest wall. In the supine position, the posterior layering of blood leads to diffuse homogeneous opacification of the hemithorax. With smaller hemothoraces, superimposed pulmonary vascular markings may be visible on the supine chest radiograph (so called *hazy* opacification). A hemopneumothorax is frequently present.

If prompt aspiration is not performed, the hematoma becomes organized with subsequent development of pleural thickening and fibrosis (fibrothorax).

▨ Computed Tomography

In the setting of acute trauma, CT may show pleural fluid of increased attenuation (i.e., 30–40 Hounsfield units) consistent with the presence of intrapleural blood and hemothorax. A fluid–fluid level may also be seen in subacute or in acute-on-subacute intrapleural hemorrhage.

CT may demonstrate an air–fluid level in hemo-/hydropneumothorax. Associated mediastinal, pulmonary and overlying chest wall injuries may be demonstrated.

Posttraumatic pleural effusion may also be due to an esophagopleural fistula, to a chylothorax secondary to thoracic duct injury or very rarely, to a cerebrospinal fluid (CSF) fistula from communication with the subarachnoid space. Biochemical analysis of aspirated pleural fluid, magnetic resonance (MR) evaluation of the thoracic spine, and upper gastro-intestinal (GI) contrast studies may provide clarification.

Pulmonary Parenchymal Trauma

Pulmonary Contusion

■ Clinical Features

Pulmonary contusion is characterized by interstitial and intra-alveolar hemorrhage, edema, and microatelectasis. These changes most frequently are found in young patients as their chest wall is more compliant and this allows the force of impact to be transmitted more readily through to the lungs. Clinical presentation with mild dyspnea, low-grade pyrexia, and hemoptysis is usual. Dramatic deterioration may occur within 36 hours of injury with progression to adult respiratory distress syndrome (see Fig. 8.**15**).

■ Radiologic Findings

The *chest radiograph* shows patchy or confluent nonsegmental opacities which usually are ipsilateral to the side of impact (Figs. 8.**10**, 8.**11**). Less commonly, con-

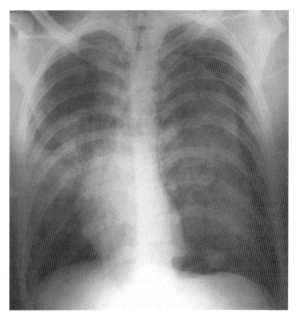

Fig. 8.**10** Pulmonary contusion and left-sided pneumothorax with contralateral mediastinal displacement.

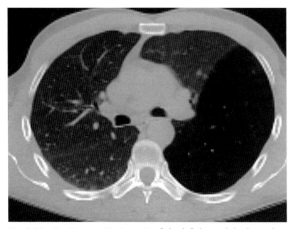

Fig. 8.**11** Posttraumatic stenosis of the left lower lobe bronchus with distal air trapping. CT shows decreased lung attenuation in left lower lobe 6 months after severe chest trauma. Bronchoscopy revealed a cicatricial stricture.

tralateral contusions are seen (contrecoup lesion). Radiographic changes appear within 6 hours of injury and tend to regress within 2–4 days. CT shows patchy ground-glass opacification and air space consolidation (Fig. 8.**12**).

Pulmonary Hematomata and Pneumatoceles

Blunt trauma may cause a shearing force which leads to a pulmonary parenchymal laceration. These lacerations alter in shape due to the elastic recoil of the lung. They then may form posttraumatic pneumatoceles which may become filled with blood to form a pulmonary hematoma (Fig. 8.**13**).

■ Radiologic Findings

In contrast to contusions, *hematomata* appear as oval, homogeneous, well-defined opacities (Fig. 8.**14**). Most hematomata regress within weeks but occasionally they may persist for months (*vanishing tumor*).

Pulmonary pneumatoceles/cysts appear as unilocular oval air-filled cavities which usually are located in the peripheral subpleural lung. They may become radiographically visible some days after injury as contusions are beginning to resolve. Occasionally, they appear within 24 hours of injury. Pulmonary cysts typically collapse and resolve completely within 4 months (Müller and Fraser 2001, Gullotta and Wenzl 1974).

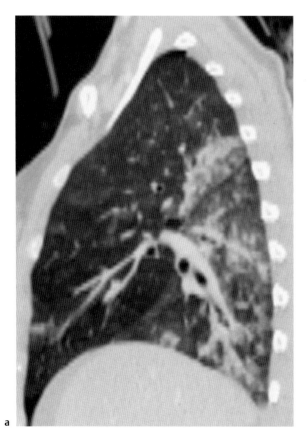

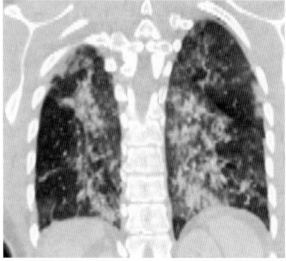

a

b

Fig. 8.**12 a, b** Pulmonary contusion following a rear-end collision, marked by posterior distribution of pulmonary changes.

Pulmonary Atelectasis

Bronchial obstruction resulting in distal atelectasis may be due to an endobronchial mucus plug or aspirated material. *Radiographs* show segmental or lobar atelectasis. Bronchoscopy is indicated to visualize and remove the obstruction.

Pneumonia in the Trauma Patient

The unconscious patient with multiple injuries is at high risk of developing aspiration pneumonia. In addition, foci of pulmonary contusion may become infected. The *chest radiograph* may show confluent airspace shadowing which is found predominantly in the posterobasal lung in cases of aspiration pneumonia.

Tracheobronchial Rupture

■ Clinical Features

Tracheal or bronchial rupture may be caused by penetrating injury or severe blunt trauma in high-velocity road traffic accidents. When due to blunt trauma, it is usually associated with severe chest-wall and pulmonary injury. Airway rupture occurs in approximately 3% of severely traumatized patients and is associated with a 30% mortality rate mainly due to associated injuries (Guest 1977). Most tears are found in the major bronchi within 2 cm of the carina.

■ Radiologic Findings

Diagnosis of tracheobronchial rupture may be difficult and is frequently delayed. Radiologic features are due to:
- Leakage of air at the site of rupture
- Altered pulmonary ventilation distally (Dee 1995 d)

Features of *air leakage* include pneumothorax found in 60 to 100% of cases (Hood 1959, Taskinen 1989) and pneumomediastinum. The coexistence of a pneumothorax and pneumomediastinum is a particularly strong indicator of airway rupture. In addition, while a pneumothorax may result from rib fractures, the presence of a pneumomediastinum in the traumatized patient is a more specific sign of airway disruption (Dee 1995 d).

Altered pulmonary ventilation results in atelectasis. While atelectasis is a common finding in severely traumatized patients when associated with bronchial rupture it tends to be persistent and unresponsive to normal therapeutic measures. An unusual but charac-

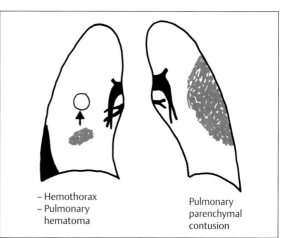

Fig. 8.**13**   Pulmonary hematoma and contusion.

Labels in figure:
– Hemothorax
– Pulmonary hematoma

Pulmonary parenchymal contusion

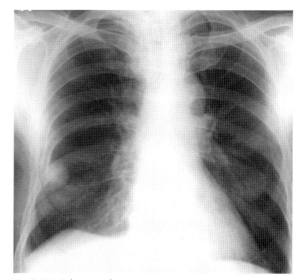

Fig. 8.**14**   Pulmonary hematoma.

teristic sign of airway rupture is the "fallen lung" sign (Kumpe et al. 1970). In the presence of a large pneumothorax, the atelectatic lung falls inferolaterally from the hilum in cases of airway disruption. When the airway is intact, atelectasis is towards the hilum.

Pulmonary Torsion

Torsion of the lung is very rare and most commonly occurs in young children. The lung rotates 180° at the hilum; the lung base then lies in the superior hemithorax while the lung apex lies inferiorly. In most cases, the affected lung rapidly becomes atelectatic. Occasionally, only one lobe undergoes torsion, producing an atypical pattern of lobar atelectasis (Müller and Fraser 2001).

Adult Respiratory Distress Syndrome (Shock Lung, Da Nang Syndrome, Stiff Lung Syndrome, Oxygen Lung, Transfusion Lung)

Clinical manifestations of adult respiratory distress syndrome (ARDS) include severe dyspnea, a restrictive pattern of ventilatory impairment due to decreased pulmonary compliance, severe hypoxemia, and extensive airspace shadowing, which may progress to pulmonary fibrosis.

ARDS has a guarded prognosis with a mortality rate of 50 to 70% (Kauffmann et al. 1983). In the traumatized patient, ARDS may result from hemorrhagic shock, severe pulmonary contusion, or fat embolism. Septic shock, acute pancreatitis, heroin overdose, disseminated intravascular coagulation (DIC), and transfusion reactions may also result in ARDS. The pathogenesis is not fully understood but may be related to disseminated thrombosis in the pulmonary capillaries, capillary membrane permeability disturbances due to endotoxins such as histamine, serotonin, and oxygen radicals, as well as disturbances in surfactant production. Diagnosis is based on the clinical history, radiographic findings, and blood gas analysis. Severe degrees of respiratory compromise are frequent and necessitate mechanical ventilation.

■ Pathology

In acute ARDS, the lungs are heavy, red, and have a tense, rubbery consistency. Histologic examination shows pulmonary microthrombosis together with alveolar and interstitial hemorrhage and edema. The pathology is that of diffuse alveolar damage (DAD) and the following stages have been described (Greene 1987): In the first 24 hours, there is capillary congestion, endothelial cell swelling, and microatelectasis (stage 1). There is fluid leakage into the interstitium and alveoli together with fibrin deposition and development of hyaline membranes from day 2 through to day 5 (stage 2). Proliferation of type II pneumocytes occurs from 5 to 7 days postinjury and is associated with microvascular destruction and progressive interstitial fibrosis (stage 3). Necrotizing pneumonia with abscess formation supervenes in a small proportion of cases.

■ Radiologic Findings

■ Chest Radiograph

Initially, the chest radiograph may be normal. From 12–72 hours posttrauma, the chest radiograph shows loss of vessel definition with bilateral, widespread patchy opacification resembling noncardiogenic pulmonary edema. Later, there is progression to confluent opacification with visible air bronchograms.

There is usually good correlation between the radiographic severity of pulmonary change and the arterial PO_2 (Hansell 1995). Intubation and mechanical ventilation may lead to a transient radiographic improvement with subsequent further deterioration.

■ Computed Tomography

- The lungs may be normal in attenuation in early ARDS. Ground-glass opacification which may progress to dense consolidation is characteristically seen in the mid-to-lower lung zones and in a dependent distribution (Fig. 8.**15**).
- Ground-glass opacification and consolidation in association with traction bronchiolectasis and bronchiectasis are seen with disease progression. These changes may progress to eventual lung honeycombing. These findings correlate with some degree of fibroproliferative change.
- Ichikado evaluated the prognostic value of thin-section CT findings in ARDS and found that CT abnormalities indicative of fibroproliferative change were predictive of a poor prognosis in patients with clinically early-stage disease (Ichikado et al. 2005).
- Desai studied CT abnormalities at long-term follow-up of ARDS survivors. A reticular pattern with a striking anterior distribution was the most prevalent finding and was seen in 85% of patients. The extent of this pattern correlated independently with the total duration of mechanical ventilation but related most strongly to the duration of pressure-controlled inverse-ratio ventilation (Desai et al. 1999).

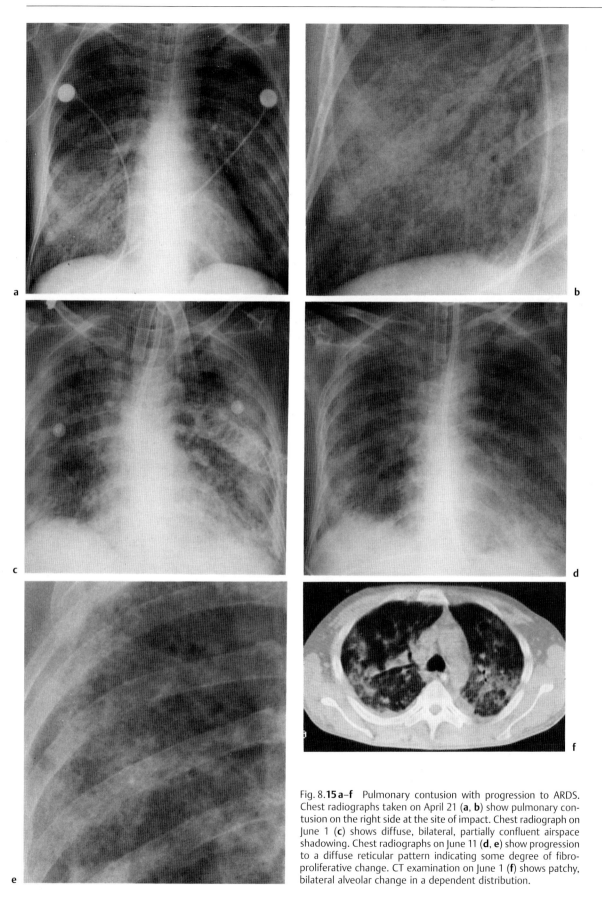

Fig. 8.**15 a–f**   Pulmonary contusion with progression to ARDS. Chest radiographs taken on April 21 (**a**, **b**) show pulmonary contusion on the right side at the site of impact. Chest radiograph on June 1 (**c**) shows diffuse, bilateral, partially confluent airspace shadowing. Chest radiographs on June 11 (**d**, **e**) show progression to a diffuse reticular pattern indicating some degree of fibroproliferative change. CT examination on June 1 (**f**) shows patchy, bilateral alveolar change in a dependent distribution.

Mediastinal Injuries

Pneumomediastinum

■ Clinical Features

Pneumomediastinum is characterized by air within the connective tissue planes of the mediastinum. The most common cause is traumatic rupture of alveoli with dissection of air along the bronchovascular interstitium and its forced entry into the mediastinal connective tissue by respiratory excursions. Less frequent but important causes include tracheobronchial and esophageal rupture and penetrating neck injuries.

■ Radiologic Findings

The *chest radiograph* shows gas bubbles and linear collections of air in the mediastinum. The combined parietal and visceral layers of the mediastinal pleura may be elevated appearing as a hairline shadow running parallel to mediastinal structures and the heart. There is frequently associated deep cervical and chest-wall emphysema (Fig. 8.**16**).

Dissection of air along tissue planes within the mediastinum may be more obvious on the lateral radiograph (Dee 1995 d), and with relatively small quantities of air, the only radiographic feature may be a band of hyper-

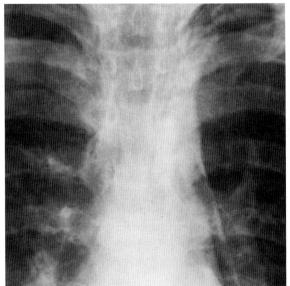

a

b

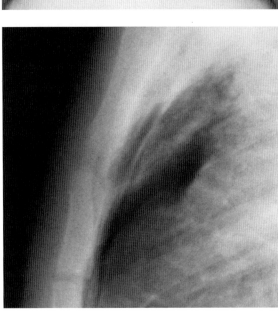

c

Fig. 8.**16 a–c** Pneumomediastinum with sternal fracture. Note the separation of the mediastinal pleura from the left heart border on the frontal radiograph (**a**, **b**) and the presence of air in the retrosternal region on the lateral view (**c**).

transradiancy in the retrosternal space. Other radiographic signs include air dissecting deep to the thymus, which is specific for pneumomediastinum, and the "continuous diaphragm" sign (Levin 1973) due to air tracking between the inferior aspect of the heart and adjacent hemidiaphragm.

CT is highly accurate in detecting pneumomediastinum and is of value when the chest radiograph is equivocal, particularly in cases of suspected tracheobronchial or esophageal rupture (Armstrong et al. 1995).

Traumatic Aortic and Great Vessel Injury

Blunt injury to the aorta or its major branches is associated with severe decelerating trauma and while a relatively rare injury, is a common cause of mediastinal hemorrhage. Ninety-five percent of aortic transactions/traumatic aortic injuries (TAI) occur in the region of the isthmus usually at the level of the ligamentum arteriosum. The mobile aortic arch is sheared off the more fixed descending aorta at this site. The ascending aorta is involved in 5% of cases (Lundell 1985) and 1% of partial ruptures are found in the descending aorta at a site distal to the isthmus (Dee 1995 d).

Twenty percent of patients survive the first hour; they have injuries which fall short of complete transection as the integrity of the adventitial layer is maintained. The risk of progression to complete rupture remains high with only 2% of patients surviving indefinitely and developing chronic pseudoaneurysm (Fig. 11.**9**).

■ Radiologic Findings

The *chest radiograph* is the initial screening examination and a normal radiograph has been reported to have a negative predictive value of 98%. However, an abnormal chest radiograph is a poor predictor of injury with only 10 to 20% of angiograms being positive for traumatic aortic injury in this patient group (Sturm 1990).

Radiographic features (Fig. 8.**17**) result from the presence of mediastinal hematoma and include:
- Diffuse widening of the mediastinum with obliteration of the aortic contour.
- Inferior displacement of the left main bronchus to >40° below the horizontal.
- Tracheal and esophageal displacement to the right side.
- Posterior gravitation of blood may result in widening of the paravertebral stripe.
- Leakage into the left pleural cavity results in hemothorax and extrapleural blood extending over the lung apices forms the characteristic apical "cap."

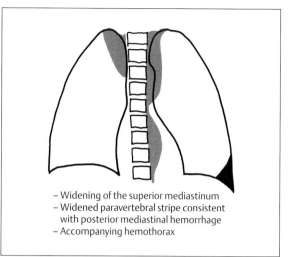

- Widening of the superior mediastinum
- Widened paravertebral stripe consistent with posterior mediastinal hemorrhage
- Accompanying hemothorax

Fig. 8.**17**   Mediastinal hemorrhage.

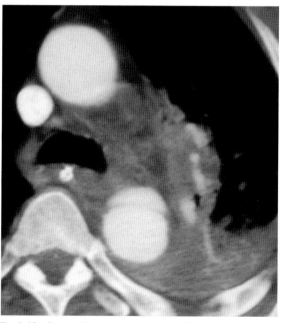

Fig. 8.**18**   Traumatic aortic injury. Axial CT image shows mediastinal hematoma and left-sided hemothorax and an intimal flap is noted within the proximal descending thoracic aorta.

While *aortography* has remained the standard of reference for diagnosis of aortic trauma, conventional *nonhelical CT* has allowed detection of periaortic hematoma and has a superior negative predictive value to the chest radiograph for exclusion of aortic injury (Morgan 1992, Raptopoulos 1992). CT signs suggestive of TAI include the presence of mediastinal hematoma, aortic contour deformity, intimal flaps, intraluminal debris, pseudoaneurysm, and pseudo-coarctation (Fig. 8.**18**). However, it has been continued practice at many institutions to proceed to aortography in patients at high risk of TAI when the CT study is negative.

The role of CT in evaluation of this patient group may have changed with the arrival of single-slice helical CT in the early 1990s and of multi-detector row CT (MDCT) in the late 1990s. This technology allows acquisition of a "volumetric" data set in contradistinction to the "conventional" CT examination. Parker et al. evaluated the role of helical CT in the evaluation of TAI and found the sensitivity and negative predictive value of CT to be equivalent to that of aortography at 100% (Parker et al. 2001). More recently, Bruckner et al. have reported results of a retrospective analysis of all patients undergoing aortography for blunt aortic injury between 1997 and 2004 at their institution. CT in those patients evaluated in the final years of the study was performed on MDCT technology. They reported a sensitivity of 100%, specificity of 40%, positive predictive value (PPV) of 15%, and negative predictive value (NPV) of 99%. They concluded that while sensitivity and NPV were excellent, there were a high number of equivocal CT studies which still necessitated subsequent aortography (Bruckner et al. 2006). Both of these studies suggest that if helical/MDCT is normal, it may be reasonable not to proceed to aortography even in patients who have sustained significant trauma and who are at high risk of TAI. Further studies are needed to determine the accuracy of MDCT particularly 16- and 64-slice technology in intrinsic evaluation of the aorta in this setting.

Traumatic Diaphragmatic Rupture

■ Clinical Features

Diaphragmatic injuries occur in 0.8–8% of patients after blunt trauma. This injury was initially believed to be more common on the left side but some have suggested that both leaflets are affected with equal frequency (Waldschmidt 1980). Traumatic diaphragmatic injury remains a diagnostic challenge and the high frequency of associated injury including pelvic fractures, thoracic aortic injury, splenic and hepatic lesions may distract attention from this lesion (Iochum et al. 2002, Mirvis et al. 2000, Shanmuananthan et al. 2000). Imaging diagnosis of diaphragmatic injury is even more important today as increasing numbers of splenic and hepatic injuries are being treated conservatively.

Intrathoracic herniation of bowel may occur soon after trauma or may develop over a prolonged interval (progressive diaphragmatic rupture). Unrecognized tears on the left side lead to hernias which have a particular predisposition to strangulation (Flower 1992).

■ Radiologic Findings

It has been reported that initial *chest radiographs* allow diagnosis of 27–60% of left-sided but just 17% of right-sided injuries (Shanmuganathan et al. 1999). The chest radiograph may show *localized contour deformity* and *apparent elevation of the soft tissue–lung interface*.

More specific radiographic signs include intrathoracic herniation of a hollow viscus including stomach, colon, and small intestine with or without focal constriction of the viscus at the site of the tear (collar sign [Fig. 8.**19**]) and visualization of a nasogastric tube above the diaphragm on the left side (Iochum et al. 2002). In the setting of acute trauma, associated rib fractures and hemothorax are frequent. Upper gastrointestinal contrast studies may demonstrate gastric/intestinal herniations through left-sided tears. Tears of the right hemidiaphragm frequently are associated with a pleural effusion and may be demonstrated at sonography.

Helical CT has been shown to be more valuable than conventional CT in the diagnosis of diaphragmatic injury (Iochum et al. 2002). A sensitivity of 71%, specificity of 100%, and accuracies of 88% for left-sided and 70% for right-sided injuries have been reported for helical CT (Shanmuganathan et al. 2000, Killeen et al. 1999) vs. sensitivities of 14–61% and specificities of 76–99% for conventional CT (Gelman et al. 1991, Murray et al. 1996, Worthy et al. 1995).

CT signs of diaphragmatic injury include:
- *Direct discontinuity of the hemidiaphragm/diaphragmatic defect* has been reported to have a sensitivity of 71–73% and appears to be the most sensitive sign (Murray et al. 1996, Worthy et al. 1995).
- *Intrathoracic herniation of intra-abdominal contents* has been reported to have a sensitivity of 55% and a specificity of 100% (Murray et al. 1996).
- The *"collar" sign* is a waist-like constriction of the herniating viscus at the site of diaphragmatic tear and has been reported to have a sensitivity of 36% on conventional and 63% on helical CT (Murray et al. 1996, Killeen et al. 1999).
- The *"dependent viscera" sign*. When a patient with a ruptured hemidiaphragm lies in the supine position for CT examination, the herniated viscera are no longer supported posteriorly by the hemidiaphragm and move to a dependent position against the posterior ribs. This sign was observed by Bergin in 90% of positive cases (Bergin et al. 2001).

Magnetic resonance imaging with breath-hold acquisitions and its capacity for multiplanar image acquisition allows good visualization of the diaphragm but this is rarely possible in the setting of acute severe trauma.

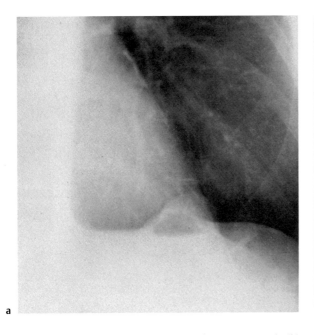

a

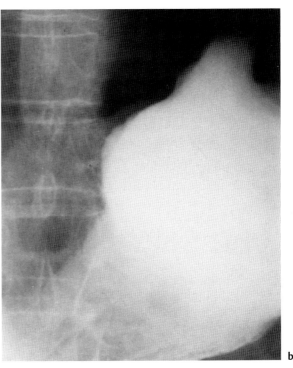

b

Fig. 8.**19a, b** Radiograph (**a**) and upper GI contrast study (**b**) show herniation of part of the fundus of the stomach into a traumatic diaphragmatic defect.

9 Diseases of the Pleura, Diaphragm, and Chest Wall

Diseases of the Pleura

Pleural Effusion

A pleural effusion is a pathologic fluid collection within the pleural cavity. Normally 10–15 mL of fluid is present and this serves as a lubricant between the parietal and visceral pleural layers. Pleural effusions may reach volumes of up to a few liters and these large effusions result in compression of the underlying lung, contralateral displacement of the mediastinum, and depression of the hemidiaphragm.

Goals of Diagnostic Imaging
Detection of the effusion and differentiation from other pathological pleural processes such as tumor and fibrous thickening. The mobility of the fluid with postural change and its computed tomography (CT) attenuation value may help in differentiation.

Detection of underlying pulmonary, cardiac, and abdominal pathology including pneumonia, bronchial carcinoma, pulmonary embolism, left ventricular failure, and hepatic cirrhosis (Tables 9.1 and 9.2).

Further evaluation of a pleural effusion may require thoracentesis with biochemical, cytologic, and bacteriologic analysis of aspirates.

Table 9.**1** Etiology of pleural effusions in the U.S. (from R. W. Light: *Pleural Diseases*, 1983)

Heart failure	500 000
Bacterial pneumonia	300 000
Malignant tumors	200 000
• Lung	60 000
• Breast	50 000
• Lymphoma	40 000
• Miscellaneous	50 000
Thromboembolism	150 000
Viral pneumonia	100 000
Hepatic cirrhosis with ascites	50 000
Gastrointestinal disease (e. g., pancreatitis)	25 000
Collagen diseases	6 000
Tuberculosis	2 600
Asbestosis	2 000
Mesothelioma	450

Table 9.**2** Causes of pleural effusion

Vascular
O Pulmonary infarction
M Heart failure
O Constrictive pericarditis

Inflammatory
O Tuberculosis
M Parapneumonic effusion (viral, mycoplasma, bacterial, fungal)
O Collagen diseases (SLE, rheumatoid arthritis)
O Postinfarction Dressler's syndrome
O Whipple disease
O Mediterranean fever
O Recurrent familial polyserositis

Neoplastic
M Bronchial carcinoma
O Lymphoma
O Metastatic pleural adenocarcinoma
O Mesothelioma

Iatrogenic
O Intrapleural infusion (e. g., due to faulty catheter placement)
M Postthoracotomy
M Radiotherapy

Traumatic
O Hemothorax
O Esophageal rupture
O Chylothorax

Mediastinal
M Superior vena caval obstruction
M Aortic rupture
O Esophageal fistula (e. g., carcinoma)
O Thoracic duct fistula (filariasis, carcinoma)
M Ruptured dermoid cyst

Subphrenic Abdominal
O Pancreatitis
O Subphrenic abscess
O Cirrhosis with ascites
O Meigs' syndrome (ascites associated with ovarian tumor)

Miscellaneous
O Asbestosis
O Nephrotic syndrome
O Myxedema
O Uremia
O Spontaneous pleural hemorrhage due to coagulopathy
O Congenital lymphedema (Milroy)

M = diseases in which the chest radiograph generally shows other changes besides pleural effusion. O = diseases in which pleural effusion may be the only radiographic finding (from Light).

■ Pathology

Pleural effusions may be classified according to their composition:

- *Pleural transudate*: Clear fluid with a specific gravity of less than 1.016 and a protein content of less than 3 g/dL. The Pandy test is negative. Left ventricular failure is the most common cause of a transudate. Ascites in hepatic cirrhosis, nephrotic syndrome, and myxedema may also cause transudative effusions.
- *Pleural exudate*: An opaque fluid with a protein content of more than 3 g/dL, a specific gravity of greater than 1.016, and a positive Pandy test. The microscopic identification of cellular elements such as granulocytes, lymphocytes, erythrocytes, and malignant cells narrows the differential diagnosis. Parapneumonic effusions are most common and are usually secondary to pulmonary infections. Tuberculous exudate is distinguished by its high lymphocyte content. Malignant pleural effusions are also exudates although malignant cells may not always be detected on cytologic evaluation.
- *Empyema*: This suppurative intrapleural exudate is usually either parapneumonic or postpneumonic. Less commonly it may result from transdiaphragmatic extension of a liver abscess.
- *Hemothorax*: Bleeding into the pleural space may be secondary to trauma, aortic rupture, or pleural malignancy. Occasionally, it is seen in thromboembolic disease when complicated by pulmonary infarction.
- *Chylothorax*: A turbid, milky fluid containing microscopic chylomicrons is an uncommon cause of a pleural effusion. It may be seen in neoplastic and traumatic fistulae of the thoracic duct (Table 9.3) and is also associated characteristically with pulmonary lymphangiomatosis (LAM).
- *Bilious and cerebrospinal fluid (CSF) pleural effusions*: Both are extremely rare. Bilious effusions are seen posthepatic and after diaphragmatic lacerations. A traumatic fistula to the spinal subarachnoid space allows CSF to enter the pleural space.

■ Clinical Features

Effusions are frequently asymptomatic but may cause pleuritic chest pain and splinting of the hemidiaphragm with decreased respiratory excursion. Large effusions may result in dyspnea. On auscultation, breathing sounds are diminished.

Table 9.3 Causes of chylothorax (modified from Reeder and Felson 2003)

Traumatic
Tumor invasion (bronchial carcinoma, mesothelioma, Hodgkin's disease, etc.)
Filariasis
Left subclavian vein thrombosis
Lymphangioma, lymphangiomatosis, lymphangioleiomyomatosis
Iatrogenic (postthoracic surgery)
Idiopathic

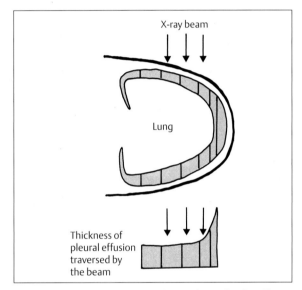

Fig. 9.1 Pleural effusion on PA chest radiograph. The effusion surrounds the entire lung base but it is visible as a meniscus only when it is tangential to the x-ray beam (from Greene, McLoud, and Stark 1977).

■ Radiologic Findings

░ Chest Radiograph

The shape of the effusion results from:

- The adhesive and cohesive forces between the pleura and the effusion.
- Elastic recoil which decreases lung volume while preserving its shape and proportions and especially.
- Gravity, which accounts for the dependent distribution of the effusion.

Pleural fluid is mobile and therefore its distribution is position-dependent. This accounts for its varying radiographic appearances (Figs. 9.1–9.3).

Upright position:

- The lateral chest radiograph shows homogeneous opacification of the posterior costophrenic angle with

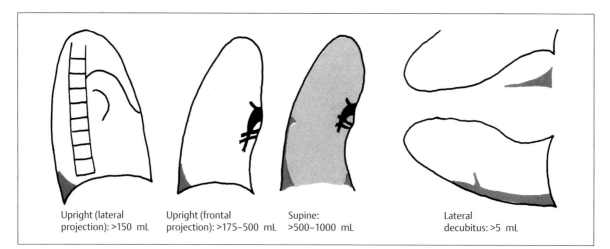

Upright (lateral projection): >150 mL	Upright (frontal projection): >175–500 mL	Supine: >500–1000 mL	Lateral decubitus: >5 mL

Fig. 9.**2**   Limits of detectability of pleural effusion (from Moskowitz 1973).

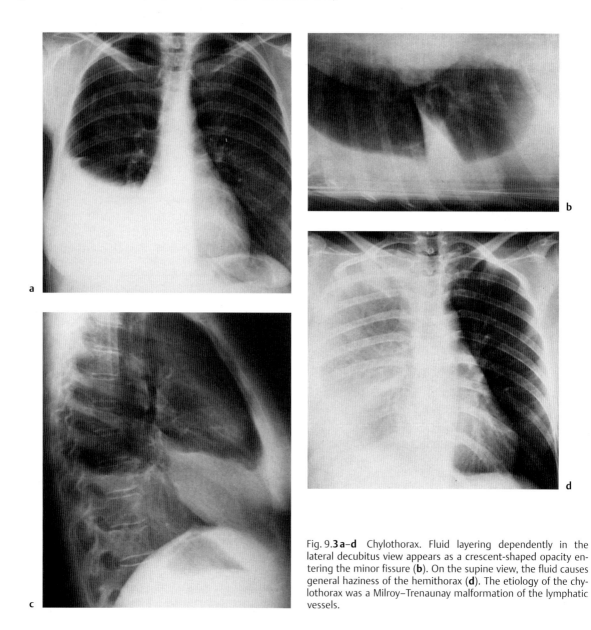

Fig. 9.**3a–d** Chylothorax. Fluid layering dependently in the lateral decubitus view appears as a crescent-shaped opacity entering the minor fissure (**b**). On the supine view, the fluid causes general haziness of the hemithorax (**d**). The etiology of the chylothorax was a Milroy–Trenaunay malformation of the lymphatic vessels.

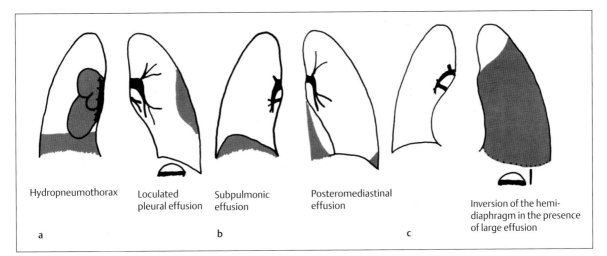

Fig. 9.**4 a–c**   Variants of pleural effusion.

a superiorly concave meniscus. At least 100 mL of fluid is present before an effusion becomes visible. Smaller effusions collect between the diaphragm and the undersurface of the lung and may only be seen on decubitus views. For clinical purposes, a significant effusion is excluded if both posterior costophrenic angles are clear.

- The posteroanterior (PA) chest radiograph shows obliteration of the costophrenic and cardiophrenic angles if the effusion is greater than approximately 175 mL. The meniscus is concave toward the lung and becomes thinner superiorly. Opacification of the mediastinal pleural space is lower and less marked because of fusion of the pleural layers at the pulmonary ligament.

Supine position:
Effusions are only visible on supine radiographs when they exceed 500 mL.

Manifestations include:
- The diaphragmatic contour is obscured
- Opacification of the lateral costophrenic angles
- Generalized "haziness" of the hemithorax
- Apical caps may indicate pooling of fluid in the upper zones

In contrast to pneumonia or atelectasis, the pulmonary vessels are well defined with small to moderate effusions and there is no evidence of an air bronchogram.

Lateral decubitus position:
Fluid collects between the lateral chest wall and the lung, producing a band of opacification which may enter the minor fissure.

Postmortem studies have shown that as little as 5 mL of fluid may be detected on the lateral decubitus view (Moskowitz et al. 1973). If the depth of the effusion

("band" thickness) is less than 1 cm, then the effusion is small.

Atypical forms of pleural effusion (Figs. 9.4, 9.5):
- *Loculated effusion:* Adhesions between the visceral and parietal pleura result in development of loculated collections along the inner aspect of the chest wall. En face, they may appear as ill-defined round opacities but tangentially they produce a semicircular opacity whose margins form an obtuse angle with the chest wall. This helps to distinguish them from peripheral pulmonary tumors, which usually form an acute angle with the chest wall.
- *Interlobar effusion* (Figs. 9.6, 9.7): This may develop in the minor or major fissures. Chest radiographs show a biconvex, spherical, or elliptical homogeneous opacity. An effusion in the right minor fissure should be distinguished from right middle lobe atelectasis. The following features help in differentiation:
  - The effusion is biconvex while lobar atelectasis is flat or concave.
  - Only atelectasis obliterates the right cardiac border and
  - Atelectasis obscures the interlobar fissure but an effusion preserves the contour of the fissure as a linear structure in its peripheral portion.
  Conventional tomography allows more accurate differentiation based on the homogeneity of the effusion versus the heterogeneity of atelectatic lung. However, today CT is usually performed when there is diagnostic difficulty.
- *Posteromedial loculated effusion:* The fluid column is higher and wider toward the mediastinum. This results from volume loss in the lower lobe and thus lower lobe atelectasis is included in the differential diagnosis.
- *Subpulmonic effusion.* Occasionally up to a liter of fluid may accumulate between the diaphragm and

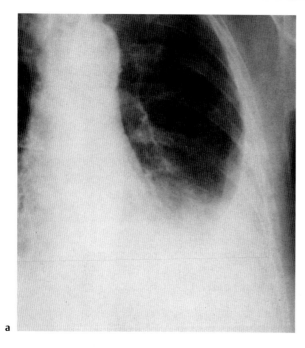

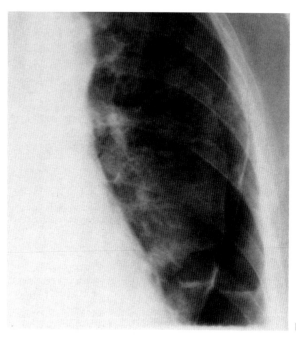

a

b

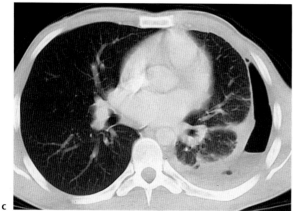

c

Fig. 9.**5 a–c**   Malignant pleural effusion in breast carcinoma (**a**). Hydropneumothorax developed following thoracentesis (**b**). CT shows visceral pleural thickening and fluid extending into the major fissure (**c**).

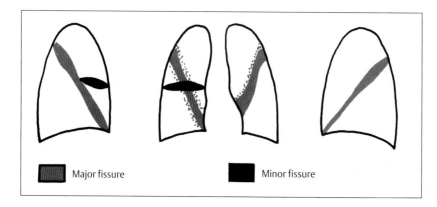

Major fissure   Minor fissure

Fig. 9.**6**   Interlobar effusions.

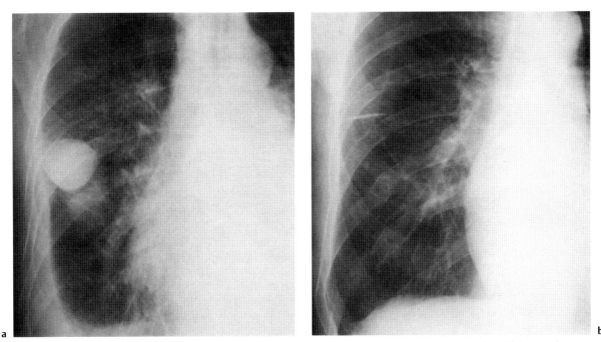

a   b

Fig. 9.**7 a, b**   Fissural effusion appears as a round opacity in the minor fissure in a patient with congestive heart failure. Radiograph post treatment shows minimal residual fissural thickening.

lung without spill into the costophrenic sulcus. Reasons for this phenomenon are not fully understood. Radiographs show elevation of the lung–soft tissue interface or apparent elevation of the hemidiaphragm. The "dome" has a relatively lateral peak and then shows a steep lateral downslope. When the subpulmonic effusion is left-sided, the distance between the inferior surface of the left lung and the gastric bubble measures more than 2 cm. The lateral decubitus view will show fluid layering along the dependent chest wall.

- *Inversion of the diaphragm*: Large effusions may cause inversion of the hemidiaphragm. Radiographs show inferomedial displacement of gastric and colonic gas. During inspiration, the diaphragm contracts and this reduces the volume of the hemithorax. This leads to significant dyspnea and paradoxical diaphragmatic motion.

Ultrasound

Most pleural fluid collections are an- or hypoechoic and have a sharp echogenic line delineating the visceral pleura and lung. Occasionally, tumors of the chest wall, particularly lymphoma and neurogenic tumors, are also hypoechoic and may be mistaken for fluid (Rosenberg 1983). Diagnostic needle aspiration therefore may form part of the evaluation when there is diagnostic difficulty.

Thin mobile strands of fibrin within the effusion usually indicate an exudate rich in protein. A profusion of septa within a collection (honeycomb pattern) predicts difficulties with tube drainage; this may be a feature of

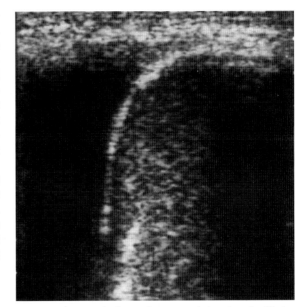

Fig. 9.**8**   Ultrasound shows large anechoic pleural effusion bordering echogenic linear hemidiaphragm.

empyema, hemothorax, and exudates caused by pleural malignancy (McLoud et al. 1991, Fig. 9.**8**).

Computed Tomography

CT does not allow differentiation between transudates, exudates, and chylous effusions (Naidich et al. 1984, Rawkin et al. 1980). Acute intrapleural hemorrhage may be identified by the presence of a fluid–fluid level or because of the high attenuation of the collection (McLoud et al. 1991, Fig. 9.**3**).

■ Magnetic Resonance Imaging (MRI)

Pleural fluid collections characteristically have low T1- and high T2-signal intensity. While MRI does not allow differentiation between exudates and transudates in vivo (Davis et al. 1990), subacute and chronic hemorrhage may be recognized by their high signal intensity on both T1- and T2-weighted images (Tshcholakoff et al. 1978).

Pneumothorax

■ Pathology

Pneumothorax is characterized by air in the pleural space and may result from a defect in the visceral pleura that allows communication between the pleural space and bronchoalveolar air. Transthoracic and transdiaphragmatic fistulae in patients with pre-existing pneumoperitoneum are less common causes of pneumothorax. In most cases, the pleural tear closes spontaneously due to a decrease in lung volume. Occasionally, a check-valve mechanism may develop leading to a tension pneumothorax with severe pulmonary atelectasis, mediastinal shift, and life-threatening compression of mediastinal vessels.

A pneumothorax may be traumatic, iatrogenic, or spontaneous in etiology.
- *Traumatic pneumothorax* is described on p. 203.
- *Iatrogenic pneumothorax* may result from trauma to the visceral pleura during thoracentesis or during central venous line insertion. Pneumothoraces are also associated with positive-pressure mechanical ventilation.
- *Spontaneous pneumothorax.* A number of pulmonary diseases lead to pleuropulmonary fistulae (Table 9.**4**). Subpleural bullae are the most common cause and these are usually found at the apices. Spontaneous pneumothorax is much more common in males than in females; it is especially common in tall, thin patients. This probably reflects the increased gravitational stress on the apices in the upright position.

Table 9.**4**   Causes of pneumothorax

Traumatic
- Rib fracture
- Stab wound

Iatrogenic
- Thoracentesis (e. g., subclavian catheter)
- Percutaneous lung biopsy
- Positive-pressure ventilation
- Tracheostomy

Spontaneous
- Subpleural emphysematous bulla
- Pneumatocele
- "Cystic" lung disease(e. g., PLCH, AIDS-related cystic lung disease)
- Cystic fibrosis
- Pneumonia with abscess formation

Esophageal rupture

Pneumoperitoneum

Pneumomediastinum

■ Clinical Features

Clinical manifestations include pleuritic chest pain and dyspnea which are usually sudden in onset.

■ Radiologic Findings

The displaced visceral pleural line courses parallel to the chest wall. Pulmonary vascular markings are absent lateral to this hairline shadow (Figs. 9.**9**–9.**12**). In the upright position, the intrapleural air accumulates at the apex. In expiration, the relative volume of the pleural air collection to that of the underlying lung increases; expiratory views therefore occasionally are useful when there is diagnostic difficulty. Tension pneumothorax is associated with ipsilateral pulmonary atelectasis and contralateral mediastinal shift.

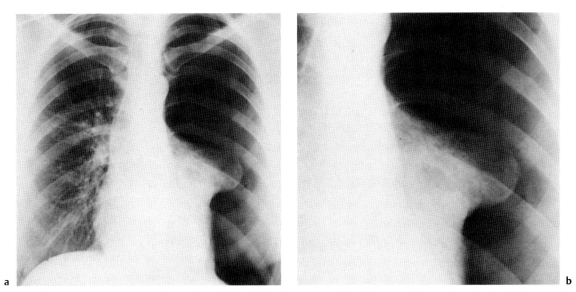

a   b

Fig. 9.**9 a, b**   Spontaneous pneumothorax. There is left-sided pulmonary atelectasis but no evidence of mediastinal displacement.

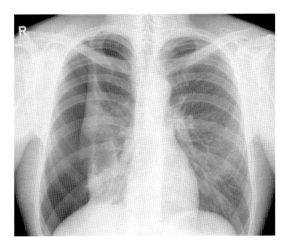

Fig. 9.**10**   Spontaneous pneumothorax with pulmonary "fixation" due to old apical pleural thickening.

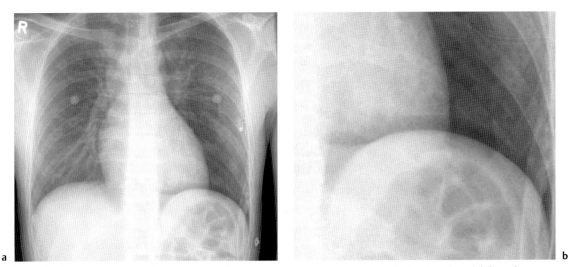

a   b

Fig. 9.**11 a, b**   Pneumothorax on radiograph acquired with patient in supine position. Air collects inferiorly and defines the contour of the left hemidiaphragm.

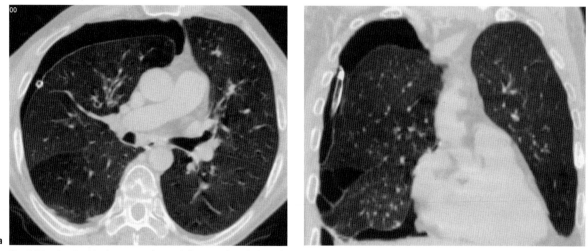

Fig. 9.**12 a, b**   Residual pneumothorax following closed pleural drainage.

Pleural Thickening and Fibrothorax

Pleural thickening is common and is usually a sequel of pleural inflammation. It may also be a delayed complication of hemothorax, pleural empyema, and recurrent pneumothorax.

Localized pleural thickening is frequently found at the bases and results in blunting of the costophrenic angles with tenting of the diaphragmatic pleura (Fig. 9.**13**). Fibrous pleural thickening is also common in the apical pleural cupola where it may be secondary to tuberculosis or represent age-related change. These "apical pleural caps" sometimes have a scalloped contour or may show slight tenting towards the lung (Fig. 9.**14**). *Pleural thickening* should be distinguished from the companion shadows of the upper ribs (see Chapter 1, p. 10) and from extrapleural linear fat deposition which usually is bilateral, symmetrical, and located predominantly along the lateral chest wall.

Fibrous pleural plaques, an indicator of past asbestos exposure, may have a ring or target configuration. Plaques may undergo hyaline transformation, calcify, or ossify (Figs. 9.**15**, 9.**16**, 9.**17 a**). These geographical opacities commonly involve the pleura of the anterolateral chest wall in the mid-to-lower zones and the diaphragmatic pleura. Computed tomography will define accurately the location and extent of pleural plaque formation (Fig. 9.**17 b**).

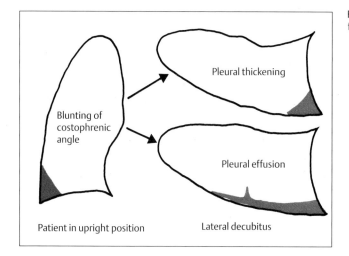

Fig. 9.**13**   Differentiation of pleural thickening from effusion on the lateral decubitus radiograph.

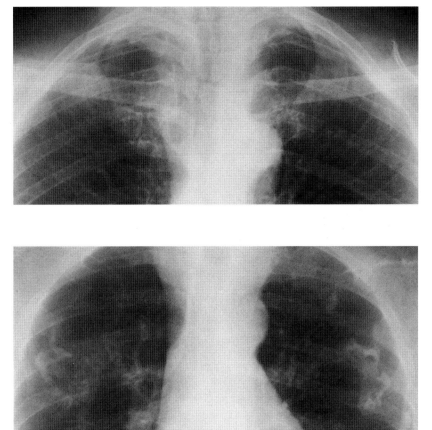

Fig. 9.**14** Apical pleural thickening. The scalloped borders and tented extension of the apical pleural cap distinguish it from the companion shadow of the second rib.

Fig. 9.**15** Calcified pleural plaques with "holly leaf" appearance.

Fig. 9.**16** Asbestos-induced pleural plaques: Chest radiograph shows bilateral calcified pleural plaque formation with involvement of the diaphragmatic pleura.

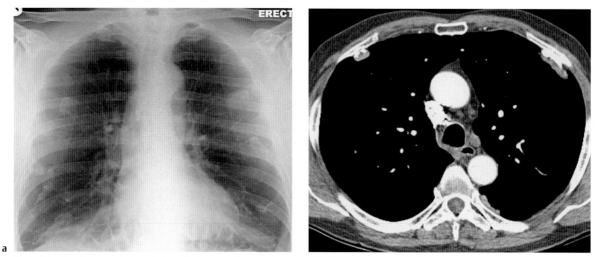

Fig. 9.**17 a, b**   Asbestos-induced pleural plaques: Chest radiograph (**a**) shows bilateral calcified pleural plaque. Axial CT image (**b**) shows characteristic distribution of plaque along anterolateral chest wall in mid-to-lower zones.

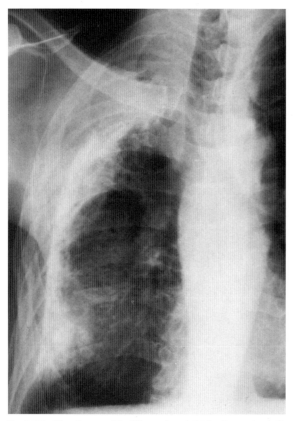

Fig. 9.**18**   Fibrothorax with diffuse pleural thickening and calcification at the pleura–lung interface.

Fibrothorax and Asbestos-Induced Diffuse Pleural Thickening

Fibrothorax results from fibrous organization of a hemothorax or empyema and is characterized by formation of a pleural peel that may be up to several millimeters in thickness and which encases the lung. Calcification is frequent at the pulmonary interface.

Pulmonary encasement prevents normal respiratory excursion and resulting unilateral hypoventilation induces reflex pulmonary vasoconstriction. This may be visible on the chest radiograph and may be confirmed by radionuclide perfusion scintigraphy.

Fibrothorax may cause significant thoracic deformity and scoliosis as well as cicatricial emphysema with pulmonary arterial hypertension (Figs. 9.**18**, 9.**19**).

Diffuse pleural thickening may result from past asbestos exposure when it may be bilateral and symmetric (Fig. 9.**20**). See also Asbestos-Induced Pleural Disease, Chapter 5, p. 140.

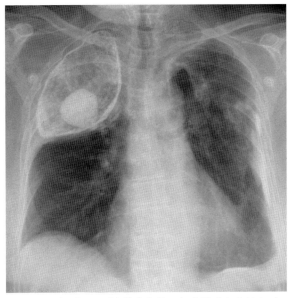

Fig. 9.**19**   Oleothorax with fibrin ball and calcified shell. Note also the left-sided pleural calcification.

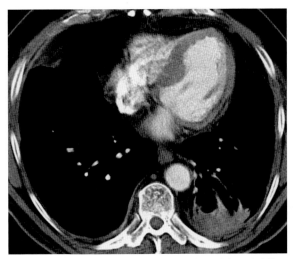

Fig. 9.**20**   Diffuse pleural thickening: CT shows bilateral diffuse pleural thickening with associated lung infolding in the left lower lobe.

Pleural Mesothelioma

Malignant pleural mesothelioma is a relatively uncommon neoplasm with approximately 120 new cases per year in Germany and approximately 500 new cases each year in the United States. However, it is the most common primary pleural malignancy and its incidence appears to be increasing. Prognosis is poor with an average survival of only 8 months. The risk of developing mesothelioma is increased approximately 300-fold in asbestos workers (Greene et al. 1977). Long thin asbestos fibers are probably the most tumorigenic and there is a particularly strong association between crocidolite fibers and development of mesothelioma.

■ Pathology

Mesothelioma usually arises in the lower hemithorax and grows along the pleural surface until it encases the entire lung. Pulmonary parenchymal, chest-wall and diaphragmatic infiltration occurs. There is usually a concomitant pleural effusion. Histologic and cytologic differentiation from metastatic pleural carcinomatosis may be difficult. Histologically, mesotheliomas may be epithelial with gland-like structures, mesenchymal with abundant collagen formation, mixed or undifferentiated in type, the epithelial variant being most common.

■ Clinical Features

The main clinical manifestations are chest pain including referred pain localized to the shoulder, dyspnea, cough, and weight loss. Thoracentesis yields serous fluid in 50% of cases and hemorrhagic fluid in the remainder of patients. In contrast to adenocarcinoma, the CEA titers are not increased but hyaluronic acid content is markedly elevated.

■ Radiologic Findings

Chest Radiograph

- *Pleural effusion* is the initial radiographic finding in 80% of cases. Drainage may be associated with a residual pneumothorax since the lung may be encased and cannot re-expand.
- *Neoplastic pleural thickening*: This encases the lung and may have a smooth or lobulated contour (Fig. 9.**21**). It sometimes becomes visible following thoracentesis and drainage of the effusion.
- *Tumor nodule*: This peripheral nodule is in contact with the chest wall. A continuum exists between nodular and lobulated tumor types (Fig. 9.**22**).
- *Rib destruction, contralateral metastatic nodules, and cardiac enlargement signifying pericardial invasion* are occasionally features of advanced disease.

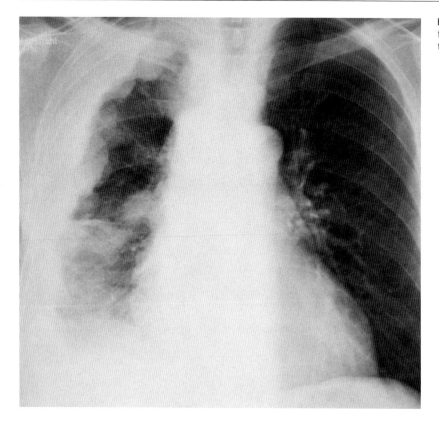

Fig. 9.**21** Mesothelioma with diffuse nodular pleural thickening in the right hemithorax.

Computed Tomography and Magnetic Resonance Imaging

Nodular pleural thickening of greater than 1 cm in thickness, involving the mediastinal pleura and forming a circumferential sheath around the lung, indicates malignant pleural disease (Leung 1990, Figs. 9.**23**, 9.**24**). The MRI findings in malignant pleural involvement have been described (Falaschi 1996). Malignant lesions were found to be hyperintense to muscle on intermediate and T2-weighted sequences in all cases.

An International Staging System has been proposed for malignant pleural mesothelioma (Rusch 1995, Patz et al. 1996, Table 9.**5**).

Tammilehto et al. assessed pretreatment CT in 88 patients. They suggested that in clinical practice it is difficult to differentiate tumor (T) from nodal involvement (N) with CT due to the "unique plate-like growth pattern of the tumor" (Tammilehto et al. 1995). Patz et al. evaluated CT and MRI findings in mesothelioma and focused on three anatomic regions; diaphragm, chest wall, and mediastinum. They found both modalities to have high sensitivity but low specificity and a high accuracy in predicting resectability (Patz et al. 1992).

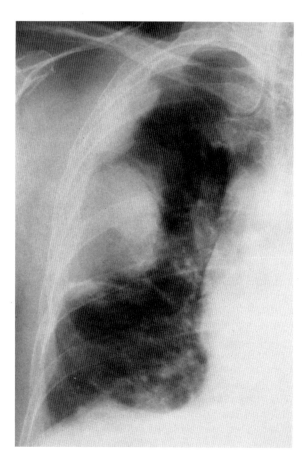

Fig. 9.**22** Nodular pleural masses in mesothelioma.

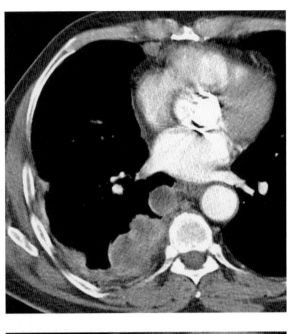

a

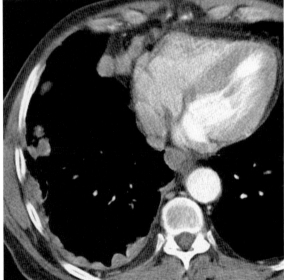

b

Fig. 9.**23 a, b** Pleural mesothelioma: Axial CT images show right-sided nodular pleural thickening with involvement of the mediastinal pleura.

Table 9.**5** International staging system for diffuse malignant pleural mesothelioma

T1 a	Tumor limited to the ipsilateral parietal pleura, including mediastinal and diaphragmatic pleura. No involvement of the visceral pleura.
T1 b	Tumor involving the ipsilateral parietal pleura, including mediastinal and diaphragmatic pleura. Scattered foci of tumor involving the visceral pleura.
T2	Tumor involving the ipsilateral pleura surfaces with: (1) Involvement of diaphragmatic muscle or (2) Confluent visceral pleural tumor (including the fissures).
T3	Locally advanced but potentially resectable disease. Involvement of all the ipsilateral pleural surfaces with at least one of the following: (1) Involvement of endothoracic fascia, (2) extension into the mediastinal fat, (3) solitary, completely resectable focus of tumor extending into the soft tissues of the chest wall, (4) nontransmural involvement of the pericardium.
T4	Locally advanced technically unresectable tumor involving all ipsilateral pleural surfaces with at least one of the following: (1) Diffuse extension into the chest wall ± associated rib destruction, (2) direct transdiaphragmatic spread of tumor to the peritoneum, (3) direct extension to the contralateral pleura, (4) direct extension to one or more mediastinal organs, (5) direct extension to the spine, (6) tumor extending to the internal surface of the pericardium ± pericardial effusion or involving the myocardium.
N0	No regional lymph node metastases.
N1	Metastases to ipsilateral bronchopulmonary or hilar lymph nodes.
N2	Metastases to subcarinal or ipsilateral mediastinal lymph nodes including ipsilateral intramammary lymph nodes.
N3	Metastases to contralateral mediastinal, contralateral internal mammary, ipsi- or contralateral supraclavicular lymph nodes.
M0	No distant metastases.
M1	Distant metastases present.

Heelan et al. compared the accuracy of CT with MRI in staging of mesothelioma with reference to the TNM (Tumor, Node, Metastasis) Staging System. They found MRI superior to CT in assessing diaphragmatic invasion, invasion of the endothoracic fascia, or solitary resectable foci of chest wall invasion. However, single-slice helical CT was available only in the final months of their study and multi-detector CT (MDCT) with its capacity for multiplanar reformats may fare better in this assessment. These authors again emphasize the limitations of both modalities in staging of mesothelioma and suggest that these are due to the complex unpredictable pattern of simultaneous local and regional spread of this neoplasm (Heelan et al. 1999).

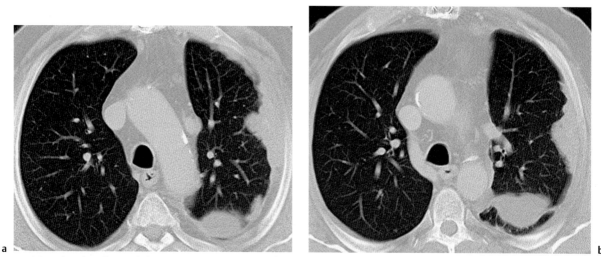

Fig. 9.24 a, b   Pleural mesothelioma: CT shows left-sided nodular pleural thickening with involvement of the superior aspect of the left major fissure.

Diseases of the Diaphragm

The fibromuscular diaphragm separates the thorax from the abdomen (Fig. 9.**25**). Diaphragmatic dysfunction is frequently a consequence of either thoracic or abdominal disease (Table 9.**6**). Primary diaphragmatic pathology is rare.

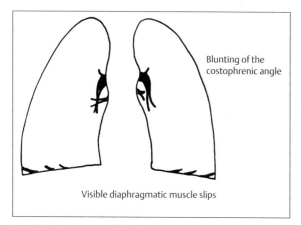

Fig. 9.**25**   Depression of the diaphragm.

Table 9.**6**   Disorders of the diaphragm

Bilateral depression secondary to pulmonary hyperinflation
- Emphysema
- Chronic severe asthma
- Bronchiolitis obliterans

Unilateral depression
- Unilateral pulmonary hyperinflation (foreign body aspiration)
- Tension pneumothorax

Bilateral elevation
- Abdominal causes (increased intra-abdominal fat in obesity, ascites, hepatomegaly)
- Restrictive ventilatory impairment

Unilateral elevation
- Intra-abdominal mass (hepatic tumor, splenomegaly, subphrenic abscess, gastric or colonic distention)
- Decreased lung volume (atelectasis, hypoplasia)
- Diaphragmatic paralysis (eventration), phrenic nerve damage

Focal contour abnormality
- Hernia (hiatus hernia, Morgagni hernia, Bochdalek hernia, traumatic diaphragmatic rupture)
- Tumors of the diaphragm
- Basal pleural tumor
- Loculated subpulmonic effusion
- Partial eventration (Fig. 9.**26**)

Subdiaphragmatic air
- Pneumoperitoneum (Fig. 9.**27**)
- Chilaiditi syndrome (Fig. 9.**28**)
- Subphrenic abscess with gas-forming organisms

Diaphragmatic Paralysis

Diaphragmatic paralysis is usually secondary to phrenic nerve dysfunction; this may result from infiltration of the nerve by bronchial or esophageal carcinoma or may be a complication of cardiac surgery. Infections which lie adjacent to the diaphragm including subphrenic abscess and lower lobe pneumonia may also lead to reduced diaphragmatic excursion. Radiographically, a large subpulmonic effusion may simulate diaphragmatic elevation.

Diaphragmatic paralysis persisting for longer than 6 months leads to muscular atrophy. It has been suggested that idiopathic diaphragmatic eventration may result from phrenic nerve palsy in early childhood (Fig. 9.**26**).

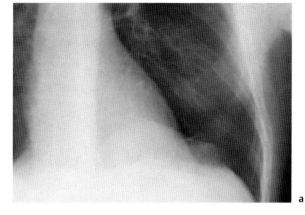

a

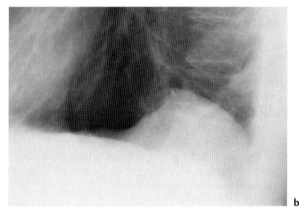

b

Fig. 9.**26 a, b** Partial eventration of the left hemidiaphragm.

■ Radiologic Findings

The chest radiograph (Fig. 9.**29**) may show:
- *Elevation of the hemidiaphragm.* The right hemidiaphragm normally lies up to 4 cm more cranial than the left hemidiaphragm since the latter is displaced inferiorly by the heart.
- *Cranial displacement of abdominal contents.* The gastric bubble, hepatic and splenic flexures move cranially.
- *Paradoxical excursion.* In inspiration, the healthy leaflet moves caudally while the paralyzed leaflet moves cranially (so called "see-saw" phenomenon). This is accentuated by sniffing (Hitzenberg sniff test). A mild degree of paresis just delays the caudad inspiratory excursion on the affected side (pseudo-paradoxical movement).
- *Dynamic mediastinal shift.* During abrupt inspiration, the intrathoracic pressure on the normal side decreases; this results in mediastinal shift towards the normal side. In expiration, the mediastinum resumes its midline position.
- *Basal discoid atelectasis.* The elevated hemidiaphragm leads to compression of the lung bases with crowding of pulmonary vessels and atelectasis.

Subphrenic Abscess

The subdiaphragmatic space acts as a sump for the peritoneal cavity particularly on the right side. Peritoneal fluid migrates here because of the intermittent suction effect of respiratory excursions and because transdiaphragmatic lymphatic vessels drain the peritoneal cavity. Subphrenic abscess formation is most commonly secondary to hollow viscus perforation (appendix, duodenum, and colon).

■ Radiologic Findings

The chest radiograph may show elevation of the hemidiaphragm. A concomitant pleural effusion is present in 80% of cases and lung base atelectasis may be seen. Subphrenic air–fluid levels are seen in 30% of cases. A medially and caudally displaced gastric air bubble is also a feature of a left subphrenic collection.

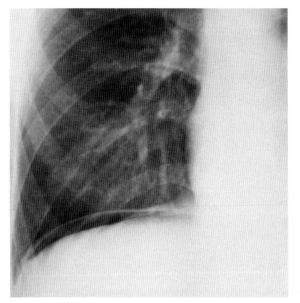

Other causes of subdiaphragmatic gas include pneumoperitoneum when signs are usually bilateral and Chilaiditi's colonic interposition between the hemidiaphragm and liver (Figs. 9.**27**, 9.**28**).

Ultrasound demonstrates both the subphrenic collection and the associated pleural effusion.

Computed tomography shows the size and exact location of the subphrenic collection and also demonstrates associated pulmonary and pleural change. CT may also demonstrate the primary intra-abdominal pathology. Abscess formation is characterized by central low attenuation with peripheral enhancement of the wall which may be quite irregular in thickness. Following localization, percutaneous CT-guided drainage may be feasible.

Fig. 9.**27**   Pneumoperitoneum in patient postabdominal surgery.

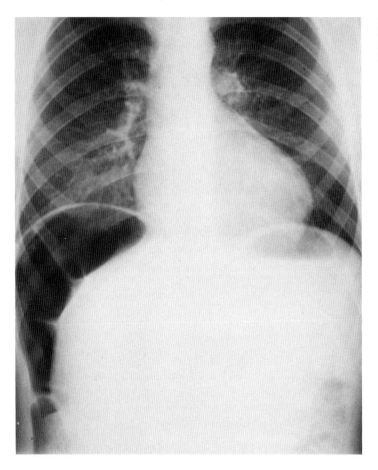

Fig. 9.**28**   Chilaiditi syndrome with hepatic flexure interposed between the liver and right hemidiaphragm. Note colonic haustral markings.

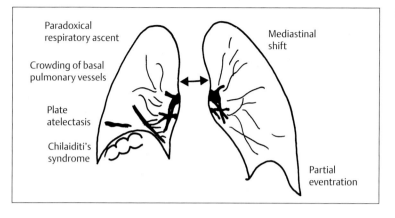

Fig. 9.**29**   Diaphragmatic paralysis.

Diaphragmatic Hernia

Diaphragmatic hernias may be classified according to the location of the defect. Herniation can occur anteriorly at the foramen of Morgagni, posterolaterally through the Bochdalek foramen, or at the esophageal hiatus (Alford 1992). Traumatic diaphragmatic ruptures may also result in herniation of abdominal contents into the thorax (Fig. 9.**30**, see Chapter 8, p. 212).

Bochdalek Hernia

The Bochdalek type of congenital diaphragmatic hernia results from a defect in the posterolateral aspect of the diaphragm. Large lesions are rare with an incidence of 1:3600 live births and 1:2200 fetuses (Saiduffin 1993). Milder forms may be an incidental finding at CT in adult patients. The Bochdalek hernia is sonographically detectable in utero. Presentation with respiratory distress in the neonatal period is common; delayed presentations are recognized (Berman 1988, Malone 1989).

In patients undergoing satisfactory surgical repair, there is still an appreciable mortality due to accompanying pulmonary hypoplasia and increased pulmonary vascular resistance with persistent fetal circulation (Alford 1992). These infants are candidates for extracorporeal membrane oxygenation (ECMO), which may be instituted before or after corrective surgery (Gross 1995).

The chest radiograph shows multiple loops of bowel within the affected hemithorax with mediastinal shift to the contralateral side. The abdominal radiograph classically has a "scaphoid" appearance. A contralateral pneumothorax, absence of contralateral aerated lung, and an intrathoracic stomach are associated with a poor prognosis (Saiduffin 1993, Fig. 9.**31**).

Computed tomography if required will confirm the diagnosis.

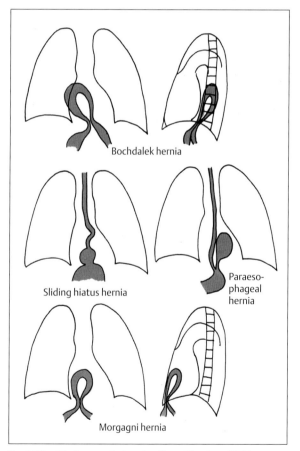

Fig. 9.**30**   Diaphragmatic herniae (from Meschan 1981).

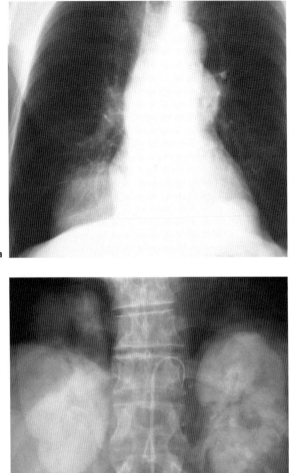

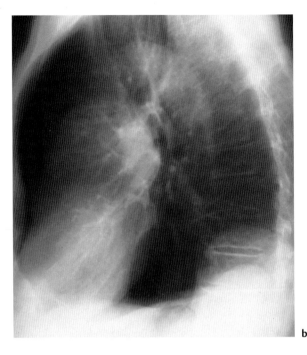

Fig. 9.**31 a–c** Bochdalek hernia with herniation of the upper pole of the right kidney.

Morgagni Hernia

Loops of small and large intestine or omentum may herniate into the thorax through the retrosternally located sternocostal trigone (the Larrey trigone). Right-sided lesions are 10-times more common than left-sided herniations.

Gas-filled intestinal loops are projected over the cardiac silhouette on the frontal *chest radiograph*. These are seen to lie anteriorly on the lateral view (Fig. 9.**32**).

Computed tomography will establish the diagnosis and may be particularly helpful in cases where only omentum has herniated into the chest.

Hiatus Hernia

Dilatation of the esophageal hiatus may result in partial prolapse of the stomach into the chest to give a hiatus hernia. The herniated viscus usually lies in either the posterior mediastinum or in the left lower hemithorax. Herniation may be reversible (sliding hernia) or may be fixed by adhesions.

The chest radiograph may show a retrocardiac opacity or apparent elevation of the hemidiaphragm. An air–fluid level is frequently seen within the herniated viscus and is highly suggestive of the correct diagnosis (Figs. 9.**33 a**, 9.**34**).

Barium swallow will confirm the diagnosis and characteristically shows an hourglass constriction of the stomach at the hernial opening.

Occasionally, a large hiatus hernia may be difficult to distinguish from eventration of the hemidiaphragm. Computed tomography may be helpful in these cases as it defines the relationship of the medial diaphragmatic crus to the stomach (Fig. 9.**33 b**, **c**). Hiatus hernia is a frequent incidental finding at CT in the elderly.

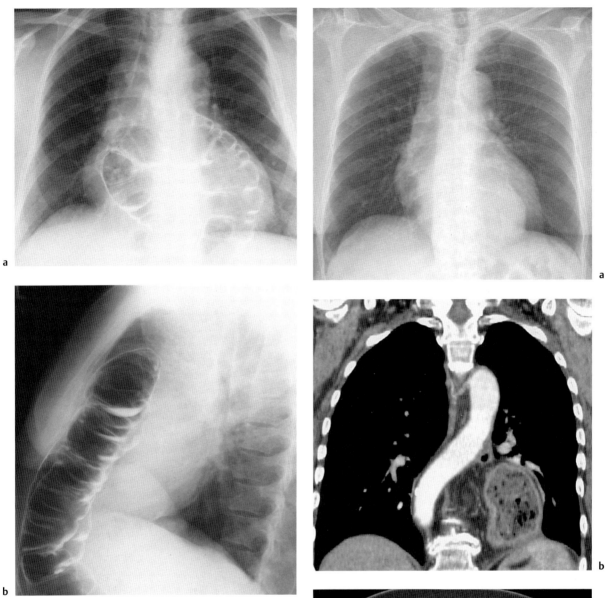

Fig. 9.**32 a, b**   Morgagni hernia diagnosed on contrast enema.

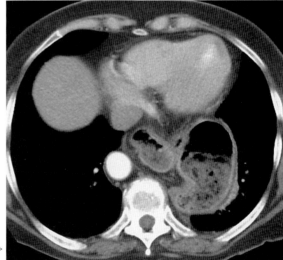

Fig. 9.**33 a–c**   Large hiatus hernia. Note the mass projected over ▷
the cardiac shadow (**a**) and the displacement of the descending
thoracic aorta (**b, c**).

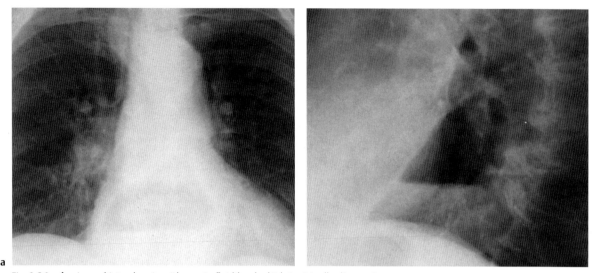

Fig. 9.**34 a, b**   Large hiatus hernia with an air–fluid level which is virtually diagnostic.

Tumors of the Diaphragm

Diaphragmatic tumors (both benign and malignant) are rare and may be an incidental finding on the chest radiograph. Histologic types include fibroma, lipoma, and sarcoma.

Benign tumors may mimic a localized eventration on the *chest radiograph*. Malignant tumors are frequently associated with a pleural effusion (Wilson 1992) and *ultrasound* will demonstrate the tumor particularly well in these cases. Helical volumetric *computed tomography* with multiplanar reformats and 3D reconstructions and *magnetic resonance imaging* will demonstrate tumor size, location, and degree of local infiltration. These modalities may also demonstrate tumor tissue characteristics and lipoma, which occasionally may contain calcium, may be identified by its characteristic CT attenuation values and MRI signal characteristics.

Diseases of the Chest Wall

Evaluation of the bony thorax and soft tissues of the chest wall is important for the following reasons:
- Chest wall abnormality may produce shadows that are projected onto the lungs on the chest radiograph and require differentiation from intrapulmonary lesions. A detailed review of the normal and abnormal bony thorax and chest wall is beyond the scope of this text. The reader, however, is referred to figures (see Figs. 9.**35**, 9.**36**) which review the principal radiographic findings.
- Pulmonary disease and cardiovascular lesions may lead to morphologic change in the chest wall and thoracic deformities may impair respiratory function (Figs. 9.**35**–9.**46**).

Examples include:
- Barrel chest in emphysema.
- Osteolytic destruction of ribs and vertebral bodies by superior sulcus tumor and bronchial carcinoma at other sites.
- Rib osteomyelitis from extension of pulmonary and pleural actinomycosis.
- Rib notching in coarctation of the aorta.
- Restrictive ventilatory impairment secondary to kyphoscoliosis.
- Upper lobe fibrosis associated with ankylosing spondylitis.

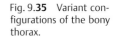

Fig. 9.**35** Variant configurations of the bony thorax.

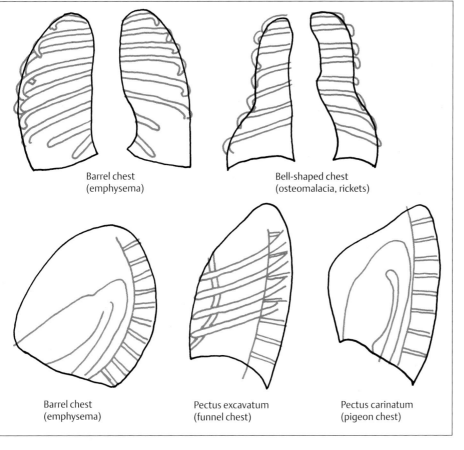

Barrel chest
(emphysema)

Bell-shaped chest
(osteomalacia, rickets)

Barrel chest
(emphysema)

Pectus excavatum
(funnel chest)

Pectus carinatum
(pigeon chest)

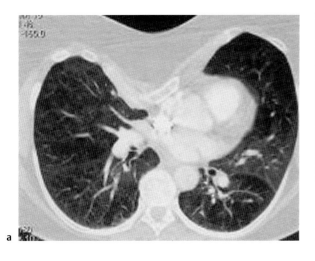

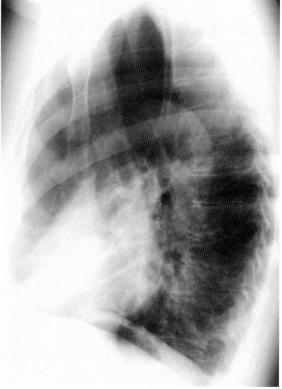

a

b

Fig. 9.**36 a, b** Pectus excavatum. Note the projection of the sternum onto the lung/mediastinum on the lateral view.

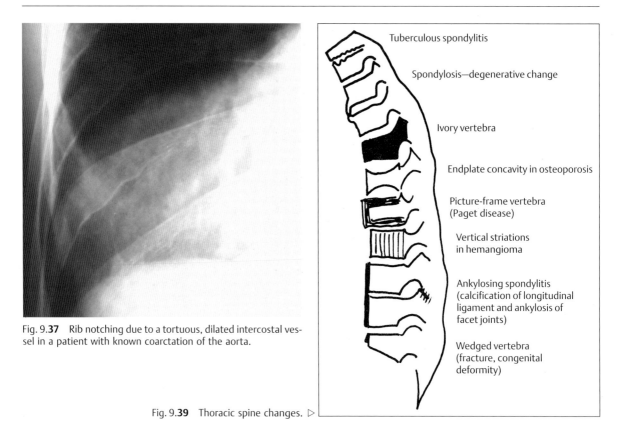

Fig. 9.**37**   Rib notching due to a tortuous, dilated intercostal vessel in a patient with known coarctation of the aorta.

Tuberculous spondylitis

Spondylosis—degenerative change

Ivory vertebra

Endplate concavity in osteoporosis

Picture-frame vertebra (Paget disease)

Vertical striations in hemangioma

Ankylosing spondylitis (calcification of longitudinal ligament and ankylosis of facet joints)

Wedged vertebra (fracture, congenital deformity)

Fig. 9.**39**   Thoracic spine changes. ▷

Fig. 9.**38**   Rib lesions and anomalies.

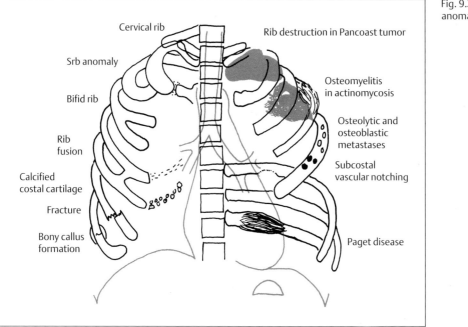

Cervical rib

Srb anomaly

Bifid rib

Rib fusion

Calcified costal cartilage

Fracture

Bony callus formation

Rib destruction in Pancoast tumor

Osteomyelitis in actinomycosis

Osteolytic and osteoblastic metastases

Subcostal vascular notching

Paget disease

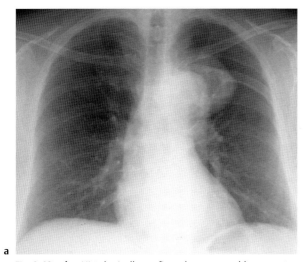

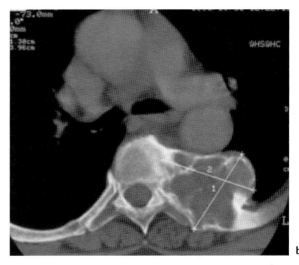

a   b

Fig. 9.**40 a, b**   Histologically confirmed aneurysmal bone cyst.

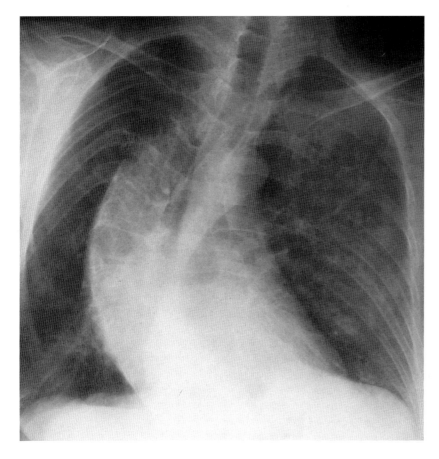

Fig. 9.**41**   Scoliosis with chest wall deformity. Note the narrowed intercostal spaces on the concave side of the curve.

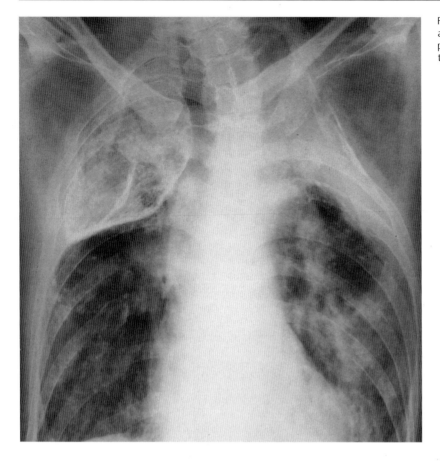

Fig. 9.**42**   Left-sided thoracoplasty and right-sided oleothorax in a patient with a history of pulmonary tuberculosis.

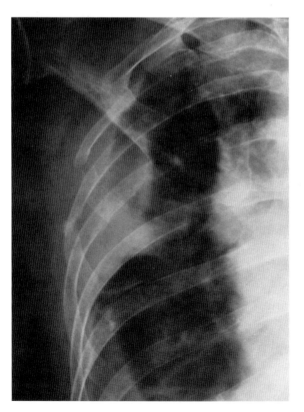

Fig. 9.**43**   Pleural mesothelioma with chest wall invasion and rib destruction.

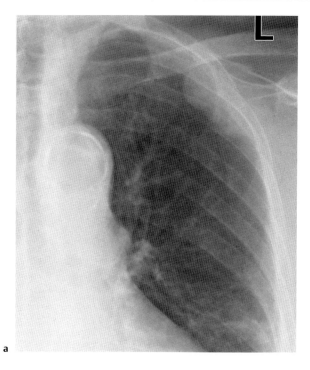

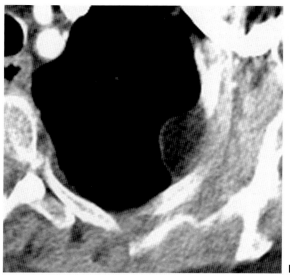

Fig. 9.**44 a, b** Extrapleural lipoma: Chest radiograph (**a**) shows low density lesion lying on left lateral chest wall. CT (**b**) shows lesion to be of negative CT attenuation consistent with fat, appearance diagnostic of an extrapleural lipoma.

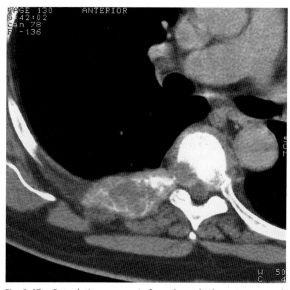

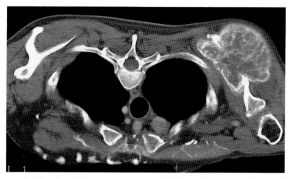

Fig. 9.**46** Scapular osteosarcoma with dilated anterior chest wall collateral vessels.

Fig. 9.**45** Osteolytic metastasis from bronchial carcinoma with rib and vertebral body destruction and with extradural soft tissue component.

10 Radiology of Cardiac Disease

Posteroanterior (PA) and lateral chest radiographs taken in inspiration are standard for evaluation of cardiac size and contour. On the PA chest radiograph, the right cardiomediastinal border is formed by the superior vena cava (SVC) and the right atrium; the left cardiomediastinal border is formed by the aortic arch, main pulmonary artery, left atrial appendage, and left ventricle (LV) (see Figs. 1.**8**, 10.**1a**).

On the lateral projection, the right ventricle is in contact with the lower sternum. More superiorly, the anterior cardiac silhouette is formed by the right ventricular outflow tract and pulmonary conus. The left atrium and left ventricle form the posterior cardiac contour (see Figs. 1.**9**, 10.**1b**).

Cardiac Size

While there is some variation in normal values, transverse cardiac diameter usually should not exceed the transverse diameter of one hemithorax or 50% of the widest transverse thoracic diameter. A more accurate determination of cardiac volume may be made from the lateral radiograph (Fig. 10.**2**) although today this has been superseded by echocardiographic assessment.

Cardiac Contour

Both congenital and acquired cardiac disease are frequently associated with specific chamber hypertrophy or enlargement resulting in alteration in the shape of the cardiac silhouette (Table 10.**1**).

Radiographic features in:
- *Left ventricular enlargement* (e.g. secondary to systemic arterial hypertension or aortic stenosis) include:
  - On the PA view transverse cardiac diameter is increased, the cardiac apex is rounded, and there is lateral convexity of the left heart border (*aortic configuration*).
  - On the lateral view, there is partial obliteration of the retrocardiac space as the heart extends up to 2 cm posterior to the inferior vena caval (IVC) shadow (Figs. 10.**3**, 10.**4c, d**).

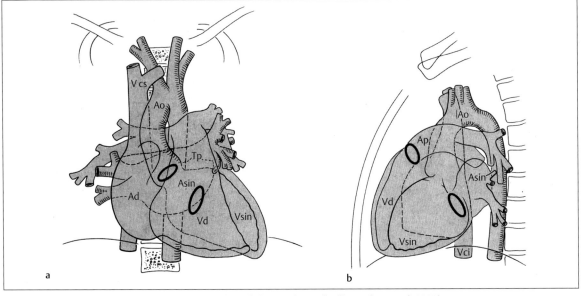

Fig. 10.**1a, b** Normal cardiac anatomy on PA and lateral chest radiographs (from Klose et al. 1991)

Ao   = Aorta
Tp   = Proximal main pulmonary artery ("pulmonary trunk")
Ap   = Pulmonary artery
Asin = Left atrium
Ad   = Right atrium

Vci = Inferior vena cava
Vd   = Right ventricle
Vcs = Superior vena cava
Vsin = Left ventricle

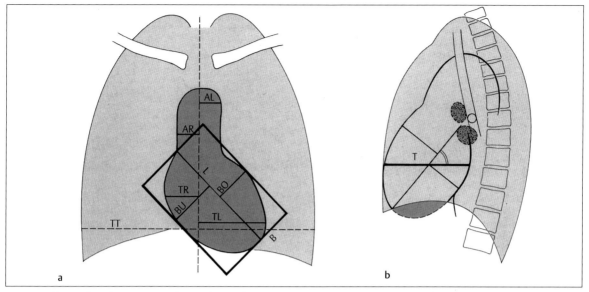

Fig. 10.**2a, b**   Cardiac dimensions on the PA chest radiograph.
Transverse cardiac diameter T = TR + TL
CT ratio = transverse cardiac diameter/transverse thoracic diameter T/TT
AL = aortic dimension to left of midline
AR = aortic dimension to right of midline (AL + AR = 1.8–3.8 cm)
L   = cardiac long axis measurement
B   = BU + BO perpendicular diagonal to L (maximum short axis measurement through the heart)

T = transverse dimension of heart in axial plane
V = relative cardiac volume
V = $0.4 \times L \times B \times T$
Normal ratio of cardiac volume to body surface area:
In women: 450–490 cm³/m²
In men: 500–540 cm³/m² (Amundsen 1959)

Table 10.**1**   Conditions which may alter heart size (modified from Higgins 1992)

Small cardiac silhouette:
- Asthenic body habitus
- Cachexia
- Emphysema (narrow, elongated heart)
- Restrictive cardiomyopathy
- Constrictive pericarditis

Normal-size cardiac silhouette despite the presence of significant lesions
- Aortic stenosis
- Arterial hypertension
- Mitral stenosis
- Hypertrophic cardiomyopathy
- Acute myocardial infarction
- Some congenital heart lesions

Large cardiac silhouette:
- Normal variant (e. g., physiologic LV hypertrophy in athletes)
- Biventricular decompensation
- Dilated cardiomyopathy
- Aortic insufficiency
- Mitral insufficiency
- Decompensated valvular stenoses
- Congenital cardiac anomalies
- Pericardial effusion (globular or triangular silhouette)

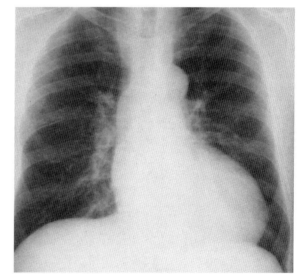

Fig. 10.**3**   Chest radiograph in aortic stenosis. Note the rounded cardiac apex, the left ventricular enlargement, and the post-stenotic dilatation of the ascending aorta.

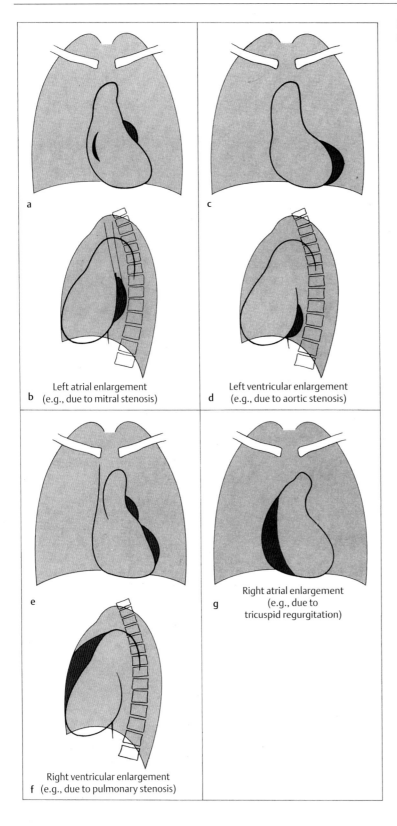

a

b   Left atrial enlargement
     (e.g., due to mitral stenosis)

c

d   Left ventricular enlargement
     (e.g., due to aortic stenosis)

e

f   Right ventricular enlargement
     (e.g., due to pulmonary stenosis)

g   Right atrial enlargement
     (e.g., due to
     tricuspid regurgitation)

Fig. 10.**4a–g**   Cardiac chamber enlargement (from Klose et al. 1991).

- *Right ventricular enlargement* (e. g., due to pulmonary arterial hypertension) include:
  - Right ventricular change may be quite marked before radiographic abnormalities become apparent. Right ventricular hypertrophy results in cardiac rotation with posterior displacement of the left ventricle. The right ventricle then forms part of the left heart border and there is characteristically some "elevation" of the cardiac apex on the PA view (Fig. 10.**4e, f**).
  - Right ventricular hypertrophy and dilatation are frequently associated with dilatation of the main and central pulmonary arteries.
- *Left atrial enlargement* (due to mitral stenosis) include:
  - On the PA radiograph, left atrial dilatation is associated with prominence or "fullness" of the left cardiac border and obliteration of the normal cardiac waist.
  - The left atrium extends posteriorly as enlargement becomes more marked and then its right border may be projected within the cardiac silhouette (double "right heart border" sign).
  - There may also be splaying of the carina to an angle of greater than 90° as the left atrium extends superiorly.
  - On the lateral view, there is narrowing of the retrocardiac space as the left atrium enlarges posteriorly (Figs. 10.**4a, b**, 10.**31**).
- *Right atrial enlargement* (e. g., due to tricuspid insufficiency) include:
  - Prominence of the right cardiac border.
  - The height of the atrial shadow exceeds 50% of the distance between the diaphragm and aortic arch (Higgins 1992, Fig. 10.**4g**).

Congenital Heart Disease

Congenital cardiac anomalies occur in 0.2 to 0.4% of the population. There is a spectrum of severity with severe anomalies being incompatible with life while other lesions may not become symptomatic until late adult life. The presence of multiple anomalies may give rise to complex hemodynamic patterns with secondary functional and structural cardiac adaptation.

Cardiac anomalies may be classified according to their hemodynamic effects, i. e., the presence or absence of a shunt.

Cardiac Anomalies without a Shunt

Cyanosis is absent but a degree of either right or left ventricular outflow obstruction is present. Isolated pulmonary valve stenosis (10–15% of all congenital heart disease), coarctation of the aorta (COA) (5–9%), and aortic valve stenosis (3–7%) are included in this group.

Pulmonary Stenosis

■ Clinical Features

Pulmonary valve stenosis (PVS) is usually congenital and results from fusion and thickening of valve cusps with formation of a diaphragm perforated by an orifice the size and position of which are quite variable. The trans-valvular systolic pressure gradient determines the severity of symptoms; the most severe end of the spectrum presents with right ventricular failure in infancy. *"Supravalvular" pulmonary stenosis* is considered to be an arteritis with segmental arterial stenosis. It is seen in Noonan's and Williams' syndrome and in congenital rubella. *Subvalvular stenosis* is frequently due to right ventricular outflow tract (RVOT) hypertrophy and the valve may be normal or dysmorphic in these patients (Boxt et al. 2003).

■ Radiologic Findings

The *chest radiograph* may show characteristic poststenotic dilatation of the main pulmonary artery extending to involve the left pulmonary artery and resulting in enlargement of the left hilum (Fig. 10.**5**). The heart is of "right ventricular" configuration with elevation, rounding, and flattening of the cardiac apex. Pulmonary vascularity is normal in most cases except in high-grade stenoses.

Echocardiography: In moderate to severe stenosis, pulmonary valve leaflets are thickened with evidence of "doming" during systole. Poststenotic dilatation of the main pulmonary artery is seen with significant degrees of obstruction. Right ventricular anterior wall thickness may be measured. Pulsed (PW) and continuous wave (CW) Doppler allow estimation of the systolic gradient across the valve. The right ventricular anterior wall thickness and the systolic gradient determine the need for surgical intervention (Grainger 1992).

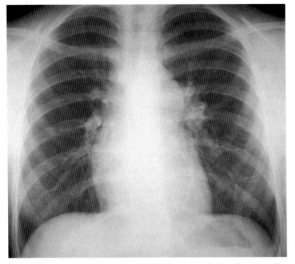

Fig. 10.**5** Congenital pulmonary valve stenosis. Chest radiograph shows poststenotic dilatation of the main pulmonary artery and left hilar enlargement.

Magnetic resonance imaging (MRI): Spin echo sequences in patients with valvular stenosis show bulging of the pulmonary valve, poststenotic dilatation of the main pulmonary artery, and a degree of right ventricular hypertrophy. The presence of associated tricuspid regurgitation is variable and is dependent on the degree of RV hypertrophy. Gradient echo (GRE) sequences show the systolic jet of signal void across the valve and allow calculation of the severity of the stenosis.

Right-heart catheterization with right ventricular injection confirms the diagnosis and demonstrates doming of the valve cusps during systole. The right ventricle is heavily trabeculated and right ventricular pressures are elevated considerably in severe stenosis.

Congenital Aortic Stenosis

■ Clinical Features

Childhood aortic valve disease encompasses a wide spectrum of abnormalities of varying severity. Severely dysplastic valves are associated with cardiac failure in the neonatal period, the so-called "critical aortic stenosis of the newborn." A congenital bicuspid aortic valve is the most frequent malformation of the aortic valve and occurs in 0.9–2% of all individuals at autopsy (Roberts 1970). These lesions do not usually become symptomatic until adult life and about one-third of these individuals eventually develop aortic stenosis (Fenoglio et al. 1977) either related to the structural abnormality or secondary to an episode of bacterial endocarditis.

■ Radiologic Findings

Chest radiograph: Features of left ventricular hypertrophy and dilatation of the ascending aorta are seen only in high-grade stenosis.

Echocardiography: Two-dimensional (2D) echocardiography shows the abnormal valve, a small valve ring, and a hypertrophied, hyperdynamic left ventricle. CW Doppler echocardiography allows estimation of the systolic gradient across the valve.

Magnetic resonance imaging demonstrates a small aortic annulus and abnormal distribution of the aortic sinuses by the unseparated valvular commissures. The valve leaflets may be thickened and leaflet doming may be evident on gradient echo sequences. These sequences also demonstrate the systolic signal void jets of stenosis. Left ventricular hypertrophy is frequent.

When there is aortic regurgitation, associated poststenotic dilatation of the ascending aorta and a degree of left ventricle dilatation may be present. GRE sequences in these cases show diastolic jets of regurgitation (Boxt et al. 2003).

The pressure gradient across the valve may be estimated from the length of signal loss across the aorta (Mitchell et al. 1989) or quantified using phase velocity mapping (Kilner et al. 1991).

Left ventriculography and aortography confirm the presence of left ventricular outflow obstruction and when appropriate balloon valvotomy may be performed during catheterization.

Left ventricular outflow obstruction may also be supravalvular and associated with infantile hypercalcemia or subvalvular due to fibromuscular hypertrophy of the left ventricular outflow tract.

Coarctation of the Aorta

■ Clinical Features

Medial hypertrophy and intimal proliferation within the aorta lead to localized stenosis which becomes hemodynamically significant when it causes more than a 50% reduction in the size of the lumen.

Two forms are recognized:
- *Infantile (preductal) COA*: In this form, the stenosis lies proximal to the ductus arteriosus which usually is patent. This may result in a right-to-left shunt with cyanosis in the lower half of the body (Fig. 10.**6**).

Fig. 10.**6a–k** Schematic representation of congenital cardiac ▷ anomalies (from Schinz et al. 1983).

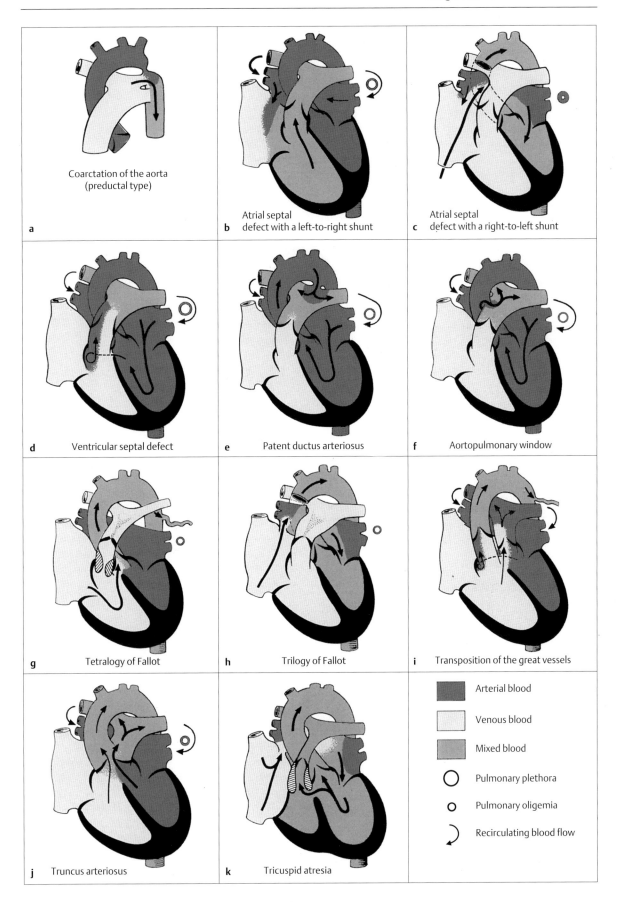

a Coarctation of the aorta (preductal type)

b Atrial septal defect with a left-to-right shunt

c Atrial septal defect with a right-to-left shunt

d Ventricular septal defect

e Patent ductus arteriosus

f Aortopulmonary window

g Tetralogy of Fallot

h Trilogy of Fallot

i Transposition of the great vessels

j Truncus arteriosus

k Tricuspid atresia

- Arterial blood
- Venous blood
- Mixed blood
- ○ Pulmonary plethora
- ○ Pulmonary oligemia
- ↻ Recirculating blood flow

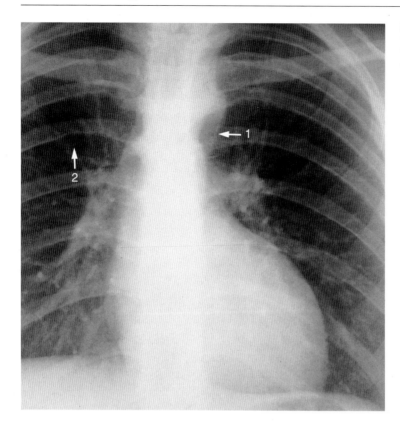

Fig. 10.**7**   Coarctation of the aorta. Note the left ventricular enlargement, the focal "notch" in the aorta giving a "reversed 3" configuration (1) and the rib notching (2).

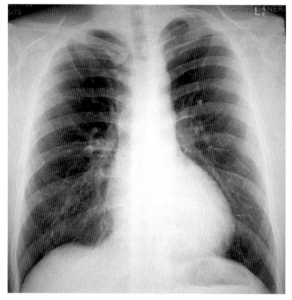

Fig. 10.**8**   Aortic coarctation: "Reversed 3" configuration of the aorta is seen.

- *Adult (postductal) COA*: In postductal or adult coarctation, systolic blood pressure in the upper limbs exceeds that in the lower limbs by at least 20 mmHg. The lower body is supplied by collateral vessels which usually have developed by late childhood. Associated anomalies including bicuspid aortic valve and aberrant subclavian artery occur in up to 75% of cases.

■ Radiologic Findings

Chest radiograph: Radiographic findings in coarctation include a high aortic arch with pre- and poststenotic dilatation (Figs. 10.**7**, 10.**8**). In the postductal type, rib notching involving the 3rd to 8th ribs is due to pressure erosion by dilated intercostal collateral vessels. In the infantile type, dilatation of the pulmonary vessels may indicate the presence of a left-to-right shunt.

Magnetic resonance imaging and *aortography* demonstrate the length and level of the coarctation segment and the degree of arterial collateralization present (Figs. 10.**9**, 10.**10**). The relationship of the origin of the subclavian arteries to the stenotic segment is important to demonstrate given the association with the aberrant subclavian artery (Boxt et al. 2003). MRI also plays a role in imaging follow-up of patients after balloon dilatation and repair of the coarctation.

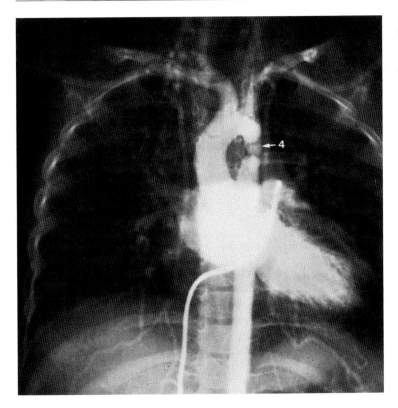

Fig. 10.**9**   Coarctation of the aorta. A catheter has been placed in the pulmonary artery, and injected contrast medium has opacified the left atrium, left ventricle, and aorta.

Congenital Cardiac Anomalies Associated with a Left-to-Right Shunt

The most common causes of a left-to-right shunt are ventricular septal defects (VSD: 20–28 % of all congenital cardiac anomalies, Fig. 10.**11**), atrial septal defects (ASD: 10–15 %), and patent ductus arteriosus (PDA: 10–15 %). Less common anomalies include Lutembacher syndrome (ASD combined with mitral stenosis) and anomalous pulmonary venous drainage (APVD).

The shunt may be at the atrial (ASD), ventricular (VSD), or arterial (PDA) level. Oxygenated blood may also be shunted from the pulmonary veins back into the right atrium (APVD). Recirculating blood volume may greatly exceed the circulating systemic volume; this leads to overload of the pulmonary circulation with resulting pulmonary arteriolar sclerosis and increased pulmonary vascular resistance. This in turn induces right ventricular hypertrophy causing further increases in pulmonary arterial pressure. Eventually right heart pressure may exceed that in the left heart chambers leading to shunt reversal (Eisenmenger reaction; see Chapter 7, p. 194).

Individuals with congenital left-to-right shunts may remain asymptomatic for many years but are at increased risk of endocarditis. Large shunts may be as-

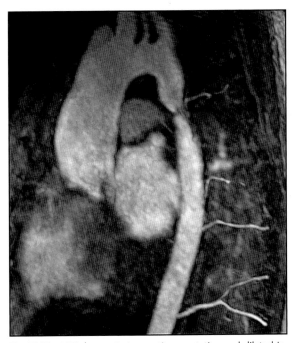

Fig. 10.**10**   MRI demonstrates aortic coarctation and dilated intercostal vessels inferior to the level of the aortic narrowing.

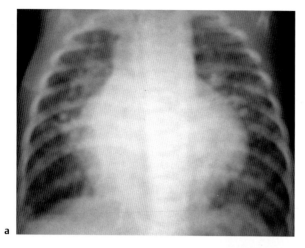

a

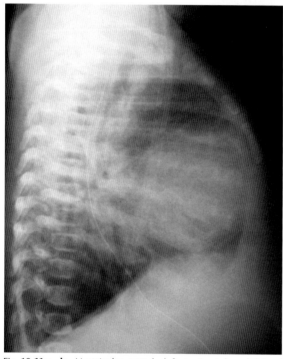

b

Fig. 10.**11 a, b** Ventricular septal defect: Frontal and lateral chest radiographs show right ventricular dilatation and marked pulmonary plethora. Echocardiography shows large VSD with left atrial and biventricular enlargement.

sociated with marked symptomatology including impaired physical development in children. Characteristic auscultatory findings include a pansystolic murmur in VSD and a continuous murmur in PDA. In advanced untreated cases, signs of right heart failure (dilated neck veins, peripheral edema, and hepatomegaly) may supervene. Cyanosis develops with reversal of the shunt.

■ Radiologic Findings

Chest radiograph: When the pulmonary to systemic shunt ratio is greater than 2:1, there is cardiomegaly (Grainger and Donner 1992) and pulmonary plethora (Higgins 1992). Other characteristic features include increased pulsation of dilated central pulmonary arteries (hilar dance) visible at fluoroscopy. The level of the shunt cannot be determined from standard radiographs although certain characteristics of the cardiac silhouette may give diagnostic clues (Fig. 10.**12**).

Atrial Septal Defect

Atrial septal defects are classified according to the site of the communication (see Fig. 10.**6 b, c**):

- An ostium secundum or fossa ovalis defect is situated in the upper part of the septum posterior to the coronary sinus and superior to the tricuspid valve. The size of the defect is variable, the mildest form being a slit-like patency of the foramen ovale that normally closes soon after birth. Significant shunts are usually greater than 2 cm in diameter, are not valvular, and will transmit blood from the left to the right atrium. Ostium secundum defects account for 80 to 90 % of all ASDs (Grainger and Donner 1992).
- An ostium primum defect involves the inferior part of the septum and is the mildest form of endocardial cushion defect. An ostium primum defect together with cleft leaflets of malformed tricuspid and mitral valves represent incomplete persistence of the arterioventricular canal. If a high VSD is also present, the combination constitutes complete persistence of the arterioventricular canal. There is mitral regurgitation with left-to-right shunting of blood. The elevation of right heart pressures results in gradual development of pulmonary hypertension.
- A sinus venosus defect is situated in the most superior part of the septum just inferior to the termination of the superior vena cava. This almost invariably is associated with aberrant drainage of the right upper lobe pulmonary vein into the inferior part of the SVC. Sinus venosus defects account for 5 % of all ASDs.

■ Radiologic Findings

Chest radiograph: If the shunt ratio is greater than 2:1, there is usually cardiomegaly. There is dilatation of the central pulmonary arteries and a variable degree of pulmonary plethora is present. The aortic arch may appear small, probably due to a degree of aortic rotation (Figs. 10.**13**, 10.**14**).

Echocardiography will demonstrate nearly all defects. When a significant shunt is present, there is evidence of right ventricular dilatation with systolic anterior motion of the interventricular septum. The four-chamber sub-

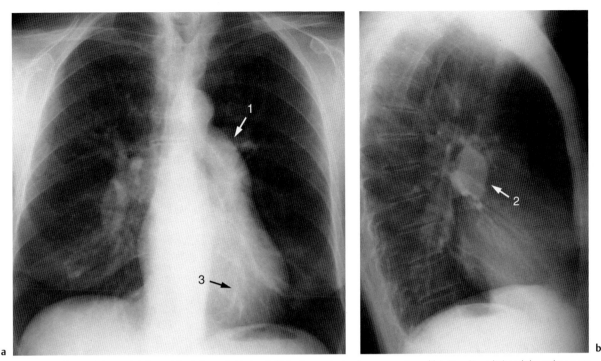

Fig. 10.**12 a, b**   Atrial septal defect with a left-to-right shunt. Note the central pulmonary artery dilatation (1 and 2) and the pulmonary plethora (3).

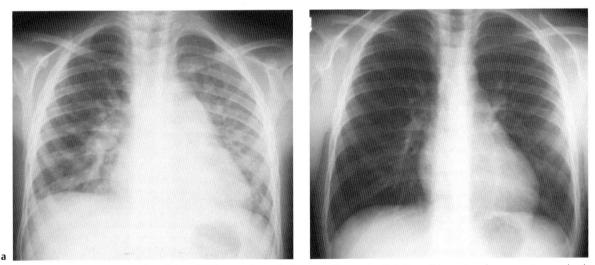

Fig. 10.**13 a, b**   Ostium secundum defect. (**a**) Chest radiograph shows cardiomegaly, dilatation of the main pulmonary artery, and pulmonary edema. Radiograph 4 years after operative closure of the defect is almost normal (**b**).

costal view will differentiate ostium secundum from primum defects (Grainger and Donner 1992).

Magnetic resonance imaging: MRI in the axial plane has 97% sensitivity and 90% specificity for detection of ASDs (Diethelm et al. 1987). Intravenous administration of gadolinium may help to demonstrate smaller and less apparent shunts (Manning et al. 1992). GRE sequences allow determination of the direction of the shunt and velocity-encoded cine (VEC) images allow some estimation of the volume of the shunt.

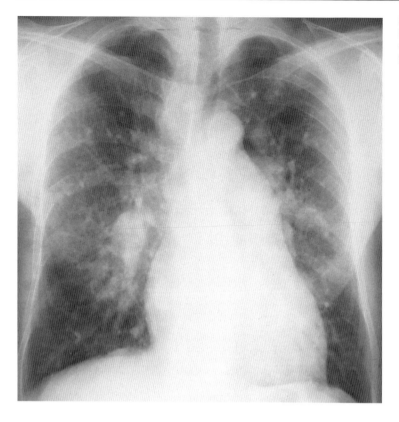

Fig. 10.**14**   Ostium primum defect with a left-to-right shunt. There is cardiomegaly, central pulmonary artery dilatation, and pulmonary plethora.

Ventricular Septal Defect

This is the most common congenital cardiac anomaly accounting for 20–28% of cases. Membranous defects are most common and occur in the upper posterior septum. Defects in the muscular septum (maladie de Roger) may be single or multiple. When multiple, they may produce a "Swiss cheese" pattern. Defects in the muscular septum are frequently quite small although the associated pansystolic murmur may be relatively loud.

The magnitude of the shunt is roughly proportional to the area of the defect. With defects smaller than 0.5 cm², systolic muscle contractions are sufficient to maintain the interventricular pressure gradient. With larger defects, the right ventricle is subjected to systemic pressures with resulting right ventricular hypertrophy. Right ventricular hypertrophy and increasing pulmonary vascular resistance lead to a reduction in the volume of the left-to-right shunt and if untreated will in time lead to its reversal (Eisenmenger reaction, see Fig. 10.**6 d**).

■ Radiologic Findings

The *chest radiograph* may be normal when just a small defect is present. Larger defects are associated with the characteristic features of a left-to-right shunt including cardiomegaly, dilated central pulmonary arteries, and pulmonary plethora.

Two-dimensional echocardiography will identify the site of the defect. Left atrial and left ventricular dilatation will be evident in moderate to large shunts. PW Doppler will confirm the presence of a shunt and Doppler color flow mapping will identify the site, extent, and direction of the shunt (Grainger and Donner 1992, Ludomirsky et al. 1986, Ortiz et al. 1985).

Magnetic resonance imaging allows diagnosis of and determination of the size of a VSD. Large defects may be readily identified on spin echo sequences as signal voids to the left of the atrioventricular rings. Smaller more distal and muscular VSDs may be difficult to demonstrate on spin echo sequences but the signal void jet of the shunted blood on GRE sequences may allow their detection.

Patent Ductus Arteriosus

This communication between the concavity of the aortic arch and the superior aspect of the main pulmonary artery constitutes an essential part of the fetal circulation and usually closes soon after birth. Persistence of this tubular connection (patent ductus arteriosus) permits passage of blood from the higher-pressure aorta into the pulmonary artery and through the pulmonary circulation thus creating a left-to-right shunt. The defect is variable in size but is seldom greater than 1 cm² in cross-sectional area. An aortopulmonary pressure gradient is maintained in the majority of cases.

Only the left heart chambers are enlarged initially as the shunt does not involve the right ventricle. Eventually, pulmonary vascular resistance increases as a result of increased pulmonary blood flow and this in turn leads to pressure overload on the right heart (see Fig. 10.6e). Eisenmenger reaction with shunt reversal occurs when pulmonary arterial pressure exceeds that of the systemic arterial circulation.

■ Radiologic Findings

The *chest radiograph* shows features of a left-to-right shunt. There is associated enlargement of structures proximal to the shunt including the left atrium, left ventricle, ascending aorta, and aortic arch (Fig. 10.15). If shunt reversal occurs (Eisenmenger reaction) then the central pulmonary arteries become more dilated and peripheral oligemia develops (Fig. 10.15). In cases of long-standing severe pulmonary hypertension with Eisenmenger reaction, calcification (Fig. 10.16) of the dilated pulmonary arteries and ductus may be seen.

Two-dimensional echocardiography will show left atrial and left ventricular dilatation. PW Doppler evaluation of the pulmonary artery confirms the diagnosis showing normal forward flow from the pulmonary valve during systole with reversed flow from the bifurcation in diastole. Doppler color flow mapping allows assessment of the overall size of the shunt (Grainger and Donner 1992, see Fig. 10.17).

Magnetic resonance imaging: Imaging in the coronal or in the parasagittal right anterior oblique (RAO) plane may demonstrate the ductal communication. However, no data are available on the sensitivity and specificity of MRI in diagnosis of PDA (Boxt et al. 2003). Furthermore, magnetic resonance (MR) evaluation of this anomaly may be limited in infants by the small size of the ductus and limited MR spatial resolution.

Aortography: Contrast medium injected into the aortic arch will demonstrate the patent ductus and opacify the pulmonary arteries (Fig. 10.17).

Total Anomalous Pulmonary Venous Drainage (TAPVD)

In TAPVD, pulmonary venous drainage is to almost any element of the sinus venosus system. This is a relatively rare anomaly accounting for approximately 2% of all cardiac malformations and is compatible with life only when a coexisting atrial septal defect is present.

TAPVD may be classified into:
- Type I: Supracardiac return is most common (55%) with pulmonary venous drainage (PVD) to the verti-

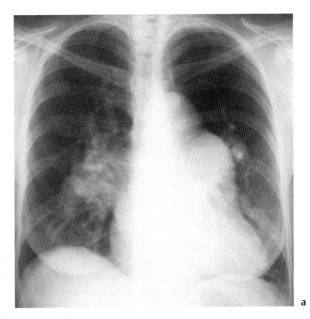
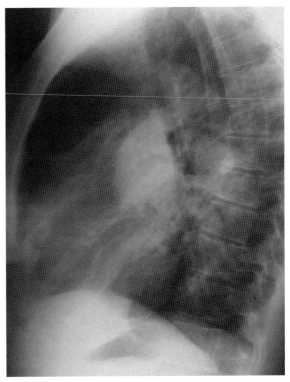

Fig. 10.15a, b Patent ductus arteriosus. Radiographs show cardiomegaly, marked central pulmonary artery dilatation, and a dilated aortic arch.

cal vein which then drains to the brachiocephalic vein and superior vena cava or with PVD to the azygos vein and then to the SVC.
- Type II: Anomalous return at cardiac level with drainage to the coronary sinus or right atrium.
- Type III: Infradiaphragmatic return with drainage to the portal system or inferior vena cava.

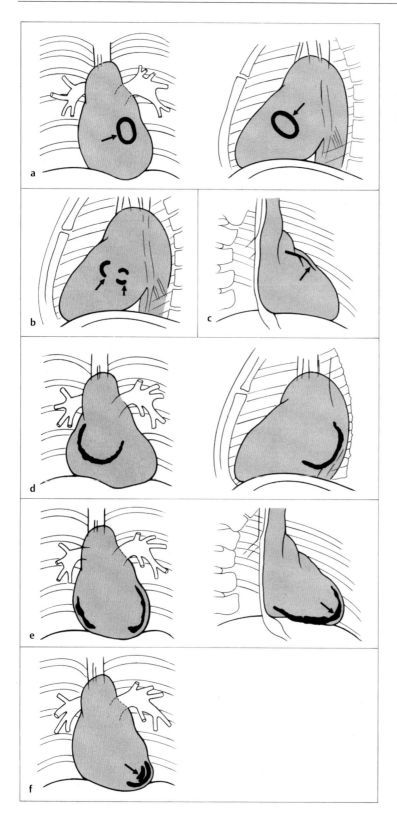

Fig. 10.**16 a–f**   Cardiac calcifications. (**a**)
Calcified mitral valve ring, PA and lateral
views. (**b**) Aortic (Ao) and mitral (Mi) valve
calcification on lateral view. (**c**) Left anterior
descending (LAD) coronary artery calcification in the RAO projection. (**d**) Calcification
in left atrial wall, PA and lateral views. (**e**)
Pericardial calcification, PA and RAO projections. (**f**) Calcified ventricular aneurysm, PA
view (from Meschan 1981).

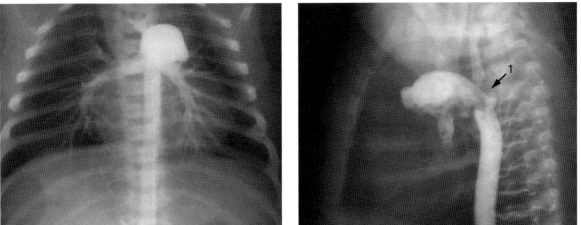

a   b

Fig. 10.**17 a, b**   Patent ductus arteriosus. Contrast medium injection into the aortic arch opacifies the pulmonary arteries through the patent ductus.

- Type IV: Drainage at multiple levels (Pearson et al. 1987).

■ Radiologic Findings

Chest radiograph: Patients with TAPVD may be divided into two groups: those with normal pulmonary vascular resistance and unobstructed venous return and those with obstructed venous return. The latter is found most commonly in type III TAPVD.

- *Type I*: The chest radiograph characteristically shows a figure-of-eight shaped mediastinum (*snowman* configuration); this represents the vertical vein, dilated left brachiocephalic vein, and SVC. If drainage is to the azygos vein, this vein may then be dilated and is seen in the right superior mediastinum.
- *Type II*: The right cardiac contour may be abnormal and this may be due to a dilated coronary sinus.
- *Type III*: There may be gross pulmonary edema in the presence of a normal-sized heart.

Echocardiography: The four-chamber view shows the characteristic features of TAPVD. The pulmonary veins unite in a venous confluence superior to the left atrium. In type I TAPVD, suprasternal views may show drainage to the SVC. In type II, a posterior four-chamber view may show dilatation of the coronary sinus.

In type III, the subcostal parasagittal view will demonstrate a descending vein originating from the pulmonary venous confluence and passing through the diaphragm in close proximity to the aorta (Pearson et al. 1987).

See also Partial Anomalous Pulmonary Venous Drainage, Chapter 2, p. 61 and Figs. 2.**22**, 2.**23**.

Congenital Cardiac Anomalies associated with a Right-to-Left Shunt

Congenital cardiac anomalies associated with a right-to-left shunt lead to central cyanosis. *Tetralogy of Fallot* is most common accounting for 10–15 % of all congenital cardiac anomalies followed by *transposition of the great vessels* (5–9 %), *tricuspid atresia* (1.2–3 %), and the *Ebstein anomaly* (0.23–1 %) (Klose et al. 1991).

When an atrial or ventricular septal defect is combined with pulmonary stenosis, the increased right heart pressure leads to development of a right-to-left shunt.

Similarly, when an atrial septal defect is combined with tricuspid stenosis or a hypoplastic right ventricle (the Ebstein anomaly), right-to-left shunting also occurs. Pulmonary flow is diminished relative to flow through the systemic circulation resulting in central cyanosis.

Tetralogy of Fallot

Tetralogy of Fallot is characterized by infundibular pulmonary stenosis, a high ventricular septal defect, and aortic override of the ventricular septum. Right ventricular hypertrophy is a consequence of these features. The degree of pulmonary stenosis determines the magnitude of the shunt and the severity of clinical symptoms (see Fig. 10.**6 g, h**). Patients may undergo a palliative shunting procedure to improve pulmonary blood flow prior to complete repair with VSD closure and infundibulectomy. A Blalock–Taussig shunt connects the subclavian to the ipsilateral pulmonary artery, a Waterston shunt connects the ascending aorta to the right pulmonary artery, and a Potts shunt connects the descending aorta to the left pulmonary artery.

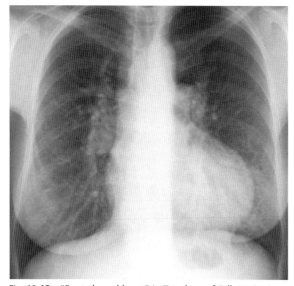

Fig. 10.**18**   "Boot-shaped heart" in Tetralogy of Fallot.

■ Radiologic Findings

The *chest radiograph* shows pulmonary oligemia. The cardiac silhouette may appear normal or have a characteristic "coeur en sabot" appearance resembling a wooden shoe depending on the severity of the right ventricular outflow obstruction. The latter is caused by right ventricular hypertrophy with cardiac rotation and by a markedly concave pulmonary bay as the main pulmonary artery is hypoplastic (Fig. 10.**18**).

Two-dimensional echocardiography will demonstrate the VSD. Long-axis parasternal views show the aortic override and parasternal short axis and suprasternal views aid in evaluation of the pulmonary valve. PW and color flow Doppler imaging show the degree of right-to-left shunting through the VSD (Grainger and Donner 1992 b).

Magnetic resonance imaging will demonstrate features of the Tetralogy. In addition, MRI may play a valuable role post shunting in evaluation of shunt patency.

Right heart catheterization: An injection into the right ventricle shows the VSD and the aortic override; these are demonstrated optimally in the left anterior oblique (60° LAO) projection. The right anterior oblique (30° RAO) projection is optimal for visualization of right ventricular outflow obstruction which is usually severe. Infundibular stenosis is most common being present in 70 % of cases. The pulmonary valve is stenosed in 60 % of patients usually in association with infundibular stenosis.

Uncorrected Transposition of the Great Vessels

Transposition of the great vessels is a cyanotic congenital heart anomaly which requires surgical correction (arterial switch) early in life. The term describes a combination of atrioventricular concordance and ventriculoarterial discordance. The anteriorly displaced aorta arises from the right ventricle while the pulmonary artery originates from the left ventricle. This creates two separate circulations which are interconnected by a bidirectional shunt (usually an ASD, less commonly a VSD or PDA, see Fig. 10.**6 i**).

■ Radiologic Findings

Chest radiograph: Cardiomegaly develops in the first weeks of life and there is associated narrowing of the superior mediastinal vascular pedicle due to superimposition of the pulmonary artery and aorta. These features lead to an "egg-shaped" cardiac silhouette. The lungs are plethoric in uncorrected transposition.

Two-dimensional echocardiography in the parasternal long- and short-axis planes shows the anteroposterior reversal of the aorta and pulmonary artery. The apical four-chamber view allows evaluation of the ventricular septum and if a VSD is present, PW and color flow Doppler imaging will demonstrate the degree of shunting from the right to the left ventricle (Grainger and Donner 1992 b).

Right heart catheterization: A contrast medium injection into the right ventricle shows the morphological right ventricle leading to the aortic valve which is situated more superiorly than is normal and to the anteriorly displaced aorta. A left ventricular injection will demonstrate the left ventricle in continuity with the pulmonary valve which lies more inferiorly than is normal (Grainger and Donner 1992 b).

Ebstein Anomaly

The malformed septal and posterior leaflets of the tricuspid valve are displaced inferiorly and attached to the wall of the right ventricle. The proximal right ventricle therefore is incorporated into the right atrium (*atrialized*) but it contracts synchronously with the right ventricle. This disordered function leads to impaired right atrial emptying. An ASD or patent foramen ovale is present in 80 % of cases and produces a right-to-left shunt resulting in cyanosis.

■ Radiologic Findings

The *chest radiograph* characteristically shows an enlarged globular-shaped heart. Right atrial enlargement accounts for the convex right lateral border while the convex left border is formed in part by the right ventricle. The vascular pedicle in the superior mediastinum is narrow, the main pulmonary arteries are inconspicuous, and there is pulmonary oligemia.

Echocardiography: The apical four-chamber view readily demonstrates displacement of the tricuspid valve leaflets into the right ventricle. The true tricuspid valve ring and the abnormal origin of the leaflets may be connected by a band of echoes representing valve tissue adherent to the ventricular wall. The degree of tricuspid regurgitation and of right-to-left shunting may be assessed with PW and color flow Doppler imaging. Evaluation of the anterior cusp is important as this may be used for "monocusp surgical repair," which aims to decrease the severity of tricuspid regurgitation (Grainger and Donner 1992 b).

Right heart catheterization confirms the diagnosis. Contrast medium injected into the right atrium demonstrates displacement of the abnormal tricuspid valve leaflets to the left of the midline. There is usually delayed emptying of the right atrium with right-to-left shunting of opacified blood through an ASD or patent foramen ovale. Right ventricular injection demonstrates the severity of tricuspid incompetence.

Acquired Heart Disease

Cardiac Failure

Cardiac failure is common, particularly in the elderly, and is characterized by inability of the heart to maintain an adequate cardiac output (Fig. 10.**19**).

Left ventricular failure leads to pulmonary edema with dyspnea and peripheral cyanosis. There is systemic venous congestion with dilatation of neck veins, peripheral edema, hepatomegaly, and ascites in right ventricular failure. Biventricular failure is frequently present.

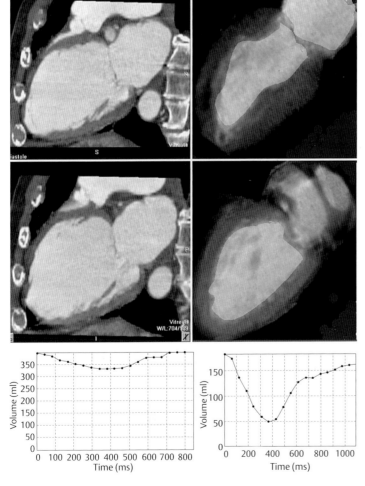

Fig. 10.**19** Left ventricular ejection fraction. *Left*: systole and diastole in cardiac failure. *Right*: systole and diastole in a normally functioning heart.

Cardiac failure may be due to:

- *Myocardial dysfunction*: A number of factors including ischemia, inflammation, and metabolic disorders may impair the contractile function of the myocardium. This leads to a decrease in the systolic ejection fraction of the ventricle.
- *Hemodynamic failure* results from severe valvular disease and other factors that impose a pressure or volume overload on the heart. Initially, the myocardium compensates with muscular hypertrophy. Eventually, the myocardial mass outstrips the coronary arterial supply leading to myogenic dilatation and overt heart failure.
- Cardiac failure due to *severe arrhythmia*: Arrhythmias disrupt the synchronization of atrial and ventricular function necessary for effective cardiac performance.

■ Radiologic Findings

See Pulmonary Edema (Chapter 7, p. 195).

Ischemic Heart Disease (IHD) and Myocardial Infarction (MI)

Ischemic heart disease is a major cause of morbidity and mortality in the industrialized world. Autopsies have shown a 50% incidence of significant coronary artery disease in men aged 45–60 years. Known risk factors include hypercholesterolemia, cigarette smoking, arterial hypertension, and diabetes mellitus. The clinical correlate of IHD is angina pectoris.

Atherosclerosis: There is initial deposition of cholesterol foci within the intima of the coronary arteries. This induces a circumscribed fibrous proliferation with plaque formation and this may lead to narrowing of the vessel lumen. Plaques may calcify over time. However, it is becoming apparent that noncalcified plaque may be more unstable and prone to rupture giving rise to acute coronary events.

IHD is the leading cause of myocardial infarction. Very occasionally, a coronary artery is occluded by embolus or involved in arteritis. Occlusion leads to myocardial cell necrosis in the territory of the affected vessel. In acute myocardial infarction, death may result from acute left ventricular failure, arrhythmias, ventricular rupture, septal perforation, or papillary muscle rupture. In patients who survive, myocardial infarcts heal by fibrosis.

Dressler's syndrome with pericardial and pleural effusions occasionally develops in the initial weeks postmyocardial infarction; it is thought to represent an autoimmune response to tissue antigens released by damaged myocardial cells.

Late sequelae of myocardial infarction include left ventricular aneurysms. True aneurysms involve all layers of the ventricular wall and most commonly occur in the anterolateral and apical regions. False aneurysms formed by endocardial tissue protruding through defects in the myocardium usually involve the inferior wall.

■ Radiologic Findings

The *chest radiograph* is usually normal in IHD in the absence of left ventricular decompensation. Occasionally coronary artery calcification may be seen (Fig. 10.**20**).

Approximately 50% of patients have a normal chest radiograph in the first 24 hours postmyocardial infarction. The remainder show *pulmonary edema often with a normal-sized cardiac silhouette*. Pulmonary edema is an important prognostic indicator. The mortality rate in the first 30 days has been reported to be 5% when there is no evidence of edema whereas the presence of edema has been reported to be associated with mortality rates approaching 80% (Battler 1980). Many acute complications of myocardial infarction are not visible on radiographs but are frequently associated with pulmonary edema.

In survivors of MI, a *left ventricular aneurysm* may calcify and appear as a circumscribed bulge with curvilinear calcification on the chest radiograph (Fig. 10.**21 a**).

Myocardial perfusion scintigraphy: Single photon emission computed tomography (SPECT) using thallium or technetium is currently the imaging modality most frequently used for assessment of myocardial perfusion. SPECT demonstrates perfusion defects as focal areas of decreased tracer uptake.

Ischemic myocardium shows decreased tracer uptake during exercise when perfusion is insufficient to meet the increased requirements of exercise; these defects resolve during rest/recovery.

Areas of irreversible myocardial ischemia (i. e., infarction) show decreased tracer uptake during stress/exercise and these defects persist during recovery/rest (Fig. 10.**22**).

▨ Computed Tomography (CT)

Nonelectrocardiographic (ECG)-gated Standard Helical CT of the Thorax

Coronary artery calcification may be readily visible (Figs. 10.**20 b, c**, 10.**23**) and should alert the physician to the possible presence of coronary artery disease. When there is no relevant history of IHD or renal impairment, these patients may benefit from cardiovascular risk assessment.

Non-ECG-gated contrast-enhanced helical CT of the thorax (when performed for evaluation of acute chest pain) occasionally may show *decreased myocardial enhancement* in the distribution of the occluded coronary artery in acute MI.

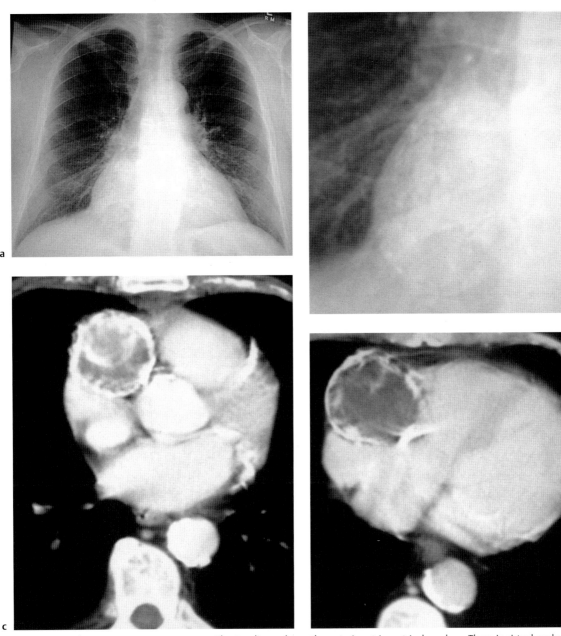

Fig. 10.**20** Right coronary artery aneurysm: Chest radiographs (**a**, **b**) show an ovoid opacity containing rim calcification overlying the right heart. CT shows aneurysmal right coronary artery within the anterior atrioventricular sulcus. There is virtual occlusion of the vessel with extensive intraluminal thrombus. Marked LAD and circumflex artery calcification are also noted (**c**, **d**).

CT findings in the patients post-MI include myocardial thinning ± LV aneurysm formation and areas of early subendocardial decreased enhancement (Fig. 10.**24**). Intraventricular thrombus may form within areas of ventricular akinesia/aneurysms. Focal areas of endo- and myocardial calcification may be secondary to old intraventricular thrombus (Fig. 10.**25a**, **b**) or represent myocardial calcification within a left ventricular aneurysm (Fig. 10.**21b**) respectively.

Dedicated ECG-gated Multi-Detector CT (MDCT) of the Heart
– Coronary artery calcium scoring: see Chapter 1, p. 29.
– MDCT coronary angiography and myocardial perfusion

For details of technique: see Chapter 1, p. 29.

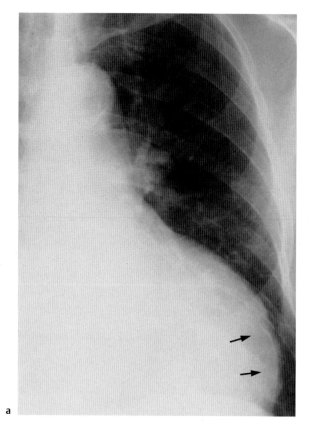

a

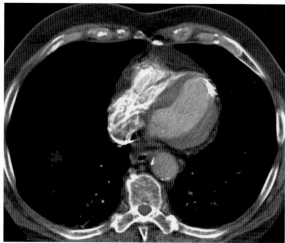

b

Fig. 10.**21 a, b**   Chest radiograph and CT show marked thinning and calcification of LV apical myocardium in a patient postmyo-cardial infarction.

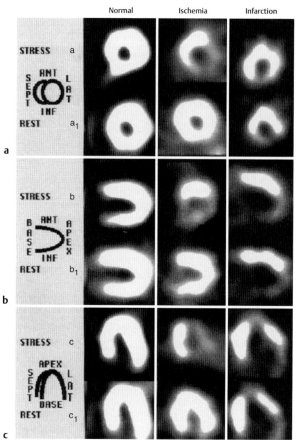

a

b

c

Fig. 10.**22 a–c**   Myocardial perfusion scintigraphy in reversible ischemia and infarction. Left ventricular myocardial uptake of thallium during stress (**a**, **b**, **c**) and during recovery (**a₁**, **b₁**, **c₁**) in three perpendicular planes of section. Homogeneous tracer up-take during stress and at rest is seen in normal subject. In patient with myocardial ischemia, focally decreased tracer uptake is seen in the laterobasal wall of the left ventricle during stress but this reverses on images acquired during recovery. Focal defect in per-fusion is irreversible in myocardial infarction.

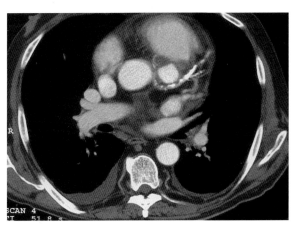

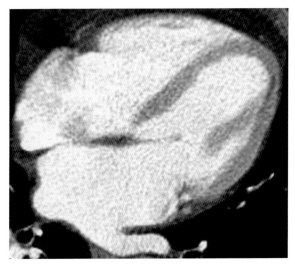

Fig. 10.**23** Axial CT image shows heavily calcified left coronary artery.

Fig. 10.**24** CT shows a crescent of subendocardial hypodensity within the LV freewall in a patient with a past history of myocardial infarction.

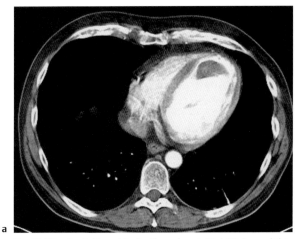

a

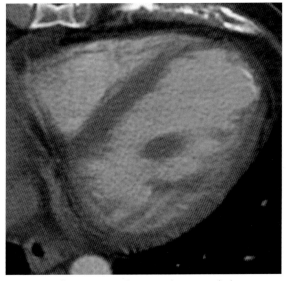

b

Fig. 10.**25 a, b** Left ventricular thrombus. Initial CT showed thinning of myocardium of left ventricular apex in patient with a past history of apical infarction. Hypodense thrombus is noted "floating" on contrast opacified blood within this hypokinetic area of the LV (**a**). Follow-up CT study acquired some weeks later postanticoagulation therapy shows resolution of thrombus with a thin crescent of calcium adherent to the apical endocardium (**b**).

MDCT in Assessment of Coronary Artery Disease

MDCT coronary angiography shows considerable promise in the assessment of asymptomatic and early-stage coronary artery disease. However, complete visualization of all segments of the epicardial coronary arteries with this technique to date has been limited by cardiac motion, the small size of the more distal vessels, and their tortuous course through standard imaging planes (Schoenhagen et al. 2004). Premedication with beta blocker therapy has been shown to give improved image quality particularly in visualization of the right coronary artery (Shim et al. 2005).

Studies using 4-slice MDCT technology report adequate visualization of 60–70% of all coronary arterial segments with a sensitivity and specificity of 91 and 84% for detection of stenoses in these adequately visualized segments in one study (Achenbach et al. 2001). Studies performed using 16-slice MDCT report improved visualization of vessel segments with similar sensitivity and specificity for detection of stenoses in adequately visualized segments to 4-slice MDCT (Nieman et al. 2002, Ropers et al. 2003). We await data from studies performed on 64-slice MDCT and further advances in CT technology.

MDCT in Acute Chest Pain/Myocardial Infarction

Ghersin et al. prospectively evaluated the role of 16-slice MDCT coronary angiography versus conventional angiography in the setting of acute chest pain syndrome. MDCT angiography was technically successful in 89% of patients and in this group, 96.9% of segments were visualized adequately. The sensitivity, specificity, positive predictive value, negative predictive value, and accuracy of MDCT in these segments was 80, 89, 52, 97, and 87%, respectively (Ghersin et al. 2006).

The improved spatial and temporal resolution of MDCT has also made possible assessment of myocardial perfusion. MDCT angiographic data is acquired during maximum enhancement of the coronary arteries and assessment of "first pass" myocardial perfusion may be possible from the same data set. Ko et al. have recently evaluated myocardial enhancement patterns in patients with acute myocardial infarction who had presented too late for thrombolysis on 2-phase contrast-enhanced ECG-gated MDCT. Subendocardial or transmural perfusion defects were seen in all but one patient on the early phase acquisition. The pattern of myocardial enhancement, however, was quite variable on late phase images in 75% of patients (Ko et al. 2006).

▓ Cardiac Magnetic Resonance Imaging (CMRI)

Evaluation of myocardial perfusion and viability: Myocardial perfusion may be evaluated with gadolinium-enhanced dynamic first-pass rest and stress studies, the latter during administration of a pharmacologic stress agent such as adenosine. Delayed imaging postgadolinium administration allows detection of regional myocardial hyperenhancement indicative of nonviable tissue. Dobutamine may also be used as a pharmacologic stress agent with assessment of resulting ventricular wall motion abnormalities.

Differences in myocardial perfusion between rest and stress suggest areas of reversible ischemia as with the scintigraphic technique. These changes can be analyzed visually or signal intensity curves may be assessed quantitatively or semi-quantitatively (Wagner et al. 2003). Prospective analyses with CMRI for the detection of coronary artery disease yielded a sensitivity of 92% and specificity of 86% using a 1-slice technique (Al-Saadi et al. 2000) and corresponding values of 94 and 83% using a 5-slice technique (Nagel et al. 1999). These correspond favorably with results of SPECT.

Revascularization of severely dysfunctional but viable myocardium may improve LV function and long-term survival. Augmentation of myocardial contractility on administration of a suitable pharmacologic stimulus such as dobutamine or absence of delayed myocardial hyperenhancement on a postgadolinium study are consistent with myocardial viability. The transmural extent of viability may also be assessed with gadolinium-enhanced CMRI and this has importance in prediction of improvement in LV function postrevascularization (Kim et al. 2000).

Myocardial infarction by definition indicates myocyte death and therefore nonviable myocardium. Acute MI may be hyperintense to normal myocardium on T2-weighted images. Thinning of the region of infarction may occur early with a resultant increase in the circumferential extent of the infarcted segment known as infarct expansion (Pirolo et al. 1986). Delayed hyperenhancement on postgadolinium sequences is consistent with nonviable infarcted myocardium (Fig. 10.**26**).

▓ Coronary Angiography

Coronary angiography currently remains the gold standard of reference for diagnosis of IHD and remains the investigation of choice in patients considered to be at moderate to high risk of significant coronary artery disease. Arterial stenoses and occlusions are readily demonstrated and the severity of each stenosis may be assessed (Fig. 10.**27**). In selected cases, it may be appropriate to proceed to coronary angioplasty ± coronary stent insertion (see Fig. 10.**45**).

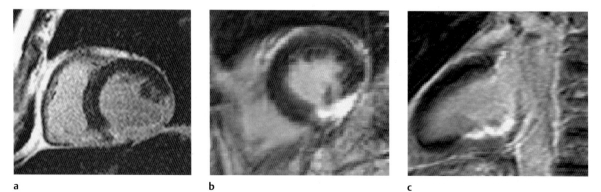

a   b   c

Fig. 10.**26 a–c**   Cardiac MR perfusion–viability study: Images show early (**a**) and late (**b**, **c**) hyperenhancement of nonviable myocardium in area of myocardial infarction.

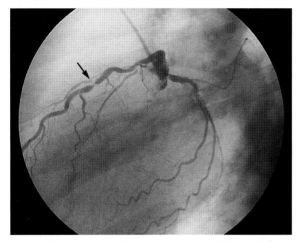

Fig. 10.**27**   Coronary angiogram in a patient with ischemic heart disease shows a high-grade stenosis in the left anterior descending (LAD) artery.

Cardiomyopathies

■ Clinical Features

Cardiomyopathies are diseases of the myocardium which do not result from pressure overload (valvular defects, hypertension, etc) or an inadequate blood supply (ischemic heart disease). The etiology is frequently unknown (primary cardiomyopathy) but some cases are secondary to exposure to toxic, infectious, or metabolic agents (secondary cardiomyopathy, Table 10.**2**).

Cardiomyopathies are classified into three main groups:
- *Dilated cardiomyopathy* is by far the most common form and is characterized by impairment in ventricular function with atrial and ventricular dilatation. Initially, there is only "forward failure" with decreased exercise tolerance. Eventually, there is frank decompensation with pulmonary edema (congestive cardiomyopathy).
- *Hypertrophic obstructive cardiomyopathy* (HOCM): There is ventricular wall thickening due to a histologically demonstrable hypertrophy of myocardial cells. The resultant loss of ventricular distensibility interferes with diastolic filling. Usually there is disproportionate hypertrophy of the septum; this may further narrow the left ventricular outflow tract leading in about one-third of cases to mitral regurgitation and left atrial dilatation.
- *Restrictive cardiomyopathy* is a rare disorder due to primary endocardial fibrosis. Involvement of the papillary muscles and chordae tendineae leads to secondary valvular dysfunction. The decreased ventricular distensibility impedes diastolic filling.

Table 10.**2**   Classification of secondary cardiomyopathies (from Schettler, 1990)

Myocarditis
- Viruses: coxsackie virus A and B, echovirus, influenza, infectious mononucleosis, poliomyelitis, mumps, measles, smallpox, varicella, psittacosis, lymphogranuloma venereum, herpes simplex, cytomegalovirus, infectious hepatitis, yellow fever
- Bacteria: diphtheria, sepsis
- Protozoons: *Trypanosoma cruzi* (Chagas disease), toxoplasmosis, amebiasis, malaria, leishmaniasis
- Parasites: trichinae, echinococcus, ascarids
- Spirochetes: syphilis, leptospirosis

Collagen diseases
- Rheumatic fever
- Systemic lupus erythematosus
- Dermatomyositis
- Scleroderma
- Ankylosing spondylitis
- Rheumatoid arthritis

Hyperimmune cardiomyopathies
- Drugs (e. g., penicillin, phenylbutazone, aureomycin, antituberculosis agents, reserpine)
- Postvaccination
- Dressler's syndrome

Toxic cardiomyopathies
- Alcohol
- Drug toxicity (e. g., cytostatic drugs, tricyclic antidepressants)
- Uremia
- Carbon monoxide poisoning

Metabolic and endocrine disorders
- Hyperthyroidism
- Hypothyroidism
- Acromegaly
- Pheochromocytoma
- Diabetes mellitus
- Hemochromatosis
- Amyloidosis
- Storage disease, lipid storage diseases, glycogen storage diseases

Neuromuscular diseases
- Friedreich ataxia
- Myotonic muscular dystrophy
- Progressive muscular dystrophy
- Myasthenia gravis

Neoplastic cardiomyopathies
- Primary and metastatic neoplasms
- Lymphatic and myeloid leukemia

Granulomatous cardiomyopathy
- Sarcoidosis

Cardiomyopathies due to physical causes
- Radiotherapy
- ECT
- Heat stroke
- Cardiac trauma

Puerperal cardiomyopathy

Nutritional disorders
- Beriberi
- Kwashiorkor
- Pellagra
- Scurvy

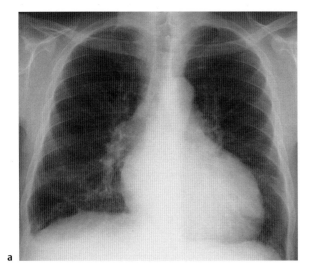

a

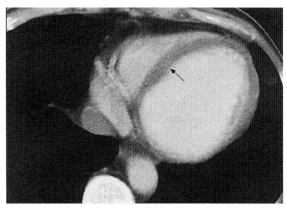

b

Fig. 10.**28 a, b**   Dilated cardiomyopathy. There is cardiomegaly and features of pulmonary venous hypertension. Axial CT image shows left ventricular dilatation.

Clinical manifestations are usually those of ventricular impairment with impaired exercise tolerance, dyspnea, and peripheral edema.

■ Radiologic Findings

The *chest radiograph* in dilated cardiomyopathy shows cardiomegaly with or without pulmonary edema and pleural effusions (Fig. 10.**28**). In HOCM, the heart may be normal in size and shape or features of left ventricular hypertrophy may be evident. In restrictive cardiomyopathy, cardiac size is usually normal but there may be right atrial enlargement and diminished pulmonary vascularity due to reduced right ventricular output.

Echocardiography: There is ventricular dilatation in dilated cardiomyopathy with uniform thinning of the myocardium. The left ventricular cavity is small in HOCM particularly at end systole and left ventricular hypertrophy is almost always present. Septal hypertrophy is most common and is frequently greater than 20 mm in thickness (normal value is less than or equal to 12 mm). Systolic anterior motion of the anterior mitral valve leaflet is characteristic of HOCM but is seen in a minority of cases (Raphael and Gibson 1992).

Computed tomography and magnetic resonance imaging: CT and MRI findings in dilated cardiomyopathy and HOCM are as described for echocardiography (Figs. 10.**28 b**, 10.**29**). MRI may be helpful in distinguishing restrictive cardiomyopathy from constrictive pericarditis. Myocardial thickening is seen in restrictive cardiomyopathy particularly when it is associated with amyloidosis (Boer et al. 1977). This condition is frequently complicated by mitral and tricuspid regurgitation.

Acquired Valvular Heart Disease

Mitral Stenosis

Mitral stenosis is characterized by restricted opening of the mitral valve as blood flows from the left atrium into the left ventricle. It most commonly results from cardiac involvement in rheumatic fever with scarring and thickening of the valve cusps and fusion of the commissures. This reduces the opening area of the mitral orifice from the normal 4–6 to 2.5 cm² (grade 1 stenosis), to 1 cm² (grade 2), or to less than 1 cm² (grade 3). The increased pressure proximal to the stenosed valve leads to:
- Dilatation of the left atrium
- Right ventricular hypertrophy and eventual right heart failure with ventricular dilatation and tricuspid insufficiency
- Raised pulmonary venous pressure with pulmonary congestion and edema

Clinically, there is frequently a history of streptococcal infection (sore throat, scarlet fever). Cardiac auscultation reveals a loud first heart sound, a presystolic crescendo murmur, and a mitral opening snap. There is frequently associated atrial fibrillation (Fig. 10.**30**) which increases the risk of systemic embolization. Dyspnea on exertion may progress to resting dyspnea and orthopnea. The lips may be cyanosed and there may be reactive dilatation of the skin capillaries (*mitral facies*).

Eventually, there is right ventricular decompensation with peripheral edema, elevated jugular venous pressure, and hepatomegaly.

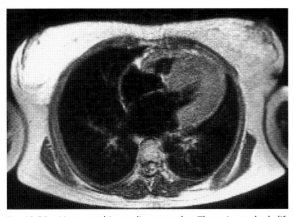

Fig. 10.**29**   Hypertrophic cardiomyopathy. There is marked diffuse thickening of the left ventricular myocardium. This patient was normotensive and had no valvular heart disease.

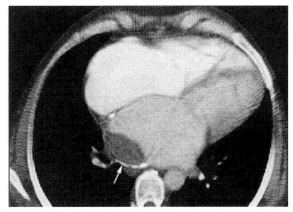

Fig. 10.**30**   CT shows left atrial thrombus in a patient with atrial fibrillation.

■ Radiologic Findings

The principal *chest radiographic* features are:
- *Left atrial enlargement* with narrowing of the retrocardiac space at the atrial level on the lateral radiograph. The frontal radiograph shows fullness of the upper left cardiac border and a double contour sign (*mitral configuration*, Fig. 10.**31**). In the elderly, calcification of the mitral annulus may be seen on the chest radiograph but this does not signify the presence of significant valvular disease (Fig. 10.**32**).
- *Features of pulmonary venous hypertension* with upper-zone blood flow redistribution. Interstitial and alveolar edema may develop with increasing degrees of pulmonary venous hypertension. Fine interstitial change in long-standing disease after multiple episodes of pulmonary edema signifies hemosiderosis due to fibrous organization of minute hemorrhages.
- *Right ventricular hypertrophy* with an increased area of sternal contact on the lateral chest radiograph and prominence of the pulmonary outflow tract.

Echocardiography shows:
- A thickened mitral valve.
- A decrease in size of the mitral orifice.
- Left atrial dilatation.
- Increased ventricular inflow velocity.
- Continuous wave Doppler allows estimation of the mitral diastolic flow velocity at the apex, and the diastolic gradient across the valve may then be calculated.

Magnetic resonance imaging may be useful when the echocardiographic data are insufficient for diagnosis or when echo findings are inconsistent with clinical data. The MR study, however, may be limited in patients with atrial fibrillation with the potential for erroneous measurements (Didier 2003).

Spin echo sequences demonstrate thickening of the valve leaflets, left atrial dilatation, and a small left ventricle. GRE sequences allow estimation of the degree of stenosis based on the size and extent of the abnormal flow jet during diastole in the left ventricle. VEC-MR allows calculation of the maximum velocity within the stenotic jet and the pressure gradient can be calculated using the modified Bernoulli equation (Heidenreich et al. 1995).

Cardiac catheterization: Both the pulmonary capillary wedge pressure (during right heart catheterization) and the pressure in the left ventricle (left ventricular catheterization) are measured and the transvalvular pressure gradient can then be calculated. Left ventricular angiography demonstrates:
- Thickened valve cusps which bow into the left ventricle in the filling phase (diastolic doming).
- A thin, turbulent jet of opacified blood entering the opacified left ventricle during diastole (*wash-in jet*).

Mitral Regurgitation

Mitral regurgitation/insufficiency is characterized by incomplete closure of the mitral valve during systole allowing blood to regurgitate from the left ventricle into the left atrium. It may be due to:
- Ruptured chordae tendineae or papillary muscle dysfunction following myocardial infarction.
- Valvular scarring and contraction secondary to bacterial or rheumatic endocarditis.
- Stretching of the mitral valve ring (functional incompetence).

Mitral valve prolapse results from elongation of the chordae tendineae and mucoid degeneration of the leaflets; this allows prolapse of the mitral valve into the left

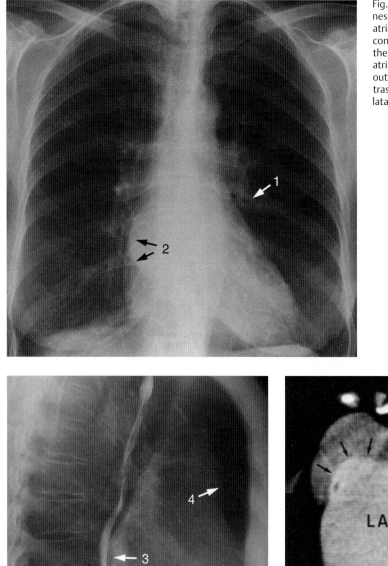

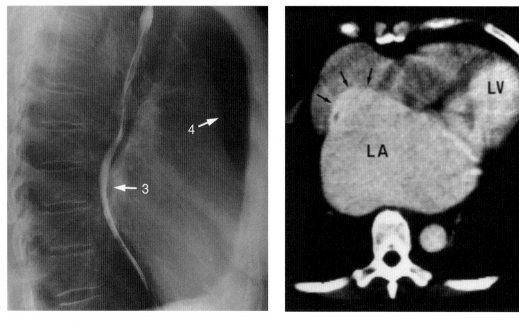

Fig. 10.**31 a–c**   Mitral stenosis. Note the fullness of the upper left heart border (dilated left atrial appendage) (1), the "double right heart contour" configuration (2), the narrowing of the retrocardiac space at the level of the atrium (3), and the prominent right ventricular outflow tract/main pulmonary artery (4). Contrast-enhanced CT shows marked left atrial dilatation.

atrium during ventricular systole. It may be present without associated regurgitation.

Regurgitation of blood during systole depends in part on the pressure within the left ventricle. The increased volume of blood flowing from the atrium to the ventricle in diastole and refluxing into the atrium during systole causes dilatation of both chambers. However, in con-

tradistinction to mitral stenosis, pulmonary venous hypertension tends to occur quite late in mitral regurgitation.

Clinical manifestations in advanced disease include pulmonary congestion with dyspnea on exertion and at rest. Cardiac auscultation reveals a diminished first heart sound and a high-frequency pansystolic murmur.

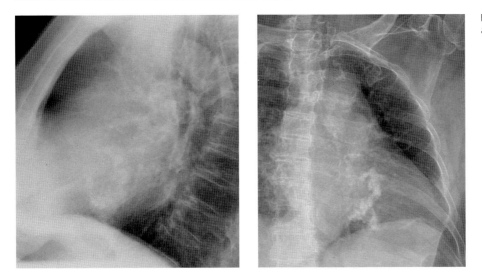

Fig. 10.**32**   Mitral annulus calcification.

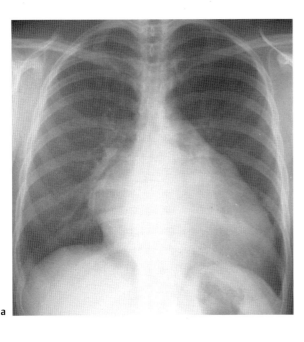

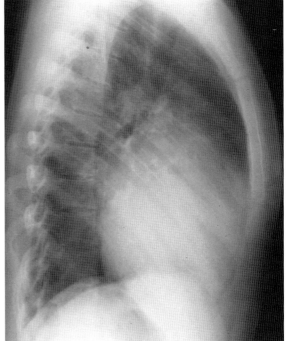

a

Fig. 10.**33 a, b**   Mitral regurgitation. Radiographs show biventricular and left atrial enlargement.

b

■ Radiologic Findings

The *chest radiograph* shows left atrial and left ventricular enlargement (Figs. 10.**33**, 10.**34**). Pulmonary venous hypertension and edema develop as the disease progresses. A useful rule of thumb is that mitral stenosis causes relatively severe pulmonary congestion and mild left atrial dilatation while mitral insufficiency causes a greater degree of atrial dilatation with less marked pulmonary venous congestion (Fig. 10.**35**). Because left ventricular output is decreased the aorta is usually small; a prominent aortic arch should raise suspicion of coexisting aortic valve disease.

Echocardiography:
- The mitral valves leaflets are thickened.
- There may be dilatation of the valve ring.
- The maximum diameter of the left atrium is greater than 40 mm.
- Ruptured chordae tendineae or papillary muscles appear as additional echoes in the region of the mitral valve.

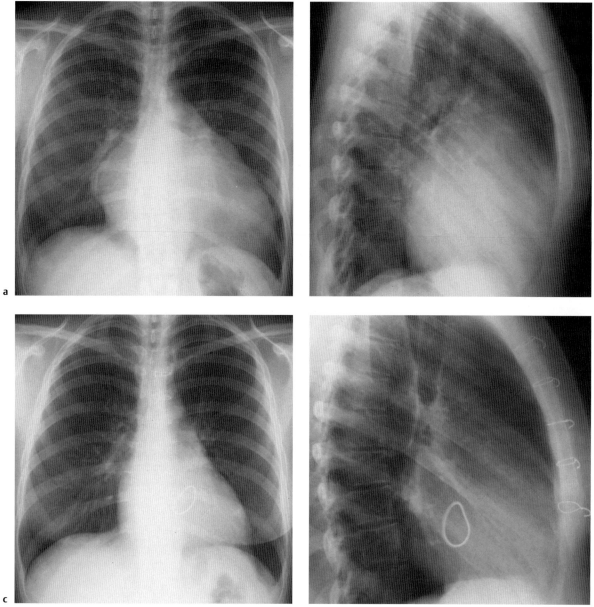

Fig. 10.**34 a–d**   Mitral regurgitation: Chest radiographs before (**a, b**) and 3 years postinsertion of mitral valve prosthesis (**c, d**).

The need for surgery is determined by the severity of symptoms, an ejection fraction of less than 60% or a LV end-systolic dimension of greater than 45 mm as determined by Doppler echocardiography (Carabello and Crawford 1997).

Magnetic resonance imaging: Spin echo sequences will show altered cardiac morphology including left atrial and ventricular dilatation. GRE sequences allow assessment of the severity of mitral regurgitation based on the area of the signal void that arises from the mitral valve. Mitral regurgitation may also be assessed with VEC-MR imaging by comparing diastolic flow across the mitral annulus with systolic outflow across the ascending aorta. These have virtually identical values in the normal individual but left ventricular inflow is increased in mitral regurgitation. The difference between the two values therefore corresponds to the volume of mitral regurgitation (Didier 2003).

Cardiac catheterization: The left ventriculogram distinguishes four grades of mitral incompetence:

Grade I: Opacified blood regurgitates to the valvular region of the left atrium.

Grade II: Contrast medium opacifies the atrium, but less than the ventricle.

Grade III: Contrast medium opacifies the atrium and ventricles equally.

Grade IV: Contrast medium opacifies the atrium and the pulmonary veins.

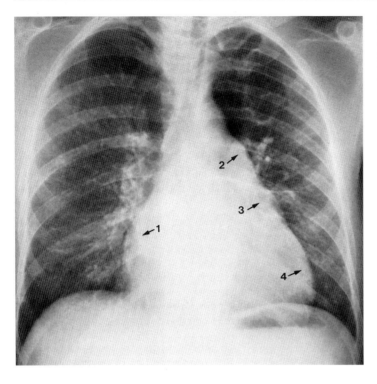

Fig. 10.**35** Chest radiograph in combined mitral valve disease. Note the "double right heart contour" sign (1), pulmonary artery dilatation (2), prominence of the atrial appendage (3), and left ventricular dilatation (4). The aortic arch is relatively small due to decreased LV output.

Aortic Stenosis

Aortic stenosis is characterized by insufficient opening of the aortic valve during ventricular systole. Causes include rheumatic endocarditis which scars and partially fuses the valve cusps. Congenital bicuspid aortic valve and aortic sclerosis which leads to stiffening and calcification of the valve may also lead to aortic stenosis. The left ventricle initially adapts to the pressure overload by concentric hypertrophy of the left ventricular myocardium and this, while reducing the volume of the chamber leads to little or no cardiomegaly. When the ventricle reaches a critical muscle mass, it exceeds its arterial supply and undergoes myogenic dilatation which increases the overall size of the heart. If this is untreated, left ventricular failure will eventually develop.

Clinically, auscultation reveals a systolic murmur which is transmitted to the carotid arteries. The disease may be virtually asymptomatic in its compensated stage but later produces angina pectoris (relative coronary insufficiency), syncopal attacks (decreased cardiac output), and dyspnea (left heart failure).

■ Radiologic Findings

The *chest radiograph* may be normal in the compensated stage or there may be poststenotic dilatation of the proximal ascending aorta. Later the typical *aortic configuration* develops with a rounded cardiac apex and left ventricular enlargement (Figs. 10.**3**, 10.**36**). Features of

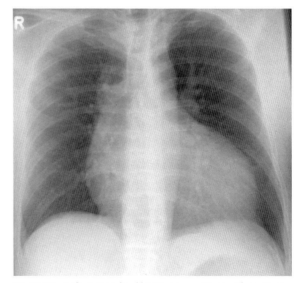

Fig. 10.**36** Left ventricular dilatation in a patient with aortic stenosis.

pulmonary venous hypertension and edema eventually supervene.

Echocardiography shows disorganization of the valve cusps with replacement by highly reflective calcium. CW Doppler allows estimation of peak systolic pressure gradient across the valve.

Magnetic resonance imaging: Spin echo sequences may show a bicuspid valve, thickening and bulging of the cusps, and dilatation of the ascending aorta. Cine GRE and VEC-MR allow assessment of the severity of the stenosis based on the size and extent of the abnormal flow jet and the maximum velocity of the stenotic jet, respectively.

Cardiac catheterization: Aortic valve calcification is seen on fluoroscopy. There is partial opening of the aortic valve during systole and a negative jet of nonopaque blood may be seen passing through the stenosed valve at aortography.

Aortic Regurgitation

Aortic regurgitation/insufficiency is characterized by incomplete closure of the valve during diastole allowing blood to reenter the left ventricle. It may result from rheumatic fever, bacterial endocarditis, or be due to syphilitic aortitis. Acute AR may be due to aortic dissection with secondary involvement of the valve ring.

Aortic regurgitation leads to increased end-diastolic volume which in the initial compensated stage is not associated with an increase in end-diastolic pressure. In more advanced disease, the left ventricle fails and end-diastolic pressure rises. This in turn is associated with functional mitral incompetence, left atrial dilatation, and pulmonary venous congestion.

Cardiac auscultation reveals an early diastolic murmur. Blood pressure amplitude is increased (water-hammer pulse). The decompensated stage presents with palpitations, tachycardia, and left ventricular failure.

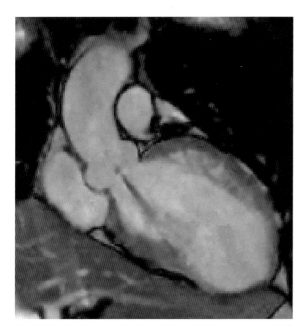

Fig. 10.**37** Aortic regurgitation. GRE cine MRI demonstrates left ventricular enlargement and the regurgitant jet from the aortic valve into the left ventricle.

■ Radiologic Findings

Chest radiograph: Left ventricular enlargement with an aortic configuration reflects adaptive dilatation rather than the myogenic decompensation seen in aortic stenosis. The degree of aortic dilatation may be more marked than is seen in aortic stenosis. Left atrial enlargement, pulmonary venous hypertension, and edema develop with increasing degrees of left ventricular failure.

Echocardiography demonstrates left ventricular hypertrophy and dilatation and allows evaluation of LV function. It may demonstrate abnormality of aortic cusps, lesions of the annulus, or dilatation of the aortic root. Color Doppler flow-mapping allows semiquantitative assessment of the severity of regurgitation based on the measurement of regurgitant jet length and width.

Magnetic resonance imaging: Spin echo sequences allow assessment of abnormal valve/valve ring morphology and size and function of the left ventricle. GRE sequences demonstrate the regurgitant jet and with VEC-MR allow calculation of the severity of the regurgitation (Fig. 10.**37**).

Cardiac catheterization and aortography: An injection of contrast medium into the ascending aorta allows grading of the degree of reflux:

Grade I: Reflux into the perivalvular region of the left ventricle.
Grade II: Opacification of the entire left ventricle.
Grade III: Virtually all the contrast medium regurgitates into the ventricle.
Grade IV: Regurgitated contrast medium is retained in the left ventricle for several cardiac cycles.

Multivalvular Disease

Involvement of two valves, usually the aortic and mitral valves, is common in patients with acquired valvular heart disease. Trivalvular disease is uncommon and four-valve involvement is extremely rare. In addition, functional incompetence of a second valve may develop as a secondary feature in advanced disease; for example in aortic stenosis, left ventricular dilatation leads to stretching of the mitral valve ring and functional mitral incompetence.

■ Radiologic Findings

Chest radiograph: Changes usually reflect the hemodynamic consequences of a combination of abnormalities that are associated with individual valve dysfunction. There is frequently marked cardiomegaly and given the frequent involvement of the mitral valve, left atrial dilatation is a common finding.

Hypertensive Heart Disease

Systemic arterial hypertension is defined as a resting arterial blood pressure exceeding 140/95–100 mmHg. It predisposes to atherosclerosis and leads to pressure overload of the left ventricle. Initially, this pressure overload evokes compensatory hypertrophy of the left ventricular muscle (concentric hypertrophy). Later relative coronary insufficiency develops, leading to myogenic dilatation with decreased ventricular output and eventual pulmonary edema.

■ Radiologic Findings

The *chest radiograph* is initially normal. Later, there is left ventricular dilatation and a rounded cardiac apex (*aortic configuration*). The lateral chest radiograph shows narrowing of the retrocardiac space at the level of the ventricle (see Fig. 10.**4c**, **d**). Coexisting aortic atherosclerosis leads to thoracic aortic ectasia and tortuosity and intimal calcification.

Echocardiography and *MRI* will show a concentric increase in left ventricular wall thickness and allow evaluation of ventricular function. Left ventricular dilatation is seen in decompensated hypertensive heart disease.

Cardiac Neoplasms

Primary cardiac tumors are rare and most cardiac neoplasms result from infiltration by adjacent malignant pulmonary or mediastinal tumors. The most common primary cardiac tumor is myxoma which is amenable to surgical excision. It most commonly arises from the interatrial septum and grows within the left atrium where it may lead to venous inflow stasis, pulmonary venous hypertension, and pulmonary edema (Fig. 10.**38**).

Other primary cardiac tumors including rhabdomyoma, myosarcoma, liposarcoma, and fibrosarcoma are very rare (Fig. 10.**39**).

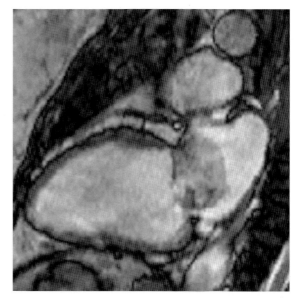

Fig. 10.**38**   Left atrial myxoma. MRI demonstrates hypointense lesion lying within the left atrium adjacent to the mitral valve.

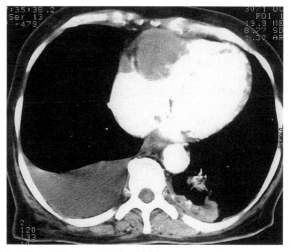

Fig. 10.**39**   Right ventricular rhabdomyoma.

Imaging the Heart Post-Intervention and Surgery

Cardiac Pacemakers

Single-chamber permanent pacemakers with an electrode in the right ventricle (VVI) are common. This type of device senses the ventricle (V), stimulates it as needed (V), and inhibits the impulse if it senses a satisfactory intrinsic rate (I) (Figs. 10.**40**, 10.**41**).

If the atrial impulse is to be used as a trigger in patients with AV block, a dual-chamber pacing system with electrodes in both the right atrium and right ventricle (DDD) may be inserted (Fig. 10.**42**).

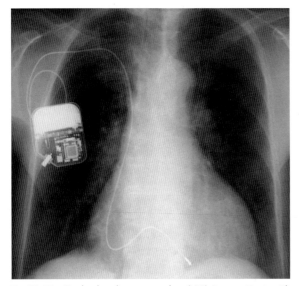

Fig. 10.**40** Single-chamber pacemaker (VVI) in a patient with atrial fibrillation.

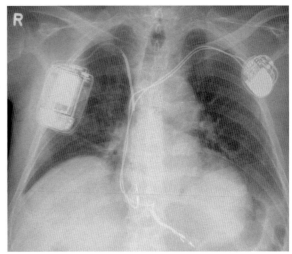

Fig. 10.**42** Dual-chamber pacemaker (DDD) with atrial and ventricular leads. Defibrillator is also present.

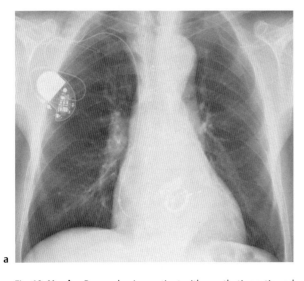

a

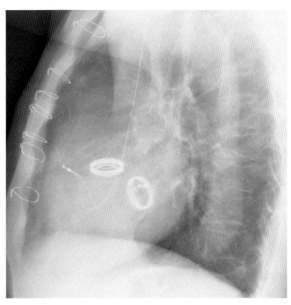

b

Fig. 10.**41 a, b** Pacemaker in a patient with prosthetic aortic and mitral valves.

■ Radiologic Findings

The *chest radiograph* documents the position of the pacemaker within the chest wall and the position of the electrodes within the cardiac chambers. Fluoroscopy can demonstrate a "floating electrode" when the electrode tip loses its endocardial attachment.

Coronary Artery Bypass Graft (CABG) Surgery

A bypass graft (venous or internal mammary artery) is interposed between the aorta and coronary artery in patients with significant coronary artery stenoses or occlusions.

■ Radiologic Findings

The *chest radiograph* shows the cerclage wires used to reapproximate the sternotomy and surgical clips at the sites of bypass (Fig. 10.**43**).

Coronary Stents

Coronary artery stenoses are frequently dilated with a balloon-tipped catheter at coronary angioplasty. Restenosis at these sites may be prevented by placement of a coronary stent. The metallic mesh of these stents can be visualized on chest radiographs and at CT (Figs. 10.**44**, 10.**45**).

ECG-gated MDCT coronary angiography particularly with 16- or 64-slice technology may be valuable in noninvasive assessment of stent patency.

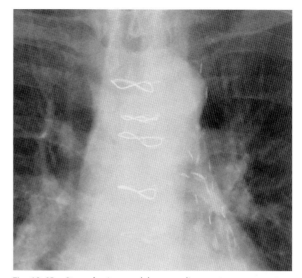

Fig. 10.**43**   Sternal wires and bypass clips postcoronary artery bypass grafting (CABG) surgery.

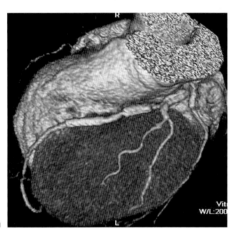

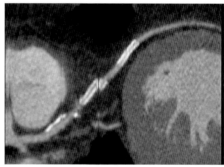

Fig. 10.**44 a, b**   Double stent in LAD coronary artery. Surface-rendered 3D reconstruction (**a**) and maximum intensity image along the course of the vessel (**b**).

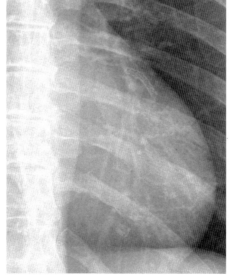

Fig. 10.**45 a, b**   Left coronary stent on chest radiograph.

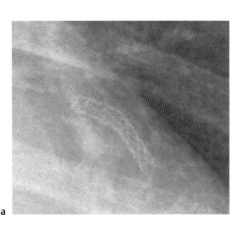

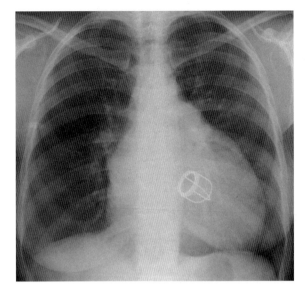

Prosthetic Heart Valves

The earliest prosthetic valve in clinical use was the Starr–Edwards ball-valve prosthesis (Fig. 10.**46**). A large number of mechanical valves and bioprostheses are available today.

The median sternotomy wires, the mechanical valve prosthesis, or the metallic ring of a bioprosthesis are visible on the chest radiograph.

Fig. 10.**46**   Combined mitral valve disease treated with a Starr–Edwards ball-and-cage valve.

Pericardial Disease

The pericardium envelops the heart and the origins of the great vessels. Its visceral layer (epicardium) is fused with the myocardium and this glides on its parietal layer (pericardium) during cardiac contraction.

Pericardial Effusion

Pericardial effusions greater than 200 mL in volume may interfere with cardiac filling (cardiac tamponade). Effusions may represent inflammatory exudate (e. g., tuber-

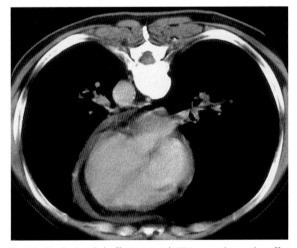

Fig. 10.**47**   Pericardial effusion. Axial CT image shows the effusion separated from the myocardium by a hypodense layer of epicardial fat.

culous), transudate (LV failure), hemorrhage (infarction, trauma), or malignant involvement of the pericardium.

■ Radiologic Findings

Chest radiograph: There is cardiomegaly and the cardiac silhouette is globular or triangular in shape. Pulmonary blood flow is often diminished due to compression of the right heart chambers; gross cardiomegaly in the absence of pulmonary edema should raise the suspicion of a pericardial effusion. The lateral chest radiograph occasionally shows a double fat stripe as the interposed pericardial stripe (soft-tissue density) is widened by the effusion.

Echocardiography, *CT*, and *MRI* all clearly demonstrate the effusion, echocardiography being the most frequently used modality in clinical practice (Fig. 10.**47**).

Constrictive Pericarditis

Inflammation and fibrosis may lead to pericardial thickening and obliteration of the pericardial cavity. The thickened pericardium, which may calcify, interferes with diastolic heart filling. These changes tend to have a more profound effect on the right than the left heart chambers resulting in systemic venous congestion with hepatomegaly, ascites, and peripheral edema.

■ Radiologic Findings

Chest radiograph: The heart is normal in size and pericardial calcification may be visible. Fluoroscopy shows diminished cardiac pulsation.

Echocardiography and cine *MRI* show restricted cardiac filling and diminished cardiac pulsation. Absence of myocardial thickening helps to distinguish constrictive pericarditis from restrictive cardiomyopathy. MRI also allows estimation of pericardial thickness (normal thickness is less than 4 mm).

Computed tomography may show pericardial thickening ± calcification (Fig. 10.**48**).

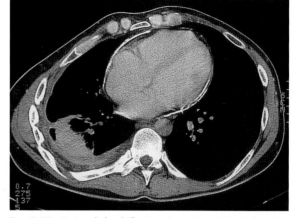

Fig. 10.**48**   Pericardial calcification in patient with clinical features of constrictive pericarditis. Pleural thickening and lung infolding is an incidental finding.

Pericardial Cysts and Diverticula

These fluid-filled lesions lie in close proximity to or in contact with the pericardium. While a pericardial cyst is separate from the pericardium, a diverticulum communicates with the pericardial sac. Pericardial cysts are most commonly found in the right cardiophrenic angle. Diverticula tend to arise from the pericardium which envelops the right atrium. Both lesions are incidental findings and have no pathologic significance.

■ Radiologic Findings

Chest radiograph: Both pericardial cysts and diverticula appear as smooth, well-defined, soft-tissue opacities which are contiguous with the cardiac silhouette.

Echocardiography, *CT*, and *MRI* show thin-walled anechoic, fluid density or signal intensity lesions, respectively in a characteristic paracardiac location (Fig. 10.**49**).

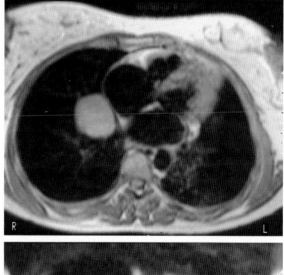

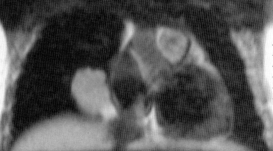

Fig. 10.**49a, b**   Pericardial cyst. Spin echo MR shows hyperintense contents of the cyst.

11 Diseases of the Mediastinum

The mediastinum is bordered anteriorly by the sternum, posteriorly by the thoracic vertebral column, and laterally by the mediastinal pleura. Its contents include the heart, esophagus, trachea, thyroid gland, thymus, major nerves, and vascular structures.

Mediastinal Displacement

Complete mediastinal displacement results in asymmetric pulmonary expansion.

More localized mediastinal displacement results in unilateral extension of a pleuropulmonary recess across the midline. These localized displacements frequently result from pulmonary atelectasis and usually involve the anterior or posterior mediastinum (Fig. 11.1).

Mediastinal displacement may be fixed when the differential diagnosis includes:

- Scoliosis
- Fibrothorax/pleural neoplasia
- Pulmonary atelectasis
- Pneumonectomy

or dynamic when there is mediastinal shift during the respiratory cycle and when the differential diagnosis includes:

- Tension pneumothorax
- Unilateral pulmonary hyperinflation (e. g., due to foreign body aspiration)
- Unilateral diaphragmatic paralysis

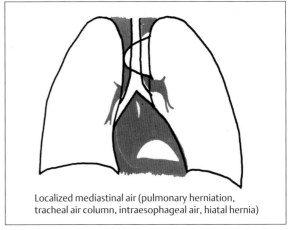

Localized mediastinal air (pulmonary herniation, tracheal air column, intraesophageal air, hiatal hernia)

Fig. 11.**1** Air in the mediastinum.

Air in the Mediastinum

Air in the Esophagus and Stomach

Occasionally, swallowed air may be identified within the esophagus; it is recognized by visualization of the left esophageal wall separate from the azygoesophageal stripe. Megaesophagus, esophageal diverticula, hiatus hernia, and communicating esophageal duplication cysts may also appear radiographically as air-containing lesions.

Pneumomediastinum

Air from ruptured alveoli dissects along the peribronchovascular connective tissue planes into the adjacent mediastinum (Figs. 11.**2**, 11.**3**). Alveolar rupture is usually a consequence of marked increases in intra-alveolar pressure during mechanical ventilation, severe bouts of coughing, or acute exacerbations of asthma. Blunt chest trauma with rupture of the esophagus or tracheobronchial tree will also result in pneumomediastinum (Table 11.**1**).

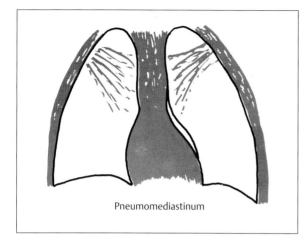

Fig. 11.**2**   Pneumomediastinum.

Table 11.**1**   Causes of pneumomediastinum

Traumatic	Pulmonary contusion and pneumothorax
	Bronchial rupture
Spontaneous	Acute exacerbation of asthma
	Pneumonia (especially in children)
	Acute mediastinitis with gas-forming organisms
	Spontaneous esophageal rupture (Boerhaave syndrome)
Iatrogenic	Tracheotomy
	Positive-pressure ventilation

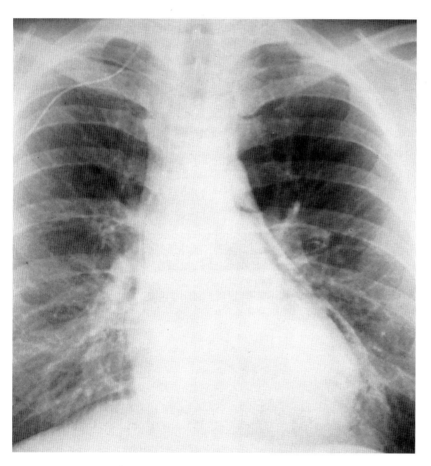

Fig. 11.**3**   Pneumomediastinum. Air column separates the visceral from the parietal layers of the mediastinal pleura.

Frequently, there is associated deep cervical and subcutaneous chest wall emphysema. Occasionally, a large pneumomediastinum may lead to impaired systemic venous return and respiratory compromise.

■ Radiologic Findings

See Chapter 8, p. 210.

Non-Neoplastic Mediastinal Widening

Mediastinal widening is a common radiographic finding. Anteroposterior (AP) supine views taken in shallow inspiration or expiration lead to foreshortening of mediastinal structures and to apparent widening of the mediastinum. Causes of *pathologic mediastinal widening* include mediastinal hemorrhage and inflammation, esophageal, aortic and vascular dilatation, and lymph node enlargement.

Acute Mediastinitis

Acute mediastinitis is a serious though rare pathologic process with a mortality rate approaching 50%. Initial diffuse purulent inflammation progresses to abscess formation and these are frequently multiple. Mediastinitis may be secondary to esophageal perforation or postoperative infection. Less commonly it results from direct spread of infection from the retropharyngeal space, lung, or from suppurative mediastinal lymph nodes.

These patients tend to be very ill with severe retrosternal chest pain and pyrexia. When esophageal perforation is present, there is associated dysphagia and deep cervical emphysema.

■ Radiologic Findings

The *chest radiograph* shows mediastinal widening with obliteration of fat planes, an accompanying pneumomediastinum, and associated unilateral or bilateral pleural effusions.

In diffuse mediastinitis, *computed tomography* (CT) shows diffuse soft tissue infiltration of the mediastinum with loss of the normal fat planes. When there is progression to abscess formation, gas bubbles and air–fluid levels may be seen within discrete collections (Armstrong 1995).

Upper gastrointestinal contrast swallow using low osmolar water-soluble contrast medium will show leakage of contrast into the mediastinum from an esophageal perforation.

Chronic Mediastinitis

Chronic mediastinitis is a granulomatous inflammatory disorder which may progress to fibrosis. Known causes include tuberculosis and in the United States, histoplasmosis. However, many cases are of unknown etiology. Idiopathic mediastinal fibrosis may be of autoimmune etiology and there may be an association with retroperitoneal fibrosis (Ormond disease).

Patients may initially be asymptomatic. Symptoms usually result from stenosis or occlusion of the superior vena cava or from extrinsic narrowing of the esophagus and tracheobronchial tree.

■ Radiologic Findings

The *chest radiograph* usually shows mediastinal widening ± calcification in cases of histoplasmosis. Other findings are determined by the severity of the obstructive phenomena and include pulmonary oligemia if a pulmonary artery is involved. Narrowing of the trachea and major bronchi may also be seen.

Computed tomography will demonstrate soft tissue infiltration of the mediastinum and there may be airway and vascular encasement. Dilated collateral vessels also may be present.

Diseases of the Thoracic Aorta

The thoracic aorta runs cranially in the anterior mediastinum (ascending aorta) from its origin at the aortic valve, curves posteriorly over the left main bronchus to form the aortic arch, and passes caudally to the diaphragm (descending aorta). The normal diameters based on CT data are:
- Aortic root: 3.7 ± 0.3 cm.
- Ascending aorta: 3.3 ± 0.6 cm.
- Descending aorta: 2.4 ± 0.3 cm.

The aortic isthmus lies just distal to the origin of the left subclavian artery at the level of the ligamentum arteriosum.

Aortic Anomalies

Coarctation of the aorta has been discussed in Chapter 10, p. 244.

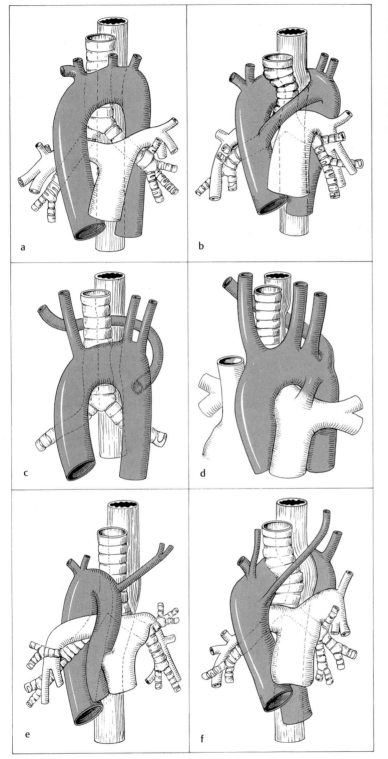

Fig. 11.**4a–f** Aortic and great vessel anomalies (modified from Schinz 1983). **a** Normal left-sided aortic arch. **b** Double aortic arch. **c, d** Left aortic arch with an aberrant right subclavian artery. **c** Right sub-clavian artery crossing the mediastinum be-tween the trachea and esophagus. **d** Right subclavian artery crossing behind the esophagus.
e Right aortic arch, anterior type. **f** Right aortic arch, posterior type.

Other common anomalies include (Figs. 11.**4**–11.**6**):

- *Left-sided aortic arch with aberrant right subclavian artery*. This is usually asymptomatic but may cause dysphagia (dysphagia lusoria) in the elderly when the

subclavian artery becomes ectatic. When aneurys-mal, the artery may present as a superior mediastinal mass.

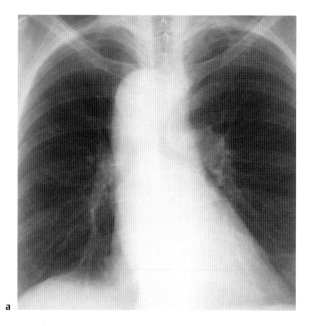

a

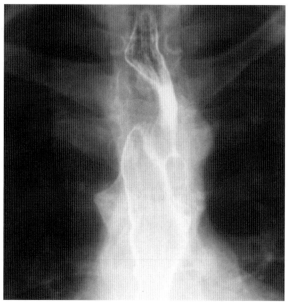

c

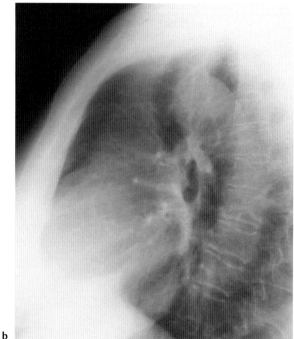

b

Fig. 11.**5 a–c**   Right aortic arch, posterior type. Note the displacement of the trachea (**b**) and the indentation of the esophagus (**c**). This patient had presented clinically with dysphagia lusoria.

- *Right aortic arch with aberrant left subclavian artery* is the most common right arch anomaly and is usually asymptomatic. A right paratracheal soft-tissue shadow is seen on the frontal radiograph and the aberrant subclavian artery produces a retroesophageal impression on the barium-filled esophagus at contrast swallow.
- *Mirror image branching of a right-sided aortic arch* is associated with congenital heart disease in over 90% of cases.

Aortic Ectasia

Loss of normal vessel elasticity results in aortic dilatation and ectasia; associated changes may be found in the aortic valve. This degenerative process is common in the elderly and eventually may result in aneurysmal dilatation (Higgins 1992, Fig. 11.**7**).

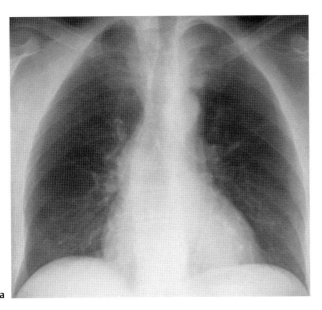

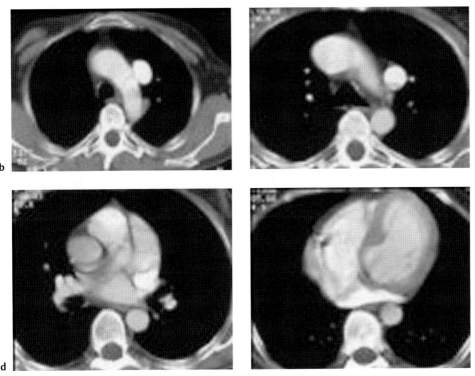

Fig. 11.**6 a–e**   Persistent left superior vena cava. Note the low density widening of the superior mediastinum on the chest radiograph (**a**). CT defines the course of the persistent left SVC through to the coronary sinus (**b–e**).

Thoracic Aortic Aneurysm and Dissection

An aneurysm is a saccular or fusiform dilatation of the aortic lumen to greater than 5 cm in diameter. It may be due to atherosclerosis (especially in individuals with systemic arterial hypertension), aortitis in patients with syphilis, some vasculitides including Takayasu's disease and cystic medial necrosis in Marfan's syndrome. Inflammatory aneurysms have a predilection for the as-

cending aorta while atherosclerosis most commonly involves the descending aorta.

- *True aneurysms* are saccular dilatations involving all layers of the aortic wall.
- *False aneurysms* result from extravasation of blood through a defect in the media to beneath the adventitia (Figs. 11.**8**, 11.**9**). This may occur post trauma or be secondary to bacterial sepsis (mycotic aneurysm).

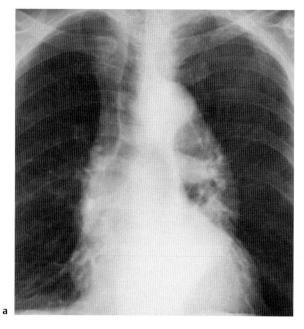

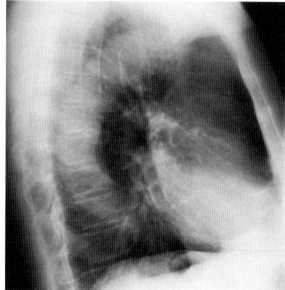

Fig. 11.**7 a, b**   Elongated, ectatic thoracic aorta.

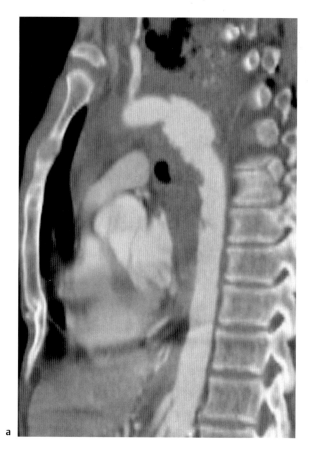

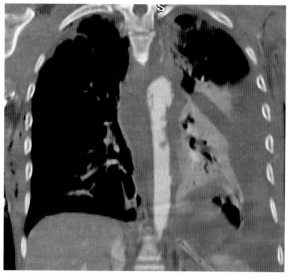

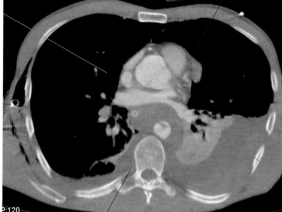

Fig. 11.**8 a–c**   Traumatic aortic injury with rupture giving hemothorax and mediastinal hemorrhage.

- *Dissecting aneurysms and aortic dissection*: Aortic dissections have been classified into three entities:
    - Classic aortic dissection due to a primary intimal tear.
    - Intramural hematoma.
    - Penetrating atherosclerotic ulcer (PAU) (Ledbetter et al. 1999, Coady et al.1999, Willens et al. 1999).

Classic aortic dissection is an emergency which requires prompt diagnosis and treatment (Pretre et al. 1997). Blood dissects between the intima and media through an intimal tear; this separates the layers and creates a false lumen that may reunite with the true lumen at a more distal level. Aortic dissections may be acute (first 2 weeks) or chronic (Crawford 1990). Sites of predilection are the proximal ascending aorta just superior to the valve ring and the region of the aortic isthmus. It is important to determine if a dissection is limited to the descending aorta (type B dissection) or if it also involves the ascending aorta and the origins of the great vessels (type A dissection, Fig. 11.**10**).

Intramural hematoma may be an early stage or a variant of aortic dissection (Yoshida et al. 2003). Many authors distinguish between aortic dissection and intramural hematoma by the presence or absence of an intimal flap (Maraj et al. 2000). Intramural hematoma is also classified as type A or B depending on its location and extent.

Ulcer–like projection/penetrating atherosclerotic ulcer. An ulcer–like projection is defined at CT and angiography as a localized blood-filled pouch protruding into the thrombosed wall of the aorta and showing the same degree of contrast enhancement as the aortic lumen. They may develop in both types A and B intramural hematoma.

Penetrating atherosclerotic ulcers, by contrast, typically involve the descending thoracic or abdominal aorta in patients with severely atherosclerotic vessels. Extensive atherosclerotic plaque may lead to medial scarring and atrophy and these changes may limit the extent of longitudinal dissection (Roberts 1981). This may explain why the rate of progression of PAU to overt dissection appears to be lower than for ulcer–like projections (Harris et al. 1994, Sueyoshi et al. 2002).

The treatment of type A dissection and probably also type A intramural hematoma is surgical while most type B lesions are initially managed conservatively with surgery being reserved for those with persistent symptoms, extending dissections, or severe ischemic complications.

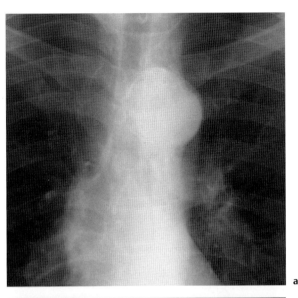

a

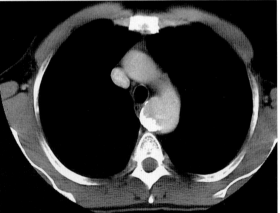

b

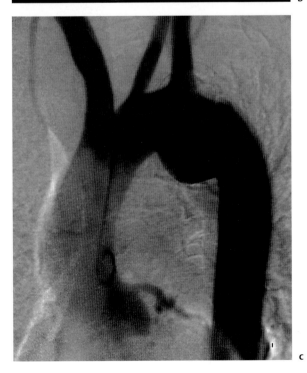

c

Fig. 11.**9a–c** False aneurysm post trauma. Crescent-shaped calcification in the region of the aortic isthmus prompted further investigation (**a**). This patient had a history of major chest trauma some 20 years earlier. CT (**b**) and aortography (**c**) show posttraumatic false aneurysm.

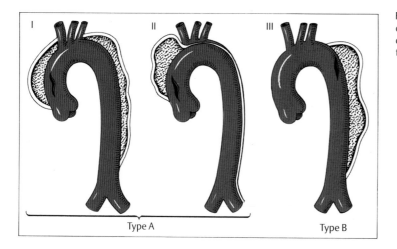

Fig. 11.**10**   Classification of thoracic aortic dissection. Types I–III in the DeBakey classification are compared with types A and B in the Stanford classification (Higgins 1992).

■ Radiologic Findings

Aortic Aneurysms

The *chest radiograph* may show saccular or fusiform aortic dilatation. There is associated intimal calcification in up to 75 % of cases. On the lateral view, partial soft-tissue obliteration of the superior retrosternal space is seen with ascending aortic aneurysms

Helical computed tomography is used most commonly for 2nd line imaging evaluation. It accurately defines the severity and extent of aneurysmal dilatation and its relationship to major branch vessels. It also demonstrates the presence of intraluminal thrombus and the diameter of the residual lumen (Figs. 11.**11**, 11.**12**).

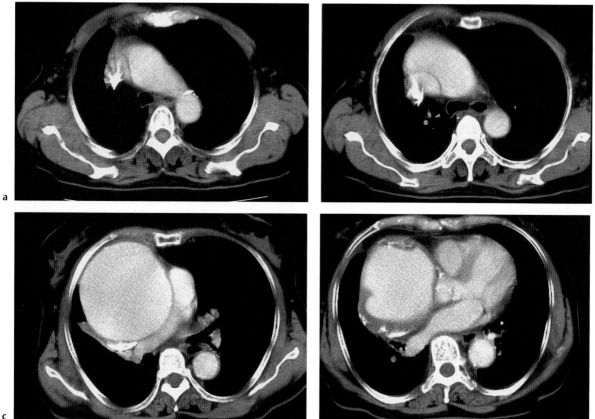

Fig. 11.**11 a–d**   Aneurysm of the ascending aorta with dissection: CT shows a large aneurysm of the ascending aorta (**a–d**) with a localized dissection of the more distal ascending aorta extending to involve the arch (**a, b**). The aneurysmal segment contains some peripheral intraluminal thrombus (**d**) and there is SVC compression (**c**).

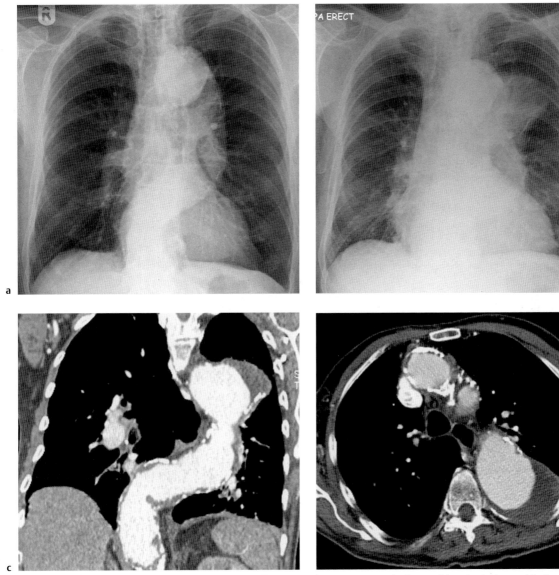

Fig. 11.**12** Initial chest radiograph (**a**) shows a dilated ectatic thoracic aorta. Chest study (**b**) acquired 4 months later shows new soft tissue opacity in the aortopulmonary window with lateral displacement of intimal calcification suggesting a vascular lesion. CT coronal reformat (**c**) and axial image (**d**) show diffuse atheromatous change with dilatation of the thoracic aorta and development of a saccular "aneurysm" containing intraluminal thrombus. There was no history of interval trauma.

Intramural Hematoma and Aortic Dissection

The *chest radiograph* may occasionally show displacement of atheromatous calcification to more than 1 cm inside the aortic contour (Earnest 1979), a feature suggestive of aortic dissection in the correct clinical setting. Leaking aortic dissection will result in mediastinal widening due to hemorrhage and hemothorax. When the dissection has extended proximally to involve the aortic root, a pericardial effusion may be present.

Computed tomography has been shown to be both sensitive and specific for diagnosis of aortic dissection (Egan 1980, Gross 1980). More recently, Yoshida et al. have reported the accuracy of helical CT in detection of

aortic dissection and intramural hematoma to be 100% (Yoshida et al. 2003).

Precontrast CT images show intramural hyperdensity with central displacement of intimal calcification in intramural hematoma.

The significance of new "ulcer–like projections" on serial CT assessment of patients with aortic intramural hematoma has been evaluated. Sueyoshi et al. found the location of intramural hematoma in the ascending aorta to be the principal predictor of development of these lesions. Seventy percent of patients who developed these ulcer–like projections then progressed to aortic enlargement or overt dissection (Sueyoshi et al. 2002).

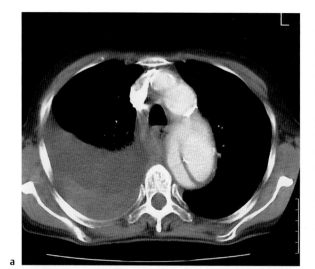

a

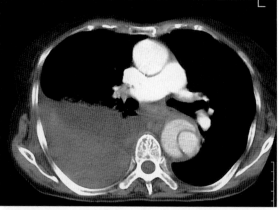

b

CT features of dissection include two lumina separated by an intimal flap; this flap appears as a curvilinear lucency within the opacified aorta (Figs. 11.**11**, 11.**13**). Differential opacification of the false lumen also may be visible and is helpful in diagnosis when the intimal flap is not seen (Armstrong et al. 1995).

Helical volumetric CT with reformatted images in selected planes defines the extent of intramural hematoma/dissection and demonstrates involvement of major branch vessels in dissection. The proximal extent of the intramural hematoma/dissection may also be defined and when it extends proximally to involve the aortic root, its relationship to the coronary sinuses ± involvement of the coronary arteries may be identified (Fig. 11.**14**).

Aortitis

Syphilitic mesaortitis is today a relatively rare entity and is characterized by aneurysmal dilatation of the ascending aorta with associated aortic regurgitation.

Takayasu arteritis is characterized by stenoses of the aorta, its main branches, and the pulmonary arteries. Less commonly, it causes saccular or fusiform aneurysms (Lui 1985) which when multiple may be found anywhere in the aorta (Armstrong et al. 1995).

Mediastinal Hematoma

Mediastinal hemorrhage may result from vascular injury caused by blunt or iatrogenic trauma. Spontaneous bleeding most commonly results from rupture of an aortic aneurysm. Vessel wall erosion by a malignant tumor very occasionally may lead to mediastinal hemorrhage.

Fig. 11.**13 a–c**   Leaking aortic dissection. Intimal dissection flap is seen within the contrast-opacified aorta and there is a right-sided hemothorax which demonstrates a blood–fluid level.

c

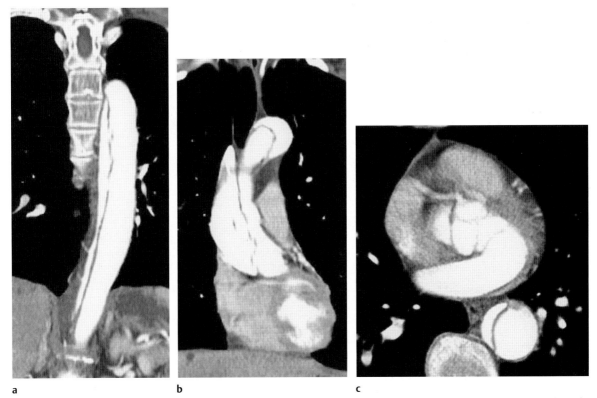

a   **b**   **c**

Fig. 11.**14 a–c** Type A aortic dissection. Coronal reformats through the aorta show a Stanford type A dissection (**a** and **b**). Axial CT image shows dissection flap extending proximally to in- volve the aortic root but with sparing of the origin of the right coronary artery (**c**). There were no ECG/EKG changes and this patient had a successful aortic root replacement.

Neoplastic Mediastinal Widening

Both benign and malignant tumors involve the mediastinum (Fig. 11.**15**). When tumors extend outside the normal mediastinal shadow on the frontal chest radiograph, the angle of interface with the mediastinum may sometimes be helpful in their differentiation from lesions arising from the adjacent lung. An obtuse angle suggests a lesion of mediastinal origin while an acute angle suggests a primary pulmonary lesion (Figs. 11.**16**, 11.**17**).

The most common mediastinal lesions are thyroid goiters and lymph node enlargement (Table 11.**2**). The normal thymus gives physiological age-related superior mediastinal widening in young children.

■ Radiologic Findings

Thyroid Goiter

Thyroid goiters showing retrosternal extension may cause a goblet-shaped widening of the superior mediastinum on the *chest radiograph* (Fig. 11.**18**). This is frequently associated with curvilinear tracheal deviation and narrowing. *Computed tomography* accurately defines the size and degree of retrosternal extension of the goiter and shows the degree of tracheal deviation and compression.

A thyroid goiter is frequently heterogeneous in attenuation due to areas of cystic degeneration and necrosis and it may contain foci of calcification (Fig. 11.**19**). The surrounding fat planes should remain intact and no significant adjacent lymph node enlargement should be evident. The presence of either of these features should raise the possibility of a thyroid neoplasm.

Radionuclide thyroid scintigraphy provides an assessment of thyroid function and in particular, determines the activity of discrete thyroid nodules. Nodules displaying increased tracer uptake (so called *hot* nodules) almost invariably are benign and while the majority of those showing no/decreased tracer uptake relative to normal thyroid parenchyma (so called *cold* nodules) are also benign, a small proportion may be neoplastic and further investigation including fine needle aspiration may be merited.

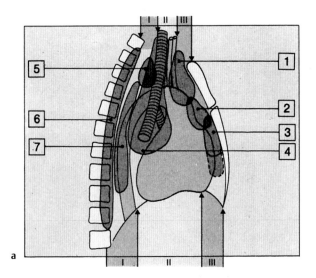

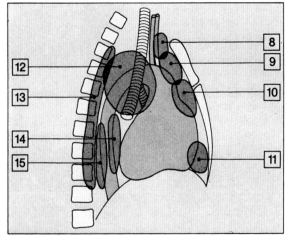

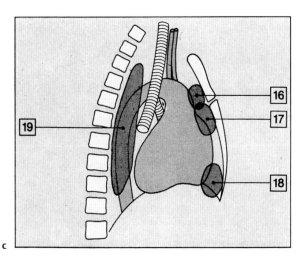

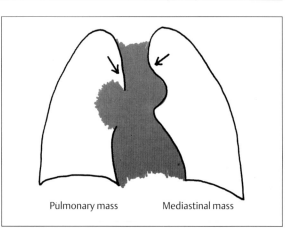

Fig. 11.**16**   Criteria for distinguishing mediastinal from pulmonary masses. A pulmonary mass may be poorly demarcated from surrounding aerated lung and its borders may form an acute angle with the mediastinum. A mediastinal mass is sharply demarcated from adjacent lung and its borders form an obtuse angle with the mediastinum.

Fig. 11.**15 a–c**   Classification of mediastinal masses from CT criteria (from O. H. Wegener: *Ganzkörper-Computertomographie.* Berlin: Blackwell; 1992)

a   *Solid masses*
 1   Retrosternal thyroid goiter
 2   Thymoma
 3   Teratoma, dysgerminoma
 4   Lymphoma
 5   Retrotracheal goiter
 6   Neurogenic tumors
 7   Esophageal tumors, fibrosarcoma
 I   Posterior mediastinum
 II   Middle mediastinum
 III   Anterior mediastinum

b   *Cystic masses*
 8   Thyroid cyst
 9   Thymic cyst
10   Cystic teratoma
11   Mesothelioma (lymphangioma)
12   Bronchogenic cyst
13   Meningocele
14   Neurenteric cyst
15   Lymphangioma

c   *Lipid-containing masses*
16   Thymolipoma
17   Dermoid cyst
18   Lipoma
19   Liposarcoma

Table 11.**2** Mediastinal masses (classified by mediastinal compartmental location) (modified from Meschan, 1981)

Anterior mediastinum	Middle mediastinum	Posterior mediastinum
Vessels: Dilated superior vena cava Persistent left SVC Aortic arch anomaly Ascending aortic aneurysm Coronary sinus aneurysm	**Vessels:** Aortic/Great vessel aneurysm Pulmonary artery dilatation Azygos vein dilatation	**Vessels:** Aneurysm descending aortic Azygos/Hemiazygos dilatation Thoracic duct cysts
Thyroid: Goiter Adenoma Carcinoma Parathyroid tumor **Thymus:** Hyperplasia Tumors **Teratoma/Germ cell tumors:** **Lymphangioma (cystic hygroma)** **Lymphoma** **Mesenchymal tumor*** **Chemodectoma**	**Lymph nodes:** Lymphoma Lymph node metastases Infectious mononucleosis Sarcoidosis Tuberculosis Histoplasmosis Silicosis **Tumors:** Vagus or phrenic nerve tumors Chemodectoma Mesenchymal tumors*	**Neurogenic:** Neurofibroma Schwannoma Neuroblastoma Pheochromocytoma Glomus tumor Chemodectoma Lateral meningocele
Sternum: Tumor Osteomyelitis	**Trachea and esophagus:** Tumor, diverticulum, megaesophagus	**Vertebral column:** Spondylosis Paravertebral abscess Extraosseous extension of metastases/ myeloma Extramedullary hematopoiesis
Cardiac: Pericardial cyst Diverticulum Effusion Epicardial fat pad **Morgagni hernia**	Bronchogenic and esophageal duplication cysts. Hiatus hernia	**Bochdalek hernia**

All compartments: mediastinitis ± abscess formation, hematogenous metastases, mesenchymal tumors,
lymph node enlargement, lipomatosis, fibrosis.
* Mesenchymal tumors include lipoma, fibroma, myoma, hemangioma, lymphangioma, chondroma, xanthofibroma,
  mixed tumors, and their malignant counterparts.

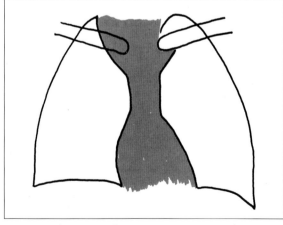

Fig. 11.**17** The "cervicothoracic" sign. Lesions in the anterior mediastinum terminate at the level of the clavicle (*left*) whereas lesions in the posterior mediastinum extend superior to the clavicle (*right*).

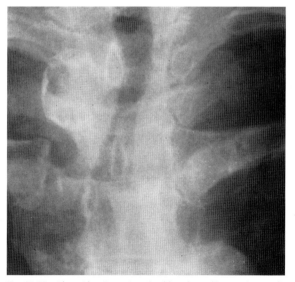

Fig. 11.**18** Thyroid goiter gives "goblet-shaped" superior mediastinal widening with tracheal narrowing. A right-sided calcified thyroid nodule is also present.

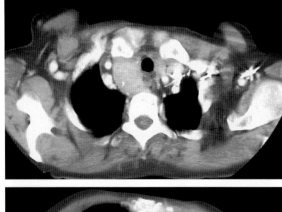

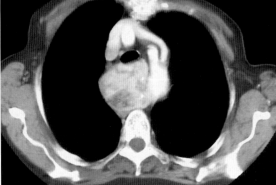

Fig. 11.**19 a, b**   Thyroid goiter with retrosternal and retrotracheal extension.

The Thymus

Thymic Hyperplasia

In infants and young children, the thymus occupies much of the anterior mediastinum and lies anterior to the great vessels. During these early years, there is considerable variation in the normal size of the gland.

Two distinct histologic types of thymic hyperplasia are recognized; true thymic hyperplasia and lymphoid hyperplasia. *True thymic hyperplasia* is defined as enlargement of the thymus which remains normally organized beyond the upper limit of normal for a given patient age. This entity is seen in patients recovering from recent "stress" including chemotherapy, corticosteroid therapy, irradiation and thermal burns (Shimosato et al. 1997, Mendelson 2001).

Lymphoid hyperplasia refers to an increased number of lymphoid follicles and this entity most commonly is seen in patients with myasthenia gravis, being present in up to 65% of cases (Mendelson 2001).

The *chest radiograph* shows superior mediastinal widening with a smooth or scalloped contour (Fig. 11.**21**). The lateral view may show obliteration of the retrosternal space and slight posterior displacement of the trachea.

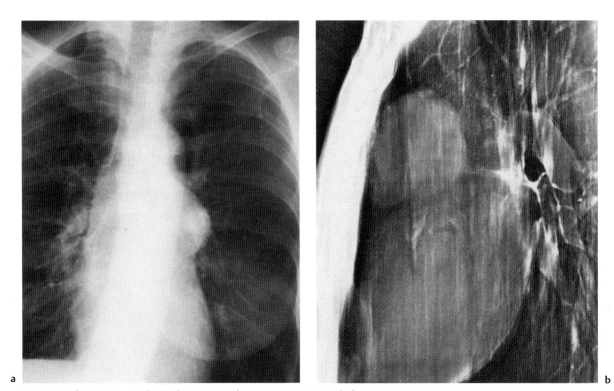

Fig. 11.**20 a, b**   Anterior mediastinal tumor. Histology was consistent with thymoma.

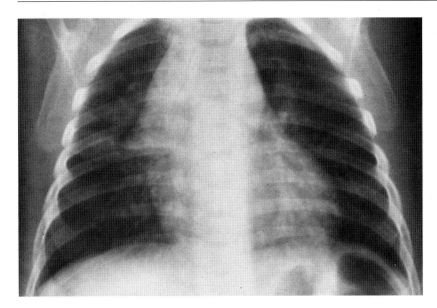

Fig. 11.**21** Thymic hyperplasia with distinctive "sail-shaped" shadow in the superior mediastinum.

Computed tomography: Axial images at the level of the aortic arch are optimal for evaluation of the thymus. In young children, the thymus is homogeneous with attenuation values close to those of adjacent soft tissues. There is a gradual decrease in attenuation values with increasing age due to fat deposition (Armstrong 1992). In thymic hyperplasia, the gland though enlarged is normal in shape.

Thymic Tumors

Thymic epithelial tumors include thymoma and thymic carcinoma (Fig. 11.**20**). These arise from thymic epithelium and demonstrate varying histologic features and biological behavior (Han et al. 2003). While a number of classifications exist, thymoma may be classified into noninvasive and invasive subtypes. Noninvasive thymoma is encapsulated completely with no microscopic evidence of extracapsular growth. Invasive thymoma shows extracapsular spread and sometimes may give pleural and occasionally more distant metastatic deposits.

Computed tomography features suggestive of invasive thymoma include invasion of mediastinal fat and/or mediastinal vessels and the presence of pleural seeding. Jeong et al. have reported a lobulated contour and mediastinal fat and great vessel invasion to be more common in invasive thymoma and thymic carcinoma (Jeong et al. 2004).

Magnetic resonance imaging (MRI): Thymoma shows signal intensity similar to muscle or normal thymic tissue on T1-weighted sequences and has heterogeneous T2 signal intensity (Han et al. 2003, Sakai et al. 1992). MRI may be useful in distinguishing thymoma from thymic cysts when this is not possible on CT due to the hemorrhagic or proteinous contents of the cyst.

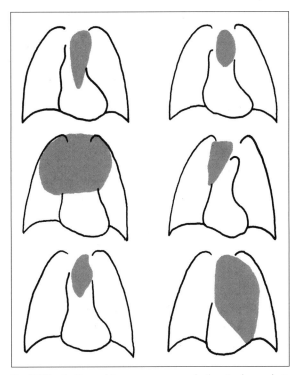

Fig. 11.**22** Radiographic appearances of thymic hyperplasia (*shaded area*) in children and adolescents (from Meschan 1981).

Positron emission tomography (PET): Sasaki et al. have suggested that PET may be helpful in distinguishing thymic carcinoma from both invasive and noninvasive thymoma. They report a sensitivity of 84.6%, specificity of 92.3%, and accuracy of 88.5% in this differentiation using a cut-off for standardized uptake value (SUV) of 5 (Sasaki et al. 1999).

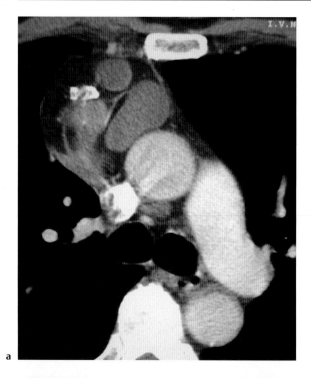

a

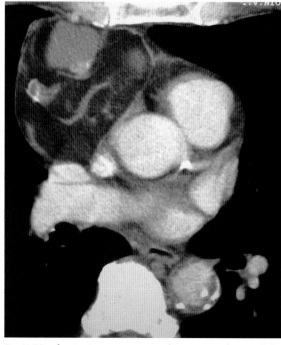

b

Fig. 11.**23a, b**   Benign teratoma. Axial CT images show well-defined anterior mediastinal mass containing areas of fat density, foci of calcification, and discrete areas of low density soft tissue.

Thymolipoma is a rare, benign tumor that is usually asymptomatic and manifests as a large anterior mediastinal mass. Histologically, it is composed of mature fat and normal thymic tissue and at CT and MRI, it appears as a fatty mass with fibrous septa (Armstrong 2000).

Thymic carcinoid is a rare primary malignant tumor of the thymus with a poor prognosis. One-third of these tumors are functionally active causing syndromes including Cushing's syndrome. CT and MRI characteristically show a large anterior mediastinal mass often with local invasion and differentiation from aggressive thymic epithelial tumors may not be possible at imaging (Armstrong 2000).

Thymic lymphoma: Lymphoma may involve the thymus as part of disseminated disease or in isolation and the nodular sclerosing variant of Hodgkin's disease is the most common histologic type. Imaging differentiation from other thymic tumors may be difficult. Distinguishing diffuse lymphomatous infiltration from thymic hyperplasia may also be problematic (Armstrong 2000, Mendelson 2001).

Mediastinal Lymph Node Enlargement

Hodgkin's disease and non-Hodgkin lymphoma, lymph node metastases from thoracic and extrathoracic malignancies, and sarcoidosis are the most common causes of mediastinal lymph node enlargement.

■ Radiologic Findings

See:
- Bronchial Carcinoma: Chapter 6, p. 157
- Hodgkin's and Non-Hodgkin's Lymphoma: Chapter 6, p. 98
- Sarcoidosis: Chapter 3. p. 91

Primary Mediastinal Tumors: Benign Teratoma and Malignant Germ Cell Tumors

Benign teratoma and malignant germ cell tumors are relatively uncommon and are thought to arise from aberrant cell nests in the mediastinum. Imaging of these tumors is initially with chest radiography, proceeding to CT and/or MRI.

Benign teratomas are frequently asymptomatic and may grow to a considerable size before detection. They are found most commonly in young adults, with a slight female predominance. The *chest radiograph* shows an anterior mediastinal mass. *Computed tomography* usually shows a thick-walled fluid-containing cyst; the attenuation of its contents may be that of fat, fluid, or soft tissue (Suzuki et al. 1983, Fig. 11.**23**).

Malignant germ cell tumors may be divided into seminoma and nonseminomatous germ cell tumors includ-

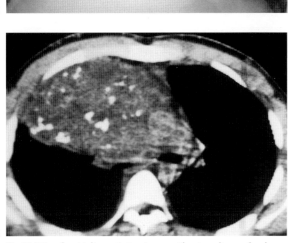

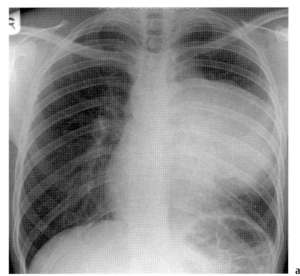

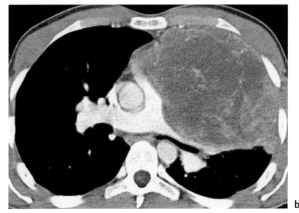

Fig. 11.**24 a, b**   Malignant teratoma. Chest radiograph shows large right-sided anterior mediastinal mass (**a**). CT shows heterogeneously enhancing soft tissue mass containing multiple foci of calcification and evidence of mediastinal invasion (**b**).

Fig. 11.**25 a, b**   Malignant teratoma. Chest radiograph shows large left-sided anterior mediastinal soft tissue mass (**a**). CT shows large heterogeneously enhancing soft tissue mass with compression of the main and left pulmonary arteries and with airway displacement and compression (**b**).

ing teratocarcinoma, embryonal carcinoma, and choriocarcinoma. These tumors grow rapidly and metastasize early and are most commonly encountered in young adult males. The *chest radiograph* characteristically shows a lobulated anterior mediastinal mass (Figs. 11.**24 a**, 11.**25 a**). *Computed tomography* demonstrates either a homogeneous soft-tissue tumor or multiple areas of contrast enhancement interspersed with regions of low attenuation representing either hemorrhage or necrosis. Scattered foci of calcification may also be present (Figs. 11.**24 b**, 11.**25 b**).

Neurogenic Tumors

Neurogenic tumors account for 20–30% of all mediastinal tumors. They most commonly arise from the thoracic nerve roots or intercostal nerves (peripheral nerve/nerve sheath tumors, neurofibroma/schwannoma). Occasionally, they arise from the sympathetic trunk (ganglioneuroma) or from paraganglionic cells (pheochromocytoma).

Neurogenic tumors typically appear as sharply circumscribed, homogeneous, round, or oval mass lesions. They are of intermediate signal intensity on T1-weighted MRI sequences, heterogeneous to hyperintense on T2-weighted sequences, and they enhance greatly postadministration of intravenous gadolinium (Figs. 11.**26**, 11.**27**). Peripheral nerve/nerve sheath tumors are frequently located in the paravertebral region and sometimes may have a "dumbbell" configuration with extradural and paravertebral/posterior mediastinal components. In these cases, there may be associated widening of the neural foramen (Fig. 11.**28**).

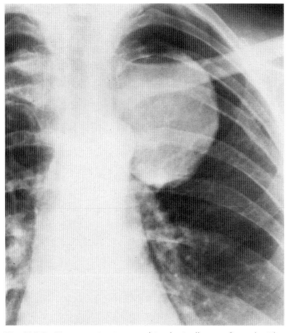

Fig. 11.**26** Neurogenic tumor histologically confirmed. The tumor mass extends superior to the clavicle indicating its posterior location. However, the aortic arch remains sharply defined suggesting that this lesion lies much more posteriorly than the aorta.

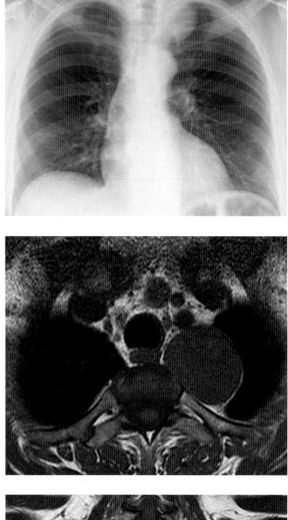

a

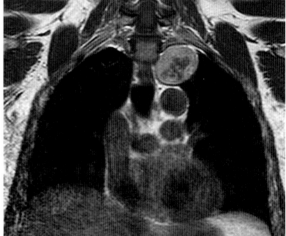

b

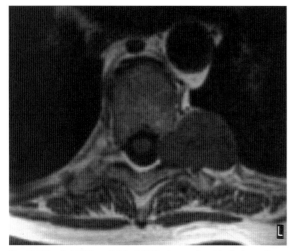

Fig. 11.**28** Axial T1-weighted MRI shows dumbbell-shaped peripheral nerve sheath tumor with paravertebral and extradural components and with expansion of the neural foramen.

c

Fig. 11.**27 a–c** Chest radiograph shows well-defined opacity lying posteriorly on the left side in the superior mediastinum (**a**). Axial T1-weighted pre and gadolinium-enhanced coronal MR images show lesion of intermediate T1 signal intensity which shows avid peripheral enhancement. Location, signal intensity, and enhancement characteristics were consistent with a peripheral nerve/nerve sheath tumor.

12 High-Resolution/Thin-Section CT Patterns in Pulmonary Disease

Computed tomography (CT) is more sensitive and more specific than the chest radiograph in evaluation of pulmonary disease. A specific diagnosis can sometimes be made from CT findings as in centrilobular emphysema. In other cases, for example ground-glass opacification (GGO), CT findings are less specific and a differential diagnosis may only be possible. This may reflect the fact that the lung's response to different insults is, in many cases, relatively isomorphic. It is, however, frequently possible to shorten the differential diagnosis when the clinical history and the duration of symptoms and radiologic findings are considered.

The following CT patterns will be considered:
- Ground-glass opacification and consolidation
- Multifocal peripheral consolidation
- Pulmonary nodules
- Intra- and interlobular septal thickening and reticular pattern
- Decreased lung attenuation and cystic lung change
- Inhomogeneous-mosaic lung attenuation

Ground-Glass Opacification— Consolidation

Ground-glass opacification reflects partial filling of the alveoli, sometimes with a degree of associated interstitial change, the latter generally being below the resolution of computed tomography. Lung attenuation is increased but this increase is not sufficient to obscure vascular markings in contradistinction to consolidation.

The difference in attenuation values between the infiltrated lung parenchyma and air-filled bronchi is larger than between normal lung and air-filled bronchi; this increased contrast leads to increased conspicuity of the bronchus, the so called "black bronchus" sign.

The differential diagnosis of pulmonary ground-glass opacification includes acute and nonacute disease processes:
- *Acute infection including Pneumocystis Jiroveci/Carinii Pneumonia (PJP; PCP)*: This infection is characteristically seen in patients with diminished cellular immunity and has been considered an index case for progression to AIDS in HIV-positive patients for many years. GGO may be uniform or inhomogeneous in distribution and may progress to frank consolidation (Fig. 12.1; see also Chapter 3, p. 87).
- *Acute Pulmonary Hemorrhage*: Acute pulmonary hemorrhage may be seen in a number of disease

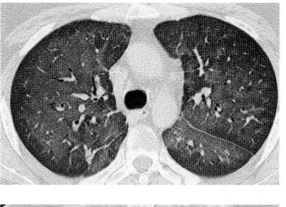

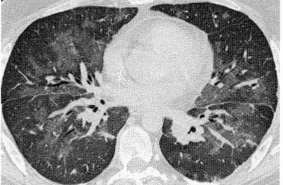

Fig. 12.**1 a**, **b** Pneumocystis pneumonia. High-resolution CT image shows bilateral ground-glass opacification with evidence of the "black bronchus" sign and with sparing of the subpleural lung.

processes including Wegener's Granulomatosis and Anti-Glomerular Basement Membrane disease. It also may be seen in hematologic disorders and particularly in the acute leukemias where it may be a manifestation of disease-induced bone marrow failure or a complication of chemotherapy-induced thrombocytopenia.
- *Pulmonary Edema*: Ground-glass opacification probably reflects a combination of interstitial and early alveolar edema. It characteristically has a dependent distribution and may involve the posterior portions of the upper lobes in patients confined to bed. "Smooth" interlobular septal thickening is also frequently present and probably reflects predominantly associated interstitial edema (Fig. 12.**2**).
- *Hypersensitivity Pneumonitis/Extrinsic Allergic Alveolitis*: Ground-glass opacification in a patchy or homogeneous distribution is a frequent finding in hy-

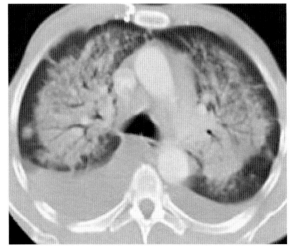

Fig. 12.**2** Pulmonary edema with bilateral pleural effusions.

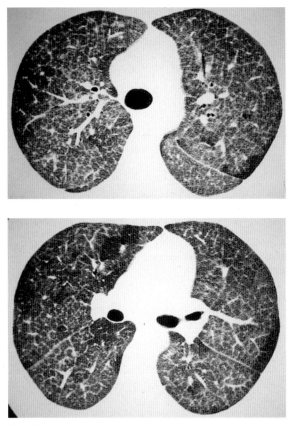

Fig. 12.**3 a, b** Alveolar proteinosis. CT images show marked septal thickening superimposed on ground-glass opacification and giving the "crazy paving" pattern.

persensitivity pneumonitis (see also Hypersensitivity Pneumonitis, Chapter 5, p. 145).

- *Respiratory Bronchiolitis-Interstitial Lung Disease (RBILD) and Desquamative Interstitial Pneumonia (DIP)*: Centrilobular nodules of GGO and GGO involv-

ing the entire secondary pulmonary lobule are manifestations of RBILD-DIP with a tendency towards more extensive and uniform change within the lobule in DIP (see also Idiopathic Interstitial Pneumonias, Chapter 3, p. 95).

- *Lymphocytic Interstitial Pneumonia (LIP)*: LIP in adult HIV-negative patients is frequently found in patients with Sjögren syndrome. Ground-glass opacification, areas of consolidation, and pulmonary cysts are frequent CT findings (see also Sjögren syndrome, Chapter 3, p. 102).
- *Alveolar Proteinosis*: The etiology of this rare disease is unknown but it may relate to a hereditary defect of surfactant production which decompensates to a pathologic state when additional infectious or toxic insults are imposed (e. g., the inhalation of tobacco smoke, silicates, aluminum, kaolin, or sawdust). Pathologically, the alveoli are filled with copious protein- and phospholipid-rich material. CT features are GGO in association with septal thickening leading to the characteristic "crazy paving" appearance (Fig. 12.**3 a**, **b**).
- *Peripheral Adenocarcinoma*: Focal areas of persisting GGO may reflect slow growing adenocarcinomas with a lepidic pattern of growth (see also Solitary Pulmonary Nodule, Chapter 6, p. 149 and Noguchi Classification, Chapter 6, p. 161).

Multifocal Peribronchial Consolidation

- *Multifocal Bronchioloalveolar Carcinoma*: Bronchioloalveolar carcinoma showing a lepidic growth pattern characteristically shows pulmonary consolidation in a peribronchial distribution.
- *Pulmonary Lymphoma*: Pulmonary lymphoma is characterized by nodular and linear areas of increased attenuation and consolidation. These changes tend to have their epicenter on the airway which may appear dilated and they correlate histologically with lymphomatous infiltration in a peribronchovascular distribution.
- *Organizing Pneumonia*: Organizing pneumonia or cryptogenic organizing pneumonia represents an organizing pneumonia and a "proliferative" bronchiolitis. High-resolution CT (HRCT) shows areas of consolidation and ground-glass opacification in a peripheral subpleural distribution (see Fig. 4.**26 a**, **b**).
- *Chronic Eosinophilic Pneumonia*: CT manifestations of chronic eosinophilic pneumonia include peribronchial consolidation that may have a peripheral subpleural distribution in up to 50% of cases.

Pulmonary Nodules

The distribution of pulmonary nodules on thin collimation/high-resolution CT images allows their classification into centrilobular, perilymphatic, and random in type.

Centrilobular nodules are characteristically a manifestation of *small airways disease-cellular bronchiolitis*, in which case they tend to be well defined and average 1–3 mm in diameter (Fig. 12.**4**; see also Small Airways Disease, Chapter 4, p. 122).

Larger less well-defined centrilobular nodules which sometimes may be of ground-glass opacification may indicate *peribronchiolar* consolidation and are seen in hypersensitivity pneumonitis and respiratory bronchiolitis-interstitial lung disease (Figs. 12.**5**, 12.**6**).

Nodules in a perilymphatic distribution are characteristically seen in *sarcoidosis*. Perilymphatic change indicates a combination of centrilobular, peribronchovascular, and perifissural nodules in keeping with the distribution of the pulmonary lymphatic channels (Fig. 12.**7**).

Nodules with a random distribution show no specific anatomic distribution within the lung (Figs. 12.**8**, 12.**9**). *Pulmonary metastases* may show a random distribution though on some occasions hematogenous metastases may demonstrate a degree of angiocentricity.

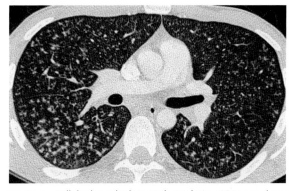

Fig. 12.**4**   Cellular bronchiolitis. High-resolution CT image shows extensive bilateral well-defined centrilobular nodules and branching structures consistent with a cellular bronchiolitis.

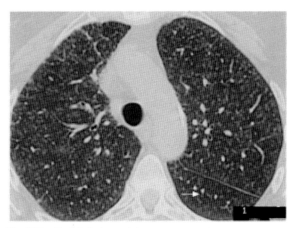

Fig. 12.**5**   Centrilobular nodules.

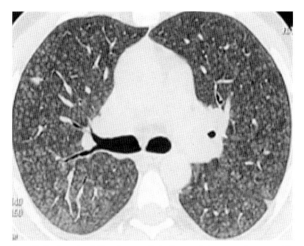

Fig. 12.**6**   Poorly-defined centrilobular nodules consistent with some degree of peribronchiolar consolidation.

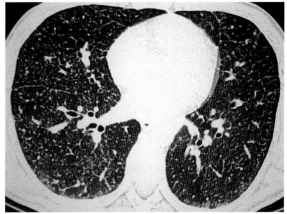

Fig. 12.**7**   Sarcoidosis. CT shows pulmonary nodules in a perilymphatic distribution. There are centrilobular and subpleural nodules and there is "beading" of the fissures and bronchovascular bundles.

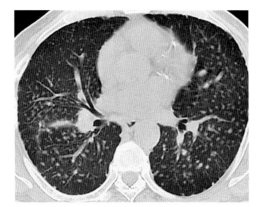

Fig. 12.8 Pulmonary nodules in pneumoconiosis.

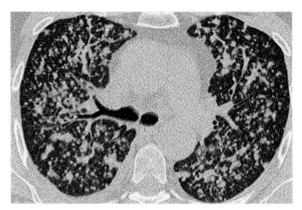

Fig. 12.9 Pulmonary metastases: CT shows bilateral profuse nodularity in no specific anatomic distribution. Histology acquired from transbronchial biopsy was adenocarcinoma.

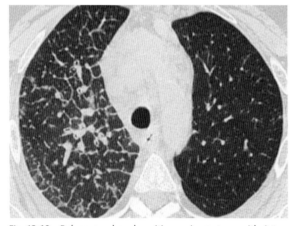

Fig. 12.10 Pulmonary lymphangitis carcinomatosa with interlobular septal thickening in the right upper lobe.

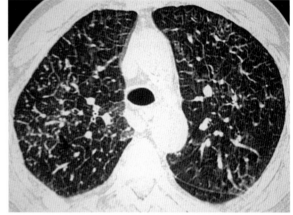

Fig. 12.11 Pulmonary lymphangitis carcinomatosa.

Intra- and Interlobular Septal Thickening and Reticular Pattern

Thickening of the pulmonary interstitium may be due to edema, inflammatory cells, neoplastic infiltration or fibrosis. The distribution of change, the relative proportions of inter- to intralobular septal thickening, the presence of accompanying features such as ground-glass opacification and traction bronchiectasis together with the clinical setting will narrow the differential diagnosis.

- *Interstitial Edema*: Smooth interlobular septal thickening tends to predominate in acute interstitial edema and is characteristically most marked in the dependent portions of the lung. There is frequently associated ground-glass opacification and the combination may give a crazy-paving pattern.
- *Subacute Pulmonary Hemorrhage*: The presence of blood within the lung parenchyma induces some

degree of organization with development of a fine reticular pattern within areas of hemorrhage 5–10 days post the acute event. Layering of blood along the septa might also account in part for this appearance. This combination of alveolar and interstitial change may also give a crazy-paving appearance.

- *Pulmonary Lymphangitis Carcinomatosa*: Pulmonary lymphangitis carcinomatosa refers to neoplastic infiltration of the pulmonary lymphatic channels. Septal thickening may be "nodular" in contradistinction to the smooth thickening of pulmonary edema. Associated centrilobular thickening is seen but ground-glass opacification occurs only in a minority of cases. There may be associated pulmonary nodular metastases and pleural effusions are also common (Figs. 12.10, 12.11).
- *Alveolar Proteinosis*: The original description of crazy paving in which septal thickening is superimposed on ground-glass opacification was in alveolar proteinosis. It is now recognized that this appearance is not

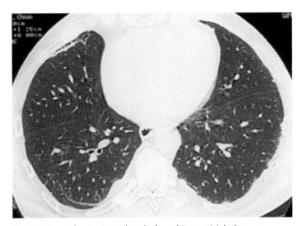

Fig. 12.**12**   Asbestosis with subpleural interstitial change.

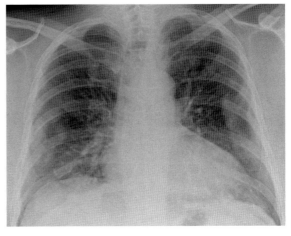

a

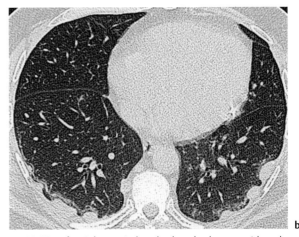

b

Fig. 12.**13 a, b**   Asbestos-induced pleural plaques with subpleural lung change. Chest radiograph (**a**) shows bilateral calcified pleural plaques. CT (**b**) shows pleural plaque formation with subpleural septal thickening giving a "subpleural line" and reticular change in the lower lobes.

specific to alveolar proteinosis and occurs in a number of other entities (see Fig. 12.**16**).

- *Idiopathic Interstitial Pneumonias*: Usual interstitial pneumonia is characterized by septal and particularly intralobular septal thickening giving rise to "fine networks," a varying degree of architectural distortion, traction bronchiectasis, and honeycombing. Distribution is characteristically subpleural and peripheral and the differential diagnosis includes other forms of idiopathic interstitial pneumonia including nonspecific interstitial pneumonia (NSIP), asbestos-induced interstitial fibrosis, and drug-induced pneumonitis (see Fig. 3.**58**).

- *Asbestosis*: Interstitial changes and fibrosis in asbestos-induced interstitial lung disease characteristically have a lower zone and peripheral distribution. The frequent presence of associated asbestos-induced benign pleural change helps in differentiation from the idiopathic interstitial pneumonias and in particular, from usual interstitial pneumonia (Figs. 12.**12**, 12.**13**).

- *Drug-induced pneumonitis*: Drug-induced pneumonitis is included in the differential diagnosis of interstitial pneumonia particularly in a lower zone distribution.

- *Connective Tissue Disease-associated Interstitial Pneumonias*: See Chapter 3, p. 100.

Decreased Lung Attenuation and Cystic Lung Change

Emphysema: CT has been shown to have high sensitivity in diagnosis of emphysema.

Centrilobular emphysema which affects predominantly the upper-to-mid zones is initially characterized by rounded areas of decreased lung attenuation which surround the centrilobular bronchovascular bundle. The extent of involvement of the secondary pulmonary lobule becomes more marked as disease progresses and uniform decreased lung attenuation with little-to-no residual intervening normal lung may be seen in severe advanced emphysema (Fig. 12.**14 a, b**).

Panlobular emphysema is characteristically seen in individuals with alpha-1 antitrypsin deficiency, tends to involve the lower lobes and in contradistinction to centrilobular emphysema, involves the entire secondary pulmonary lobule. Uniform decreased lung attenuation is seen in the lower zones. This appearance may sometimes be difficult to distinguish from the diffuse air trapping which is sometimes seen in bronchiolitis obliterans (constrictive bronchiolitis).

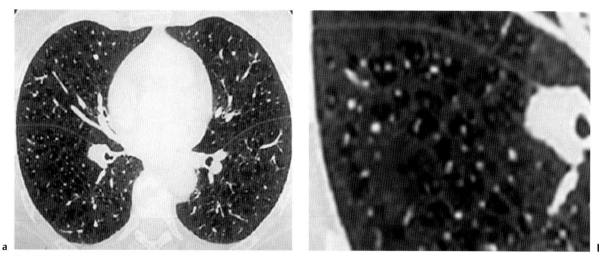

a   b

Fig. 12.**14 a, b**   Centrilobular emphysema. Emphysematous lung surrounds the centrilobular bundle with sparing of the peripheral lobule.

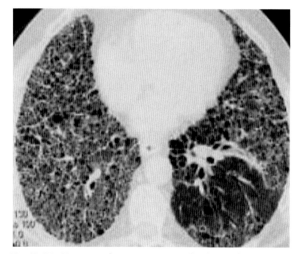

Fig. 12.**15**   Honeycombing consistent with advanced pulmonary fibrosis in rheumatoid lung disease.

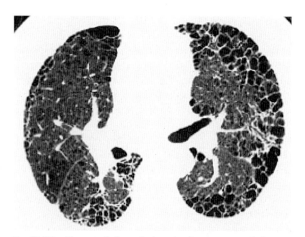

Fig. 12.**16**   Characteristic subpleural distribution of honeycombing in idiopathic pulmonary fibrosis.

- *Air trapping and constrictive bronchiolitis:* see Inhomogeneous Mosaic/Lung Attenuation (p. 299).
- *Honeycombing:* This refers to the presence of multiple cystic cavities that range from a few to several millimeters in diameter and which are surrounded by a thick fibrous wall. Honeycombing characteristically has a subpleural distribution and is frequently extensive in end-stage fibrosis, particularly in end-stage usual interstitial pneumonia (UIP) (Figs. 12.**15**, 12.**16**).
- *Cavitating Lesions:* Pyogenic lung abscess, tuberculous infection, septic pulmonary emboli, squamous cell neoplasia both primary and metastatic are among pulmonary lesions which may cavitate (Fig. 12.**17**).
- *Tuberous Sclerosis:* Tuberous sclerosis is characterized by the triad of epilepsy, café-au-lait spots, and hamartomatous lesions. Well-defined discrete cystic lesions may be seen scattered throughout the lungs (Fig. 12.**18**).
- *Pulmonary Langerhans Cell Histiocytosis (PLCH):* CT changes in PLCH range from peribronchial and peribronchiolar nodularity in early-stage disease through cavitatory nodules and thick-walled cysts to thin-walled and confluent cysts with fibrosis in advanced disease. Changes are most marked in the upper-to-mid zones with relative sparing of the basal lung (Fig. 12.**19**).
- *Lymphangiomyomatosis (LAM):* LAM is characteristically seen in premenopausal females. Cystic lung changes are similar to those seen in PLCH but tend to have a more diffuse distribution (Fig. 12.**20**). There may be an associated chylothorax.
- *Lymphocytic Interstitial Pneumonia:* Discrete air-filled cysts scattered through the lungs is a described finding in LIP (see Fig. 3.**72**).
- *Cystic Lung Disease in Acquired Immunodeficiency Syndrome:* Cystic lung disease tends to occur in

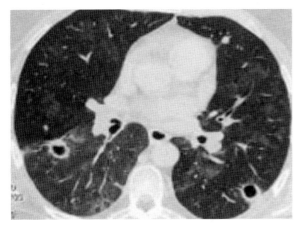

Fig. 12.**17**   Cavitating septic pulmonary emboli.

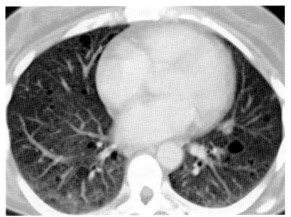

Fig. 12.**18**   Tuberous sclerosis: CT shows bilateral scattered air-filled cysts in a patient with known tuberous sclerosis.

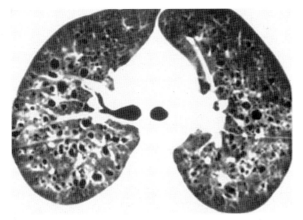

Fig. 12.**19**   Pulmonary Langerhans cell histiocytosis with many thick-walled cysts.

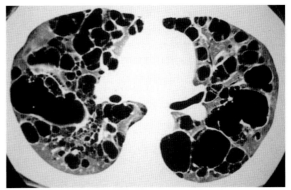

Fig. 12.**20**   Lymphangiomyomatosis: CT shows cysts of varying size and shape in the lung bilaterally.

patients who have had recurrent episodes of PJP-PCP and appearances may be indistinguishable from advanced PLCH (see Fig. 3.**46**). Cystic disease in this setting predisposes to development of pneumothorax.

Inhomogeneous-Mosaic Lung Attenuation

Inhomogeneous lung attenuation is usually due to one or a combination of the following:

- *Ground-glass opacification in an inhomogeneous patchy distribution* (Fig. 12.**21**).
  1. Infiltrated secondary pulmonary lobules are interspersed with areas of normal lung giving inhomogeneous lung attenuation.
  2. Pulmonary vessel density and vessel caliber tend to remain uniform throughout both infiltrated and normal lung.

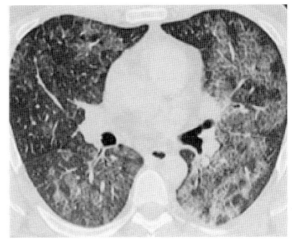

Fig. 12.**21**   Hypersensitivity pneumonitis with inhomogeneous lung attenuation due to patchy distribution of ground-glass opacification.

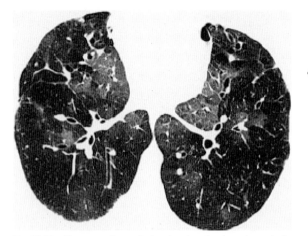

Fig. 12.**22** True mosaic perfusion in chronic thromboembolic pulmonary hypertension.

- *True mosaic perfusion in chronic thromboembolic pulmonary arterial hypertension* (CTEPH; Fig. 12.**22**).
  1. Pulmonary vascular stenoses and occlusions lead to nonuniform pulmonary perfusion and an inhomogeneous pattern of lung attenuation.

  2. Vessel caliber and vessel density are decreased within areas of decreased lung perfusion.
  3. Differences in attenuation do not become more pronounced in expiration.
- *Constrictive bronchiolitis and air trapping* (Fig. 12.**23 a, b**).
  1. Areas of air trapping are interspersed with areas of normal lung. This gives inhomogeneous lung attenuation on images acquired in inspiration.
  2. Vessel caliber and vessel density both may be decreased within the areas of air trapping due to reflex vasoconstriction.
  3. Differences in attenuation become more pronounced on images acquired in expiration with the normal increase in attenuation in areas of normal lung while areas of air trapping remain of decreased attenuation.

When areas of *ground-glass opacification* are seen in association with air trapping, sarcoidosis and hypersensitivity pneumonitis should be considered (see Fig. 5.**26 a, b**).

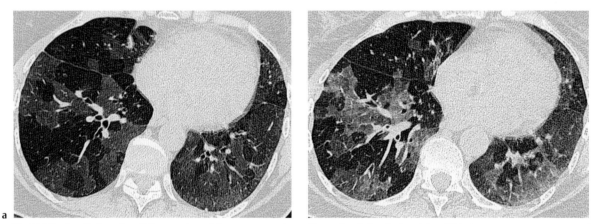

a   b

Fig. 12.**23 a, b** Air trapping: CT image shows inhomogeneous lung attenuation in inspiration (**a**) and this becomes more pronounced on images acquired in expiration (**b**).

13 Radiographic Signs and Differential Diagnosis

1. The Opaque Hemithorax (Table 13.1)

■ Diagnostic Approach

Complete opacification of a hemithorax frequently indicates the presence of significant disease. The differential diagnosis includes:
- Inflammatory or neoplastic unilateral pulmonary infiltration
- Unilateral pulmonary atelectasis or agenesis
- Pneumonectomy
- Pleural disease and most commonly the presence of a large pleural effusion

The *chest radiograph* shows the opaque hemithorax, any associated mediastinal displacement, and occasionally may suggest the correct diagnosis. *Computed tomography* (CT) ± *bronchoscopy* are standard 2nd line investigations for further assessment.

Comparison of the volume of the opaque hemithorax to that of the unaffected side is important when considering the differential diagnosis (Fig. 13.**1**):
- An increase in the volume of the hemithorax is recognized by contralateral mediastinal displacement, widening of the intercostal spaces, and depression of the hemidiaphragm. A large opaque hemithorax may indicate either a massive pleural effusion or a large

Table 13.**1** The opaque hemithorax

Pleural effusion
Pleural thickening and fibrothorax
Pleural mesothelioma and metastatic pleural carcinomatosis
Pneumonia
Atelectasis
Tuberculosis
Pulmonary aplasia, agenesis, and pneumonectomy
Diaphragmatic hernia
Thoracic scoliosis and chest wall deformity

intrathoracic mass. While a pleural effusion may lead to complete opacification of the hemithorax in the supine position, some aerated lung is usually visible at the apices on upright views.
- Ultrasound will show the presence of an effusion and allow image-guided diagnostic aspiration. Computed tomography, however, is the imaging modality of choice for assessment of underlying pulmonary and mediastinal abnormality.
- A decrease in the volume of the hemithorax is manifest by ipsilateral mediastinal displacement,

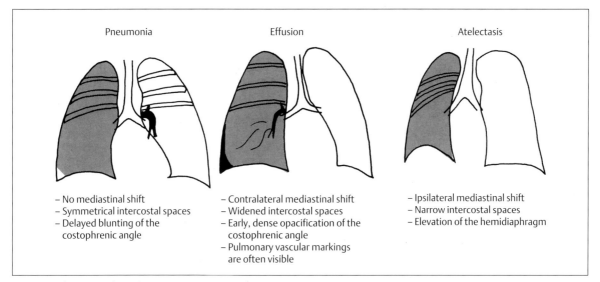

Pneumonia
- No mediastinal shift
- Symmetrical intercostal spaces
- Delayed blunting of the costophrenic angle

Effusion
- Contralateral mediastinal shift
- Widened intercostal spaces
- Early, dense opacification of the costophrenic angle
- Pulmonary vascular markings are often visible

Atelectasis
- Ipsilateral mediastinal shift
- Narrow intercostal spaces
- Elevation of the hemidiaphragm

Fig. 13.**1** The opaque hemithorax.

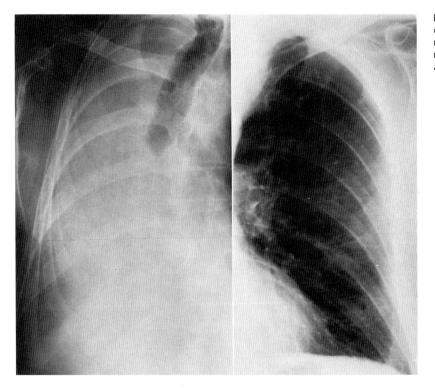

Fig. 13.**2**   Right lung atelectasis secondary to central bronchial carcinoma. There is occlusion of the right main bronchus and ipsilateral mediastinal displacement.

narrowing of the intercostal spaces, and elevation of the hemidiaphragm. A small opaque hemithorax may indicate a restrictive pleural process, pulmonary atelectasis, pulmonary hypoplasia, or past pneumonectomy. A fibrothorax may show a rind of calcification at its pulmonary interface. Complete lung atelectasis is most commonly secondary to central bronchial carcinoma. Pulmonary hypoplasia is associated with marked ipsilateral mediastinal displacement (see Chapter 2, p. 57).

- An opaque hemithorax of normal volume may indicate extensive unilateral pulmonary consolidation or it may be seen when a pleural effusion is associated with underlying pulmonary atelectasis.

■ Differential Diagnosis

Pleural Effusion

On upright views, the opacification is particularly marked in the laterobasal hemithorax with blunting of the costophrenic angles. The effusion may be mobile with changes in patient position.

Pleural Thickening and Fibrothorax

Empyema, tuberculous effusion, and hemothorax may resolve leaving marked fibrous pleural thickening. This may lead to severe pulmonary encasement with resulting ventilatory impairment.

Pleural Mesothelioma and Metastatic Pleural Carcinomatosis

An opaque hemithorax in pleural neoplasia may be due to the presence of an effusion and/or pleural tumor. Marked encasement of the underlying lung with resulting atelectasis may lead to a decrease in the size of the hemithorax.

Atelectasis

Complete pulmonary atelectasis results from occlusion of a main bronchus by carcinoma or less commonly by an aspirated foreign body, mucus plug, stricture, or bronchial tear. The volume of the hemithorax is reduced and there is ipsilateral mediastinal displacement (Fig. 13.**2**). A concomitant pleural effusion, however, may restore thoracic symmetry (Fig. 13.**3**).

Pneumonia

It is rare for pneumonic infiltration to involve the entire lung. A well-penetrated chest radiograph may show small residual areas of normal lung and air-filled bronchi traversing the consolidation (air bronchogram). The diagnosis is supported by clinical findings of cough, sputum production, pyrexia, and leukocytosis, and by identifying the causative organism in sputum samples or from blood cultures.

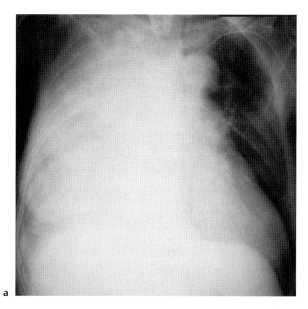

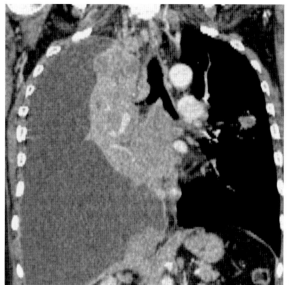

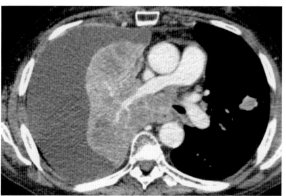

Fig. 13.**3a–c**   Opaque right hemithorax. Chest radiograph (**a**) shows opaque right hemithorax. CT images (**b** and **c**) show the large effusion with extensive abnormal soft tissue infiltrating the mediastinum and right hilum and with right lung atelectasis. Diagnosis was bronchial carcinoma and left midzone pulmonary metastasis is noted.

Tuberculosis (TB)

Tuberculous pneumonia very occasionally may involve the entire lung in children. Computed tomography in such cases will usually reveal areas of cavitation ± features of endobronchial spread.

Pulmonary Aplasia, Agenesis, and Pneumonectomy

The involved hemithorax is small and there is ipsilateral mediastinal displacement (see Chapter 2, p. 58) (Fig. 13.**4**).

Thoracic Scoliosis and Chest Wall Deformity

Extreme scoliosis with posterior unilateral rib prominence and thoracic deformity can occasionally mimic an opaque hemithorax, particularly on underexposed views. This appearance may be accentuated by the secondary ventilatory restriction and pulmonary underexpansion seen in some of these cases.

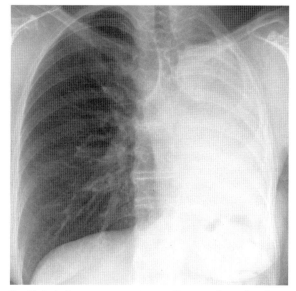

Fig. 13.**4**   Left pneumonectomy: Chest radiograph shows opaque left hemithorax with ipsilateral mediastinal displacement.

2. Lobar and Segmental Opacification

■ Diagnostic Approach

The lung is subdivided into functional anatomic units and some pathologic processes tend not to transgress lobar and/or segmental boundaries. Lobar/segmental opacification may be patchy or confluent depending on the volume of residually aerated lung.

Opacification may be due to consolidation or atelectasis. Occasionally, overlying pleural or chest wall lesions may mimic segmental opacification.

The commonest cause of lobar/segmental opacification is acute pneumonia. This can usually be diagnosed from the clinical history and characteristic radiographic appearances; these tend to resolve within days of commencing appropriate antibiotic therapy.

Diagnosis becomes more difficult and merits further evaluation when radiographic abnormality persists. Bronchial carcinoma is a frequent cause of persistent atelectasis and/or consolidation, particularly in older individuals from "at risk" categories (see Chapter 6, p. 157). Bronchial obstruction by mucus plugs, foreign bodies, and benign tumors are less common causes of persistent lobar/segmental opacification. Pulmonary infarction may also lead to segmental opacification which is slow to resolve (see Chapter 7, p. 189).

■ Differential Diagnosis (Table 13.2)

Pseudosegmental Opacities

Loculated pleural effusions, interlobar effusions, chest wall tumors, and large pulmonary angiomata and tumors occasionally mimic segmental opacities in their shape and location but they never have an air bronchogram or alveologram.

Lobar and Segmental Consolidation

An inflammatory or neoplastic process may spread within the alveolar spaces of a segment until it reaches the segmental or lobar boundary. Aerated lung is replaced by fluid and cellular infiltrate. Residually aerated alveoli may appear as small "foamy" lucencies (positive air alveologram) and residual air within the bronchi forms a pattern of branching radiolucent channels (positive air bronchogram) within the consolidation. Usually the anatomic shape of the segments remains unchanged although a slight volume increase can occur in entities such as *Klebsiella pneumonia* producing a convex border with the adjacent normal lung.

Table 13.**2**   Lobar and segmental opacification

Lobar and segmental consolidation
- Bacterial pneumonia
- Tuberculous pneumonia
- Bronchioloalveolar carcinoma
- Pulmonary infarction

Atelectasis:
Absorption atelectasis
- Bronchial carcinoma
- Endobronchial metastasis
- Benign bronchial tumors
- Bronchial mucus plug
- Postoperative atelectasis
- Bronchial rupture and hematoma
- Inflammatory bronchial stricture and extrinsic compression

Relaxation atelectasis
- Pneumothorax
- Pleural effusion
- Pleural tumor
- Scoliosis

Pseudosegmental opacities
- Interlobar effusion
- Loculated pleural effusion

Acute Lobar and Segmental Pneumonia
(Figs. 13.**5**–13.**10**)
Classic lobar pneumonia caused by pneumococci or *Klebsiella pneumoniae* has become a rarity. Because bacterial pneumonia spreads from alveolus to alveolus through the pores of Kohn, lobar and segmental boundaries create a reasonably effective barrier. Because of this, the opacity exhibits at least one sharp border, even if the consolidation does not involve the entire segment (peripheral consolidation).

Tuberculous Pneumonia
Tuberculous pneumonia has a predilection for the upper lobes and the apical segments of the lower lobes. Often there are accompanying features of past tuberculosis such as apical pleural thickening and fibrocirrhotic changes in the apical parenchyma. Any upper lobar segmental opacity persisting for weeks should raise suspicion of tuberculous pneumonia, particularly in at-risk groups of individuals.

Bronchioloalveolar Carcinoma
Some bronchial carcinomas, especially those of bronchioloalveolar type, spread within the alveoli of a lung lobe or segment and may be indistinguishable from pneumonic consolidation.

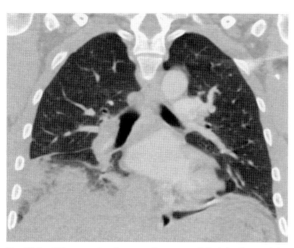

Fig. 13.**5**   CT coronal reformat shows partial right lower lobe consolidation with loss of definition of the right hemidiaphragm.

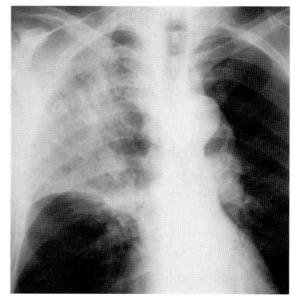

Fig. 13.**6**   Right upper lobe consolidation with a minor degree of associated atelectasis leading to slight superior displacement of the right minor fissure.

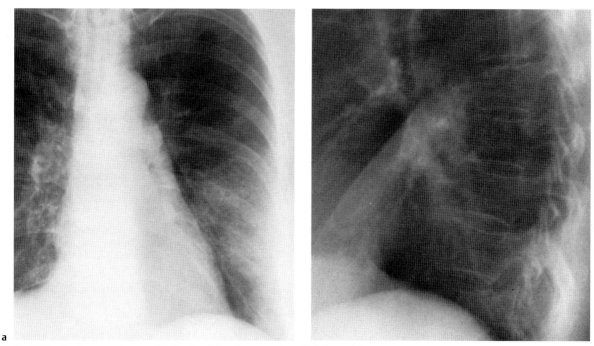

a
b

Fig. 13.**7 a, b**   Pneumonic consolidation involving the anterobasal left lower lobe.

Pulmonary Infarction

Pulmonary infarcts appear as subtle segmental opacities which occur predominantly in the subpleural lung of the lower lobes. Left ventricular failure usually is a prerequisite for the development of infarction following pulmonary embolism.

Lobar and Segmental Atelectasis

- *Absorption atelectasis* (obstructive atelectasis) in which there is initial occlusion of the bronchial lumen followed by absorption of air in the distal lung: Airway obstruction may be caused by tumor, mucus plugs, foreign bodies, inflammatory bronchial nar-

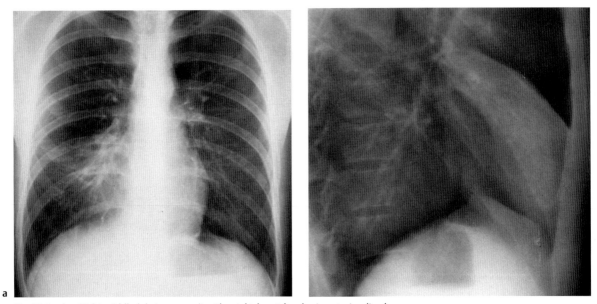

Fig. 13.**8 a, b**   Right middle lobe pneumonia. The right heart border is not visualized.

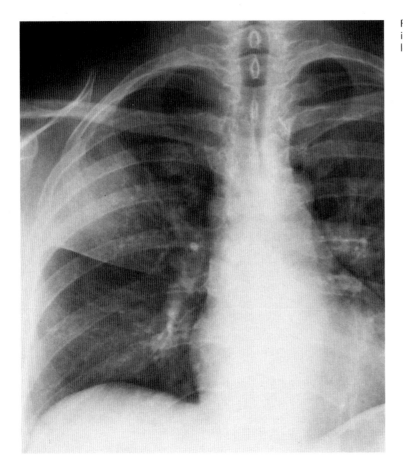

Fig. 13.**9**   Pneumonic consolidation involving the anterior segment of the right upper lobe lies adjacent to the minor fissure.

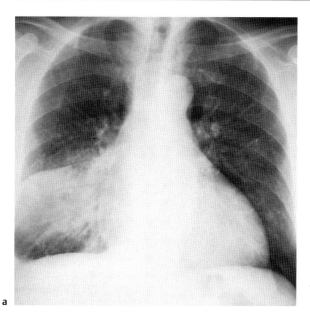

a

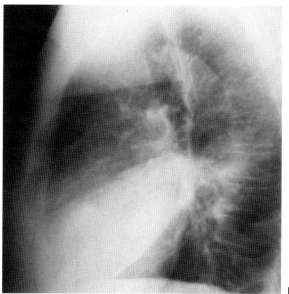

b

Fig. 13.**10a, b**   Right middle lobe pneumonia.

rowing or occlusion, or extrinsic compression (e. g., by lymph node enlargement in "right middle lobe" syndrome). In most cases there is incomplete collapse of the involved segment or lobe because of collateral air drift through the pores of Kohn.
- *Relaxation atelectasis (compression atelectasis)*: In this case lung expansion is prevented by a pneumothorax or large pleural effusion with resulting pulmonary atelectasis. This form of atelectasis may persist for a short time following aspiration of the effusion or pneumothorax.

Volume loss in a lobe tends to have a specific radiographic appearance (Fig. 13.**12**):
- Right upper lobe atelectasis is manifest as a wedge/ triangular-shaped opacity lying adjacent to the superior mediastinum (Fig. 13.**14**).
- Right middle lobe atelectasis is associated with obliteration/"loss" of the right cardiac border.
- Right and left lower lobe atelectasis lead to obliteration/"loss" of the respective hemidiaphragm (Fig. 13.**15a, b**) and in left lower lobe atelectasis, a wedge-shaped opacity may be visible in the left paravertebral/retrocardiac region.
- Left upper lobe atelectasis leads to "hazy" opacification of the left hemithorax (Figs. 13.**16a, b**, see also Fig. 6.**24a-c**).
- Lingular segment atelectasis leads to obliteration/ loss of the left cardiac border.

Atypical appearances may be due to collateral aeration of isolated boundary zones or may occur in cases where fibrous adhesions prevent uniform volume loss.

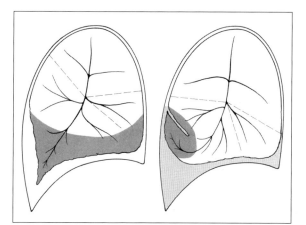

Fig. 13.**11**   Evolution of round atelectasis (from Hanke and Kretschmar 1983).

Complete atelectasis appears radiographically as a homogeneous shadow but initially some portions of the segment may still be aerated. The following radiographic features characterize atelectasis:
- The shape and location of the opacification (see Fig. 1.**33**).
- Concavity of the segmental margin. This is clearly appreciated only at sites where the segment borders on the lobar boundary or interlobar fissure.
- Hyperexpansion of adjacent lung characterized by decreased vascular markings and local hypertransradiancy.
- Displacement of interlobar fissures and vascular shadows.

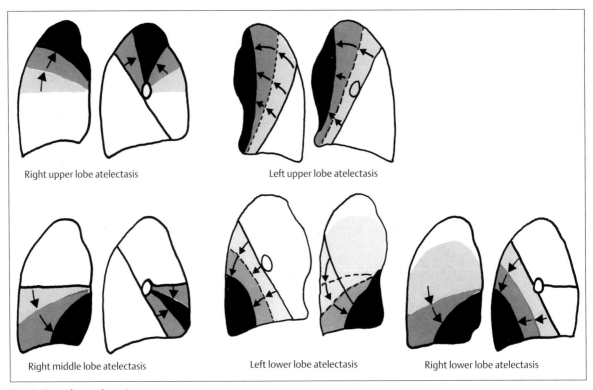

Right upper lobe atelectasis

Left upper lobe atelectasis

Right middle lobe atelectasis

Left lower lobe atelectasis

Right lower lobe atelectasis

Fig. 13.**12**   Lobar atelectasis.

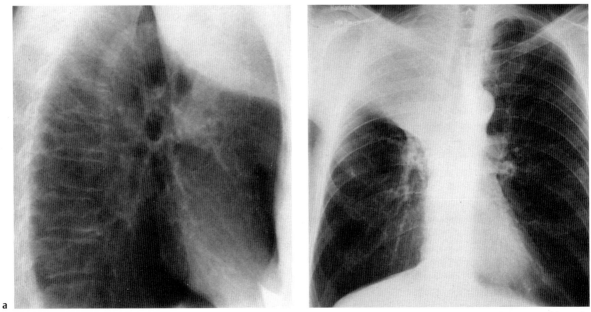

a

b

Fig. 13.**13 a, b**   Right upper lobe consolidation and atelectasis due to endobronchial tumor. There is superior displacement of the right minor fissure and the major fissure is displaced anteriorly.

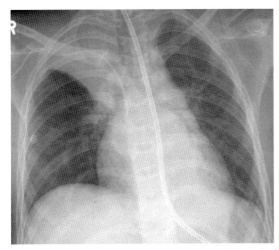

Fig. 13.**14**   Right upper lobe atelectasis due to an endobronchial mucus plug.

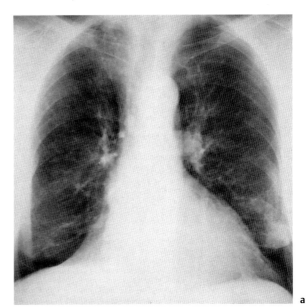

a

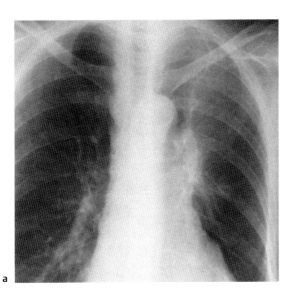

a

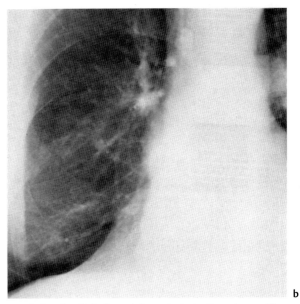

b

Fig. 13.**15 a, b**   Right lower lobe atelectasis. There is opacification of the right cardiophrenic angle with "loss" of the right hemidiaphragm.

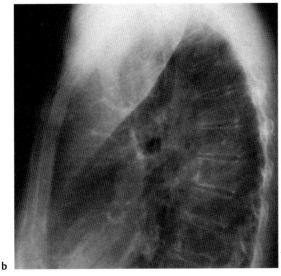

b

◁ Fig. 13.**16 a, b**   Left upper lobe atelectasis secondary to central bronchial carcinoma.

- Ipsilateral shift of the mediastinum, elevation of the hemidiaphragm, narrowing of the intercostal spaces, and transmediastinal herniation of the opposite lung. These changes are seen with lobar or complete pulmonary atelectasis.

Central Bronchial Carcinoma
Lobar or segmental atelectasis may be associated with ipsilateral hilar enlargement ± mediastinal lymph node enlargement.

Endobronchial Metastases
Breast carcinoma and other tumors occasionally metastasize to the wall of a lobar or segmental bronchus (see Fig. 6.**34 a, b**).

Benign Endobronchial Tumors
Bronchial carcinoid is the most common benign tumor to display endobronchial growth and lead to distal atelectasis. A small number of cases will develop bronchoceles distal to the obstructing tumor and branching opacities may then be the predominant radiographic finding. Other endobronchial tumors including chondroma, which occasionally shows flocculent calcification, hamartomas, and amyloid tumors are comparatively rare.

Endobronchial Mucus Plugging
This is characteristically seen in severe asthma and in patients with superimposed Allergic Bronchopulmonary Aspergillosis (ABPA).

Bronchial Rupture and Hematoma
Severe thoracic injuries may rupture a main or lobar bronchus with submucosal hematoma and distal atelectasis.

Inflammatory Bronchial Strictures and Extrinsic Compression
Inflammatory bronchial strictures may be seen in entities such as tuberculous infection and Wegener's granulomatosis.

The right middle lobe bronchus is particularly susceptible to compression by adjacent tuberculous lymph nodes resulting in distal atelectasis.

3. Opacification which does not Conform to Anatomic Boundaries

Inhomogeneous and Regionally Confluent Air Space Opacification

■ Diagnostic Approach

These are poorly-defined nonsegmental areas of consolidation which may contain air broncho- and air alveolograms. The commonest cause of nonsegmental consolidation is bronchopneumonia, which is readily diagnosed when classic presentation is combined with radiographic findings of patchy or confluent air space consolidation.

■ Differential Diagnosis (Table 13.3)

Acute Bronchopneumonia
This disease is characterized by patchy air space shadowing characteristically involving the mid-to-lower lung zones. Acute bronchopneumonia is usually due to bacterial infection (Fig. 13.**17**).

Table 13.**3** Pulmonary opacification not conforming to lobar and segmental boundaries

Inflammatory
- Bronchopneumonia
- Aspiration pneumonia
- Tuberculous pneumonia
- Fungal pneumonia (semi-invasive pulmonary aspergillosis)
- Chronic eosinophilic pneumonia
- Organizing pneumonia (OP)
- Hypersensitivity pneumonitis
- Churg–Strauss allergic granulomatosis

Edema and hemorrhage
- Pulmonary edema
- Pulmonary hemorrhage in Wegener's granulomatosis and antiglomerular basement membrane disease

Neoplastic
- Bronchioloalveolar carcinoma
- Primary pulmonary lymphoma and lung involvement in systemic lymphoma

Miscellaneous
- Radiation pneumonitis
- Silicosis

Bilateral symmetric opacification
- Pulmonary edema and hemorrhage
- Infection including pneumocystis pneumonia
- Hyaline membrane disease in the newborn
- ARDS
- Alveolar proteinosis

Aspiration Pneumonia

Aspiration pneumonia characteristically involves the dependent portions of the lung, most commonly the lower lobes. Right lung involvement is more frequent due to the more vertical course of the bronchus intermedius. Aspiration pneumonia may be complicated by pulmonary abscess formation.

Tuberculous Pneumonia

Multifocal areas of bronchocentric consolidation may be a manifestation of endobronchial spread of tuberculosis and there may be associated micronodular shadowing consistent with a cellular bronchiolitis

Fungal Pneumonia

Fungal pneumonias and particularly semi-invasive aspergillosis (Fig. 13.18) in older individuals with a mild degree of immunocompromise due to co-morbidities may manifest as patchy air space consolidation.

Pulmonary Edema

Early-stage alveolar edema may have an inhomogeneous patchy distribution in the mid-to-lower lung zones. There are characteristically features of associated interstitial edema with peribronchial cuffing and interlobular septal thickening.

Pulmonary Contusion

Patchy, confluent opacities representing sites of intra-alveolar edema and hemorrhage are seen in the traumatized lung. Pulmonary contusions typically resolve in 3 to 6 days except when infection supervenes.

Pulmonary Hemorrhage

Diffuse pulmonary hemorrhage is associated with underlying disease entities including Antiglomerular Basement Membrane Disease (AGBMD) and Wegener's Granulomatosis. Initial multifocal opacification in a peribronchovascular distribution may progress to areas of confluent consolidation.

Churg–Strauss Allergic Granulomatosis

Chest radiographs may show transient, recurrent pneumonic infiltrates in addition to pericardial and pleural effusion in patients with this systemic necrotizing vasculitis.

Pulmonary Neoplasia

Both bronchioloalveolar carcinoma and pulmonary lymphoma may be manifest radiographically as patchy air space consolidation in a peribronchial distribution.

Radiation Pneumonitis and Fibrosis

Air space consolidation characteristically conforms to the radiation portal in radiotherapy-induced pneumonitis. Consolidation over time may organize leaving some degree of interstitial fibrosis (Fig. 13.19).

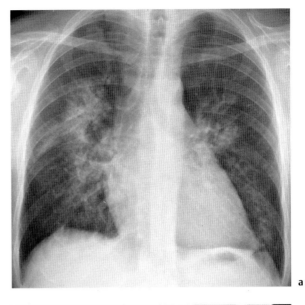

a

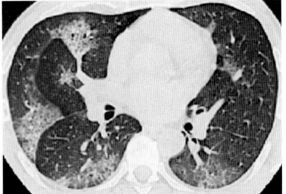

b

Fig. 13.**17 a, b**   Multifocal airspace consolidation not conforming to segmental or lobar boundaries.

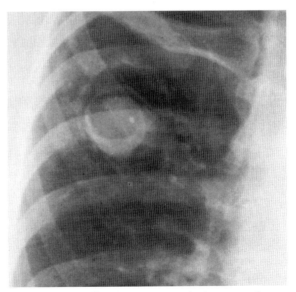

Fig. 13.**18**   Aspergilloma: Mycetoma with air crescent is seen within right upper lobe cavity.

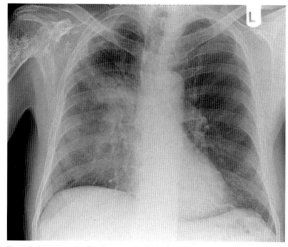

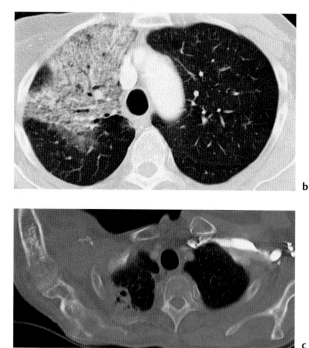

Fig. 13.**19 a–c** Radiotherapy-induced pulmonary fibrosis. Chest radiograph (**a**) shows right-sided pulmonary opacification not conforming to lobar or segmental boundaries. Patchy sclerosis in the proximal diaphysis of the right humerus is characteristic of old bone infarct. Axial CT image displayed at lung windows (**b**) shows pulmonary change consistent with fibrosis in the right upper zone. CT displayed at bony windows (**c**) shows bone infarct in right proximal humerus.

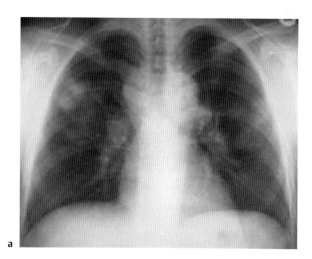

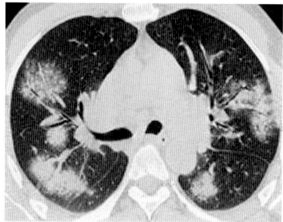

Sarcoidosis (Fig. 13.**20**)
See Chapter 3, p. 91.

Adult Respiratory Distress Syndrome
See Chapter 8, p. 208.

Bilateral Symmetric Hazy Opacification

◼ Differential Diagnosis

- Bilateral posterior pleural effusions in a supine patient (Fig. 13.**21 a**, **b**).
- Hyaline membrane disease—Acute respiratory distress syndrome in the newborn (Fig. 13.**22**).
- Adult respiratory distress syndrome—Diffuse alveolar damage (Fig. 13.**23**).
- Pulmonary infection, edema, hemorrhage (Fig. 13.**24**).
- Alveolar proteinosis (Fig. 13.**25**).

Fig. 13.**20 a, b** Sarcoidosis. The chest radiograph (**a**) shows bilateral hilar and mediastinal lymph node enlargement with areas of pulmonary consolidation. CT shows bilateral hilar and mediastinal lymph node enlargement with areas of consolidation consistent with the "alveolar" variant of sarcoidosis.

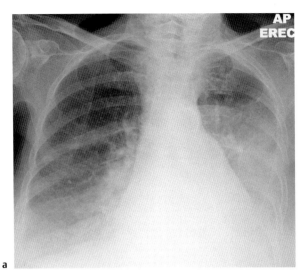

a

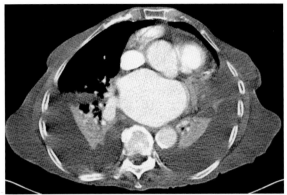

b

Fig. 13.**21 a, b**   Pleural effusions in supine patient: Hazy opacification of both hemithoraces on AP supine projection (**a**) is due to bilateral pleural effusions and underlying pulmonary atelectasis (**b**).

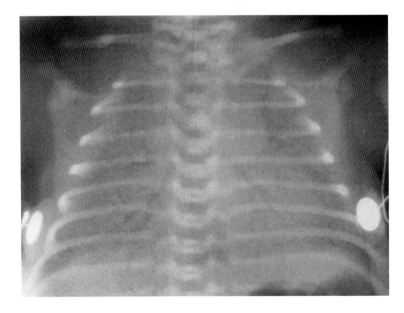

Fig. 13.**22**   Hyaline membrane disease with bilateral "ground-glass opacification" in a preterm infant. Air bronchograms are visible.

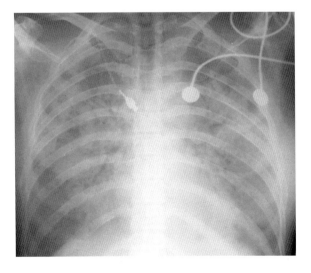

Fig. 13.**23**   Adult respiratory distress syndrome in acute pancreatitis. Initial chest radiograph shows diffuse, bilateral pulmonary opacification.

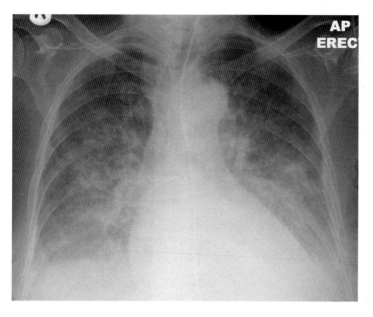

Fig. 13.**24**   Noncardiogenic pulmonary edema in a patient with renal impairment.

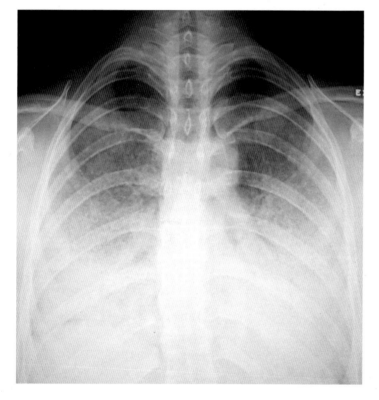

Fig. 13.**25**   Alveolar proteinosis. Chest radiograph shows "hazy" opacification of both lungs with associated interstitial thickening in patient with alveolar proteinosis.

4. Opacification involving the Upper Zone and/or Apicomediastinal Angle

■ Diagnostic Approach

Opacification of the lung apex and upper paramediastinal lung may be due to pulmonary, pleural, or mediastinal disease. Pulmonary diseases showing a predilection for the upper lobe include tuberculosis, ABPA, and pulmonary Langerhans cell histiocytosis (PLCH). Superior mediastinal widening may be due to vascular ectasia, thyroid goiter, or mediastinal lymph node enlargement.

■ Differential Diagnosis (Fig. 13.26, Table 13.4)

Vascular and Mediastinal Lesions

Vascular Ectasia
Ectasia of superior mediastinal vessels leads to mediastinal widening with a curved, sharply defined lateral border. Dilatation and elongation are particularly common in elderly patients and may involve the left brachiocephalic vein, subclavian vein, superior vena cava, and innominate artery. Computed tomography will confirm the vascular ectasia when there is diagnostic uncertainty.

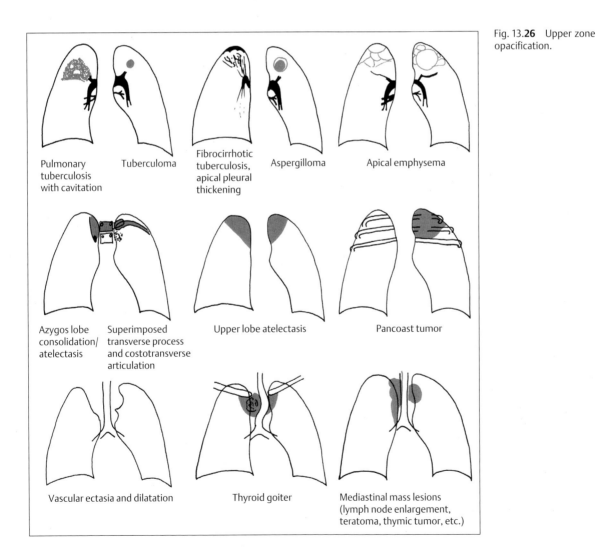

Fig. 13.26 Upper zone opacification.

Table 13.**4**   Upper zone and apicomediastinal angle opacification

Mediastinal
Vascular
- Arterial and venous ectasia/dilatation
- Aortic aneurysm

Nonvascular
- Thyroid goiter and thyroid carcinoma
- Thymic hyperplasia and thymic tumors
- Lymph node enlargement
- Benign cystic teratoma and germ cell tumors
- Peripheral nerve sheath tumors
- Bronchogenic cyst
- Lymphangioma (cystic hygroma)

Pulmonary and Pleural
- Upper lobe pneumonia and atelectasis
- Upper lobe tuberculosis
- Bronchial carcinoma including Pancoast tumor
- Aspergilloma
- Allergic bronchopulmonary aspergillosis
- Pulmonary Langerhans cell histiocytosis
- Silicosis
- Apical fibrosis in ankylosing spondylitis
- Apical pleural thickening

Miscellaneous
- Azygos vein within fissure (Fig. 13.**30**)

Aortic/Great Vessel Aneurysm

Aneurysmal dilatation of the aortic arch may produce a large mediastinal density, generally with a convex lateral border on the posteroanterior (PA) chest radiograph (see also Chapter 11, p. 283). Aneurysmal dilatation of a subclavian/anomalous right subclavian artery may lead to unilateral superior mediastinal widening.

Retrosternal Goiter and other Mediastinal Soft Tissue Lesions

There is widening of the superior mediastinum and the trachea may be narrowed or displaced. Thyroid nodules may show flocculent calcification. See also Chapter 11, p. 285.

Pulmonary and Pleural

Upper Lobe Pneumonia

Pneumonia involving the apical segment of the right upper lobe or the apicoposterior segment of the left upper lobe appears as a triangular paramediastinal opacity. Consolidation in the anterior segment of the right upper lobe abuts the minor fissure.

Upper Lobe Tuberculosis (Fig. 13.**27**)

Tuberculous infection should be excluded in all cases of persisting upper lobe consolidation (see also Chapter 3, p. 72).

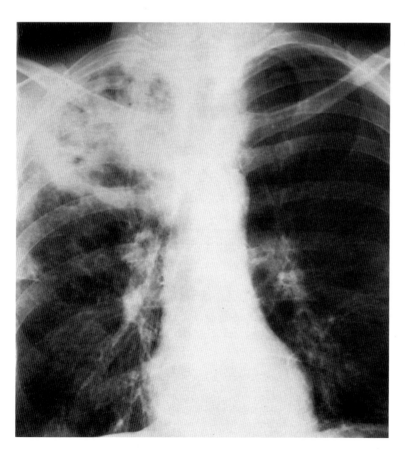

Fig. 13.**27**   Right upper lobe tuberculosis.

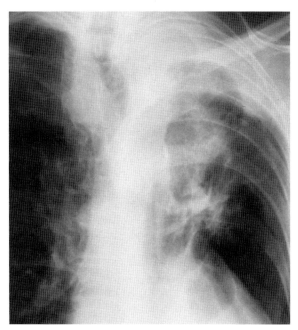

Fig. 13.**28** Radiation pneumonitis posttreatment of left hilar/upper lobe bronchial carcinoma.

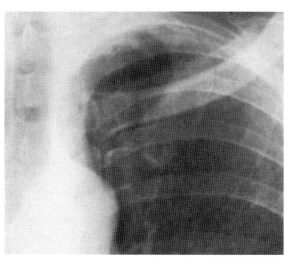

Fig. 13.**29** Apical pleural thickening.

Bronchial Carcinoma

Bronchial carcinomas may occur in the superior sulcus of the lung and infiltrate locally (Pancoast tumor). The chest radiograph may demonstrate destruction of adjacent ribs. More commonly, bronchial carcinoma arising from and occluding the upper lobe bronchus leads to distal upper lobe consolidation and atelectasis (Fig. 13.**28**).

Silicosis

Silicotic nodules sometimes may be concentrated in the upper lobes. Progressive massive fibrosis (PMF) complicating silicosis has a marked predilection for the upper lobes.

Pulmonary Langerhans Cell Histiocytosis

Early-stage nodular PLCH characteristically involves the upper-to-mid zones with relative sparing of the lung bases (see also Chapter 6, p. 154).

Mucoid Impaction (Bronchocele Formation)

Congenital bronchial atresia occurs most commonly in the apicoposterior segmental bronchus of the left upper lobe. The airway distal to the atresia is dilated and filled with mucus and appears as an elongated, partially branched opacity in the left upper lobe (bronchocele). Allergic bronchopulmonary aspergillosis also leads to mucus plugging of bronchi and characteristically colonizes dilated upper lobe bronchi.

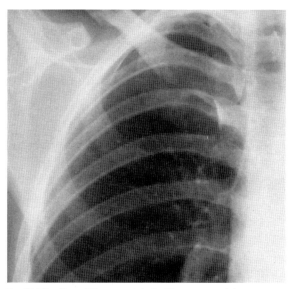

Fig. 13.**30** Pleural line associated with an azygos lobe.

Apical Pleural Thickening

An apical pleural peel may extend to involve the mediastinal pleura and reach a thickness of several millimeters (Fig. 13.**29**).

Azygos Lobe and Fissure (Fig. 13.**30**)

See Chapter 1, p. 14.

5. Lower Lung and Cardiophrenic Angle Opacification

Lower lung and cardiophrenic angle opacification may result from a variety of pulmonary, pleural, diaphragmatic, and mediastinal processes.

■ Differential Diagnosis (Fig. 13.31, Table 13.5)

Crowding of Basal Vessels
During expiration and in cases where inspiration is restricted due to obesity or ascites, compression of the basal pulmonary vessels occurs, causing a bilateral increase in basal vascular markings.

Plate Atelectasis (Fig. 13.32)
These linear opacities, which may be up to 3 mm in width and 10 cm in length, are usually seen coursing horizontally in the lower zones. There may be associated elevation of the ipsilateral hemidiaphragm.

Table 13.5   Lower zone and cardiophrenic angle opacification

Pulmonary
- Vascular crowding
- Plate atelectasis
- Lower lobe consolidation and atelectasis
- Right middle lobe consolidation and atelectasis
- Basal lung edema
- Bronchopulmonary sequestration

Pleural-diaphragmatic
- Pleural effusion
- Pleural thickening
- Pleural tumor
- Transdiaphragmatic hernias
- Tumors of the diaphragm

Mediastinal
- Epicardial fat
- Pericardial cyst
- Mediastinal tumors
- Paravertebral abscess and osteophyte formation

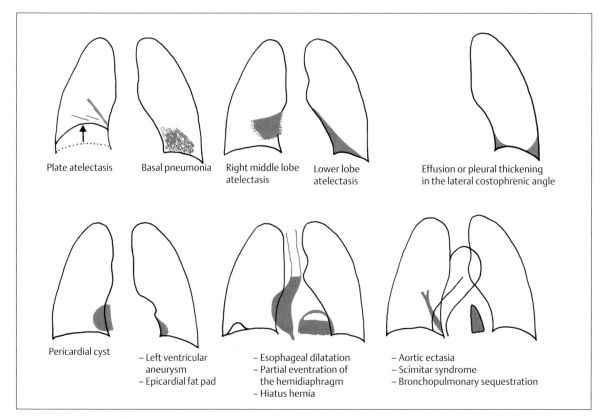

Plate atelectasis   Basal pneumonia   Right middle lobe atelectasis   Lower lobe atelectasis   Effusion or pleural thickening in the lateral costophrenic angle

Pericardial cyst   – Left ventricular aneurysm – Epicardial fat pad   – Esophageal dilatation – Partial eventration of the hemidiaphragm – Hiatus hernia   – Aortic ectasia – Scimitar syndrome – Bronchopulmonary sequestration

Fig. 13.31   Basal and cardiomediastinal opacification.

Pneumonic Consolidation

Bronchopneumonia commonly develops in dependent lung and is characterized by patchy basal opacification with typical acinar shadows of peribronchiolar consolidation. Classic lobar pneumonia may also involve the right middle and lower lobes as may aspiration pneumonia. Right middle lobe change appears as a right paracardiac opacity that obscures the right cardiac border. Lower lobe consolidation leads to loss of visibility of the ipsilateral hemidiaphragm.

Pulmonary Edema

Pulmonary edema is often basal in distribution due to the greater hydrostatic pressure in these regions. It is characterized by loss of vessel definition, interlobular septal thickening, and peribronchial cuffing and it may progress to air space shadowing (alveolar edema).

Bronchopulmonary Sequestration

Bronchopulmonary sequestrations are most commonly located in the vertebrophrenic angle. Radiographically, they may be manifest as homogeneous opacities that may reach up to 10 cm in diameter. The lateral radiograph confirms their posterior location (see also Chapter 2, p. 50).

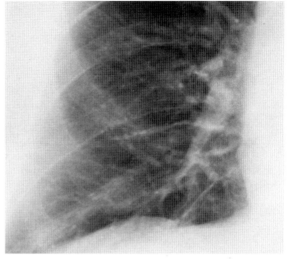

Fig. 13.**32**   Basal plate atelectasis in a postoperative patient.

Basal Pleural Effusion (Fig. 13.**33**)

In the upright position, the effusion gravitates towards the lower zones with loss of both the posterior and lateral costophrenic angles. The effusion slopes superiorly towards the lateral chest wall and has a concave interface with the lung.

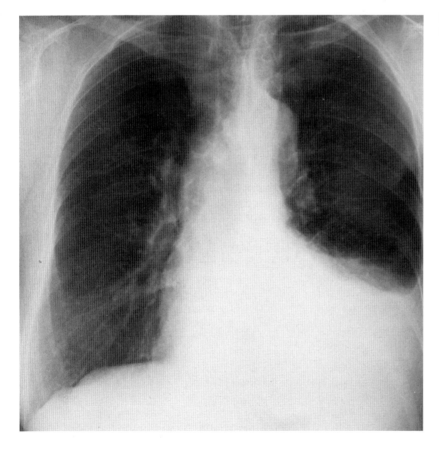

Fig. 13.**33**   Left basal pleural effusion.

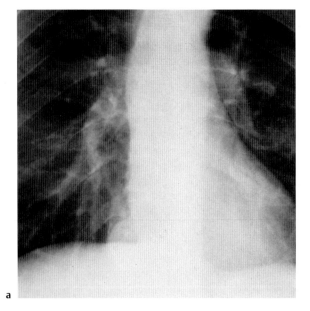

a

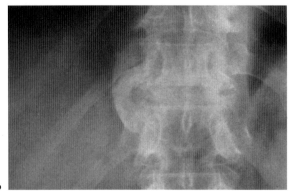

b

Basal Pleural Thickening
Basal pleural thickening may lead to blunting of the co-stophrenic angles. There may be associated tenting of the hemidiaphragm towards the lung. Ultrasound will differentiate pleural thickening from an effusion.

Diaphragmatic Hernias
Bochdalek and Morgagni herniae, particularly when they contain only peritoneal fat, may be manifest radio-graphically as soft tissue opacities in the lower zones.

Epicardial Fat Pad
The cardiophrenic angle may be obliterated by fat, especially in obese individuals. CT demonstrates negative attenuation values characteristic of lipid.

Pericardial Cyst
Pericardial cysts are well-defined relatively low density opacities that are a frequent radiographic finding and which fill the cardiophrenic angle. CT shows well-defined lesions of fluid attenuation.

Paravertebral Abscess and Osteophyte Formation
A paravertebral abscess may be secondary to septic or tuberculous (cold abscess) discitis and vertebral osteomyelitis. Lateral paravertebral osteophytes are associated with degenerative intervertebral disk change in the lower thoracic spine (Fig. 13.**34**).

Fig. 13.**34 a, b**   Round opacity in the right cardiophrenic angle is due to a large bridging osteophyte in the lower thoracic spine.

6. Pulmonary Nodules

■ Diagnostic Approach

The *solitary pulmonary nodule* is discussed in Chapter 6, p. 149.

Multiple pulmonary nodules
Pulmonary nodules are round opacities most commonly of soft tissue density that frequently have well-defined margins. Individual nodules range from < 1 to several millimeters in size.

They may be subclassified according to size:
- Macronodular opacities: 3–25 mm in diameter.
- Micronodular (miliary) opacities: less than 3 mm in diameter (*L. milium* = millet seed). A miliary opacity on the radiograph may not correspond to a single pulmonary focus even when foci of similar size can be seen histologically. A miliary pattern actually frequently results from the summation of many foci intercepted by the x-ray beam (Heitzman 1993).

Superimposed extrapulmonary lesions including skin tumors, subcutaneous abnormalities, pleural plaques, and bony enostoses may mimic the presence of lung nodules on the chest radiograph (Figs. 13.**35**–13.**37**, 13.**45**, 13.**46**). Computed tomography is occasionally necessary in these cases to make the differentiation.

The pathological correlate of nodular opacification is variable:
- *Alveolar-based nodules* (Table 13.**6**): Focal opacities may result from airspace filling with fluid, exudate, blood, or neoplastic tissue. These infiltrates must be 5–7 mm in diameter before they are visible on the chest radiograph. These nodules may be poorly de-

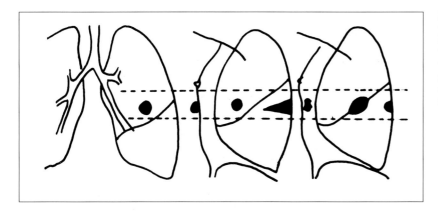

Fig. 13.**35** Rounded opacity on the frontal chest radiograph. The lateral view demonstrates the location and shape of the opacity (skin tumor, rib enostosis, pulmonary nodule, interlobar effusion, segmental infiltrate, pleural tumor) (from Rübe).

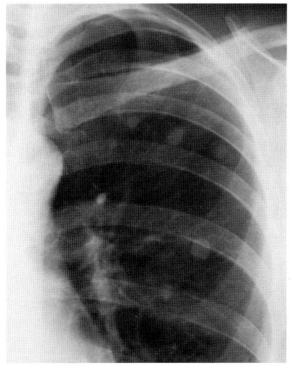

Fig. 13.**36** Multiple nodular lesions projected onto the lung in von Recklinghausen's (type 1) neurofibromatosis.

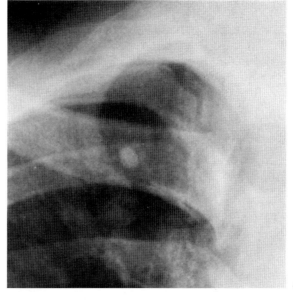

a

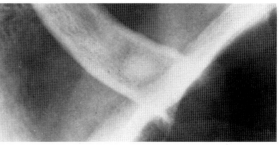

b

Fig. 13.**37 a, b** Bone island/enostosis in the right clavicle. The ▷ rotated view confirms the location of the lesion.

fined due to their irregular interface with surrounding normally aerated alveoli.

- *Interstitial-based nodules*: Granulomata and tumor nodules may be interstitial in location. The size of individual nodules is very variable but these lesions are generally sharply demarcated with respect to adjacent aerated alveoli.

Table 13.**6** Radiographic features of alveolar shadowing (from Felson)

1. Ill-defined focal opacification
2. Confluent opacification
3. Segmental or lobar distribution
4. Butterfly pattern in the perihilar lung
5. Air bronchogram and air alveologram
6. Peribronchiolar (acinar) nodular opacification

Table 13.**7**   Pulmonary nodules

Extrapulmonary opacities
- Skin lesions: nipple, neurofibromas
- Bony enostoses
- Pleural plaques
- Interlobar effusion

Pulmonary nodules
Neoplastic
- Pulmonary metastases
- Kaposi's sarcoma
- Malignant leiomyomatosis

Infection
- Miliary tuberculosis
- Endobronchial spread in 2° tuberculosis
- Histoplasmosis, blastomycosis, candidiasis, coccidioidomycosis
- Acute invasive aspergillosis

Connective Tissue Disorders and Vasculitides
- Rheumatoid nodules
- Wegener granulomatosis

Pneumoconioses
- Silicosis
- Coal worker's pneumoconiosis

Vascular
- Multiple pulmonary arteriovenous malformations
- Hemosiderosis

Hypersensitivity and Idiopathic
- Pulmonary Langerhans cell histiocytosis
- Sarcoidosis
- Hypersensitivity pneumonitis

■ Differential Diagnosis (Table 13.**7**)

Neoplasia

Metastases
These well-defined lesions show considerable variation in both individual size and number (Fig. 13.**38**). Metastases from thyroid carcinoma may produce a fine miliary pattern of nodularity while renal cell carcinoma is characteristically associated with large so called "cannonball" metastases. Metastases from osteosarcoma or chondrosarcoma will show ossification or calcification, respectively, while metastases from squamous cell primary tumors have a tendency to cavitate.

Kaposi Sarcoma
See Chapter 3, p. 98.

Malignant Leiomyomatosis (Fig. 13.**39**)
This is a rare hamartomatous lung disease arising from the vascular smooth-muscle cells of bronchi and alveolar septae. The disease can lead to respiratory failure and death within a few years. Pleural involvement is frequent, resulting in a chylous effusion. The chest radiograph shows multiple confluent opacities 5–9 mm in diameter with an accompanying honeycomb pattern.

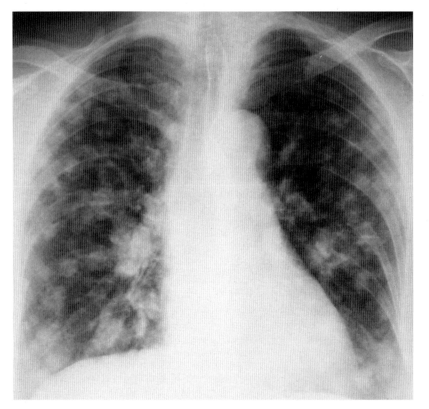

Fig. 13.**38**   Multiple pulmonary metastases from known colon carcinoma.

Infection

Multiple Pulmonary Abscesses and Septic Emboli
Pyogenic abscesses present as single or multiple, ill-defined focal opacities up to 2 cm in diameter scattered throughout the lung (see Figs. 13.**55a**, **b**, 13.**56**).

Acute Invasive Aspergillosis
See Chapter 3, p. 81.

Miliary Tuberculosis
Hematogenous spread of tuberculosis leads to diffuse fine nodular shadowing (miliary pattern) (see Fig. 13.**40**).

Secondary Pulmonary Tuberculosis
Coarse, confluent acinar shadows are seen in endobronchial spread of tuberculosis, with multiple acinonodular opacities 3–6 mm in diameter coalescing to form caseous foci of tuberculous pneumonia. A finer nodular pattern in secondary tuberculosis also indicates endobronchial spread of TB but with changes predominating within the bronchioles (*cellular bronchiolitis*). CT findings are of centrilobular nodules and branching linear opacities.

Histoplasmosis
See Chapter 3, p. 84.

Pneumoconiosis

Coal Worker's Pneumoconiosis
See Chapter 5, p. 140.

Silicosis
The nodular form of silicosis is characterized by multiple well-defined nodules 1–10 mm in diameter, often combined with pulmonary fibrosis and cicatricial emphysema.

Connective Tissue Disorders and Vasculitides

Rheumatoid Nodules
These appear as subpleural nodules 3–7 mm in diameter and their size and number wax and wane with the subcutaneous nodules and with systemic disease activity.

Wegener Granulomatosis
Typically, there are multiple nodules or masses that frequently cavitate. The patients usually are quite ill and concomitant sinusitis and hematuria may be present. The diagnosis is based on positive ANCA (anti-neutrophilic cytoplasmic antibody) titers.

Vascular

Multiple Arteriovenous Malformations
See Chapter 2, p. 61.

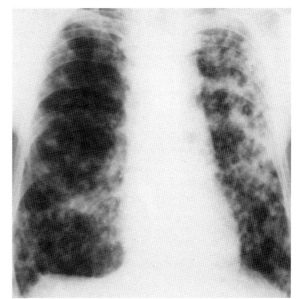

Fig. 13.**39**   Malignant leiomyomatosis confirmed at autopsy.

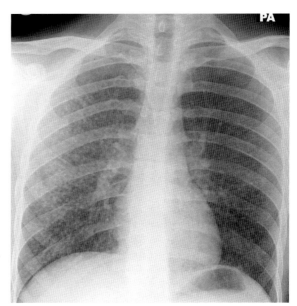

Fig. 13.**40**   Chest radiograph shows bilateral fine nodular shadowing.

Hypersensitivity and Idiopathic

Hypersensitivity Pneumonitis
Diffuse nodular shadowing may be seen in the subacute stage of hypersensitivity pneumonitis.

Sarcoidosis (Fig. 13.**41**)
The miliary stage of sarcoidosis is occasionally manifest as diffuse nodular opacification which is most marked in the perihilar lung. Hilar and mediastinal lymph node enlargement is a frequent associated finding.

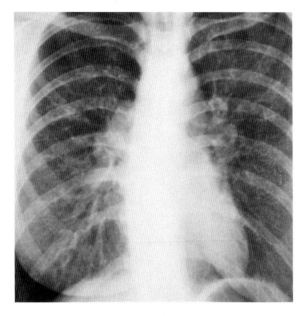

Pulmonary Langerhans Cell Histiocytosis
Radiographs in the granulomatous stage of this disease show multiple, bilaterally symmetric pulmonary nodules 1–10 mm in diameter, which are most numerous in the upper zones and with relative sparing of the lung bases.

Fig. 13.**41** Sarcoidosis with bilateral hilar lymph node enlargement and fine nodular shadowing in the perihilar lung bilaterally.

7. Linear Shadowing (Tables 13.**8**, 13.**9**)

Table 13.**8**   Vascular shadows in the lung

- Normal pulmonary vascular markings
- Pulmonary congestion
- Pulmonary plethora
- Atelectasis with "crowding" of pulmonary vessels

Table 13.**9**   Linear opacification

Chest wall
- Medial border of scapula
- Manubrium sternum
- Rib companion shadows
- Clavicular companion shadow
- Extrapleural fat deposition
- Skin folds

Pleura
- Pleural reflections
- Interlobar fissure, azygos fissure
- Linear pleural fibrosis/scarring
- Pneumothorax
- Pneumoperitoneum
- Accessory diaphragm

Pulmonary
- Atelectasis
- Parenchymal bands
- Bronchiectasis
- Kerley A lines
- Kerley B lines
- Carcinomatous lymphangitis

Pulmonary arterial and venous line shadows give the pulmonary markings which are seen on the normal chest radiograph. Vessels which normally are below the threshold of radiographic resolution become visible when dilated leading to an increase in linear markings. This is observed in cardiogenic pulmonary edema and in pulmonary plethora.

Vascular markings may appear increased when they are crowded due to pulmonary atelectasis. This "crowding" of vessels is seen at the lung bases on normal expiratory views and in elevation of the hemidiaphragm.

Large emphysematous bullae may also compress the adjacent lung parenchyma and lead to vascular crowding.

Line shadows are homogeneous linear or band-like opacities that are sharply delineated with respect to adjacent aerated lung. They have sharper margins than vascular shadows and are frequently solitary.

Line shadows may be due to (Figs. 13.**42**, 13.**43**):
- Chest wall structures projected onto the lung
- Interlobar fissures viewed tangentially
- Pulmonary scarring/fibrosis
- Discoid atelectasis
- Thickened interlobular septa (Kerley A and B lines)
- Thickened bronchial walls

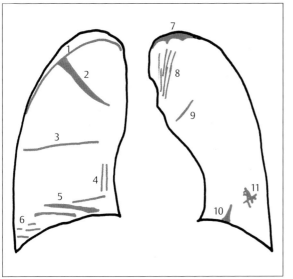

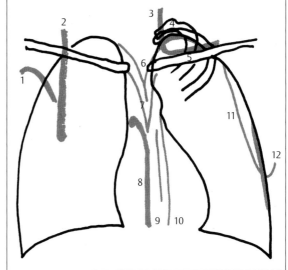

Fig. 13.**42** Linear opacification (from Teschendorf).

1	Pneumothorax	7	Apical pleural thickening
2	Atelectasis	8	Apicohilar strands of fibrous tissue
3	Interlobar fissure	9	Kerley A lines
4	Bronchiectasis	10	Pleural reflection at the major fissure
5	Plate atelectasis		
6	Kerley B lines	11	Pulmonary parenchymal bands/ scarring

Fig. 13.**43** Other causes of linear opacification (from Teschendorf).

1	Axillary fold	7	Anterior junction line
2	Skin fold	8	Azygoesophageal stripe
3	Sternocleidomastoid muscle	9	Paravertebral stripe
4	Rib companion shadow	10	Para-aortic stripe
5	Clavicular companion shadow	11	Medial border of scapula
6	Posterior superior junction line	12	Extrapleural fat deposition

Chest Wall Structures Projected onto the Lung

Medial Border of the Scapula (Fig. 13.**44**)
This line shadow projects symmetrically onto the lateral half of the upper-to-mid zones. It may be traced inferiorly to the angle of the scapula.

Manubrium Sternum
The cortex of the manubrium sternum is projected as a vertical stripe over the upper mediastinum on both sides of the trachea. This stripe may be prominent in osteoporosis.

Clavicle Companion Shadow
The upper border of the clavicle is associated with a band-like shadow approximately 4 cm in width and this represents the overlying skin seen tangential to the beam.

Rib Companion Shadow
A companion shadow is usually seen at the posteroinferior border of the left 2nd rib; this corresponds to the subclavian artery. This shadow is not strictly parallel to the rib but is continuous medially with the supra-aortic mediastinal shadow. Its smooth margins serve to distinguish it from an apical pleural cap, which generally has a wavy contour and shows tent-like extensions into the lung parenchyma.

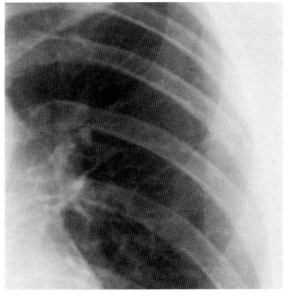

Fig. 13.**44** Vertical line shadow produced by the medial border of the scapula.

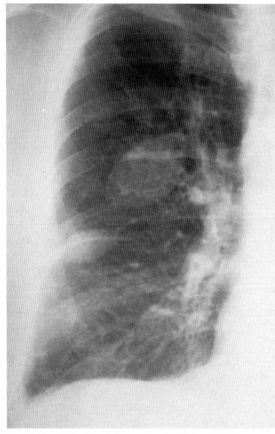

Fig. 13.**45** Typical oval shape of an interlobar effusion.

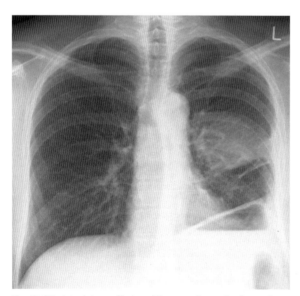

Fig. 13.**46** Interlobar effusion. Chest radiograph shows loculated left basal hydropneumothorax and interlobar effusion.

Extrapleural Fat Deposition

Fat deposition superficial to the parietal pleura may appear as a chest wall companion shadow. This is most conspicuous along the lateral chest wall.

Skin Folds

Skin folds are seen most frequently in cachectic patients who are imaged in the supine position. They appear as vertical, sharply defined linear densities. The lines often transcend the lung boundaries and this feature helps to distinguish them from pleural lines.

Linear Opacities of Pleural Origin

Interlobar Fissures

Interlobar pleural lines are visible in 15 to 20 % of chest radiographs. They are seen only when a significant part of the fissure (i. e., several centimeters in length) is tangential to the roentgen beam. These shadows are most conspicuous when they are thickened as a result of fibrosis or subpleural edema (Figs. 13.**45**, 13.**46**). The major and minor fissures are most commonly seen; intersegmental fissures are occasionally visible (see Figs. 1.**21**, 1.**25**).

Linear Pleural Scarring and Fibrosis

Areas of fibrosis secondary to pleural inflammation may be drawn into strands by the motion of the pleural layers. These usually appear radiographically as vertical or oblique lines.

Pneumothorax

The visceral pleura appears as a hairline shadow which runs parallel to the chest wall in the presence of a pneumothorax.

Pneumoperitoneum

In the presence of subdiaphragmatic free air, the hemidiaphragm appears as a thin, horizontal, superiorly convex linear density.

Accessory Diaphragm

This is a very rare anomaly in which the accessory diaphragm appears as a sail-shaped opacity traversing the right lower lobe. The radiographic appearance may be mistaken for thickening of the interlobar fissure but may be distinguished by its atypical course.

Linear Opacities of Pulmonary Origin

Segmental Atelectasis

Segmental atelectasis may give a linear shadow that is sharply defined where it borders on the interlobar fissure. Segments S3, S2, and S8 most commonly give this appearance.

Plate Atelectasis, Fleischner Lines

Plate-like or discoid atelectasis appears as a linear opacity 1–3 mm in width and 4–10 mm in length, which usually runs horizontally in the lower zones and obliquely upward and laterally in the midzones (Fig. 13.**47**). It occurs in association with elevation of the hemidiaphragm and hypoventilation (e. g., postoperative). Plate-like atelectasis is a very common radiographic finding, although the exact mechanism of its occurrence is unclear. It may relate to an infolding of the visceral pleura (Fig. 13.**48**) or a band-like area of atelectasis occurring adjacent to connective tissue septa.

Linear Pulmonary Scarring and Parenchymal Bands

Disease processes including pneumonia, tuberculosis, sarcoidosis, the pneumoconioses, and pleural inflammation may lead to contractile scarring of the lung parenchyma. These "scars" appear as linear shadows which often radiate towards the hilum. Accentuated apicohilar linear markings are frequently seen in association with upper lobe tuberculosis. There may be architectural distortion with vascular and fissural displacement and cicatricial emphysema is a common associated finding.

Pulmonary Encasement

Pleural neoplasia and particularly mesothelioma may infiltrate the interlobar fissures and encase the lung (Fig. 13.**49**).

Bronchiectasis

The chest radiograph in bronchiectasis occasionally shows parallel linear densities, which represent the parallel bronchial walls separated by an expanded lumen. Known as "tramlines," these features are most conspicuous in the paracardiac lung and are frequently associated with accentuated basohilar markings.

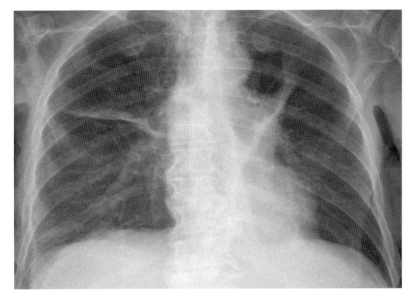

Fig. 13.**47**   Plate atelectasis due to hypoventilation.

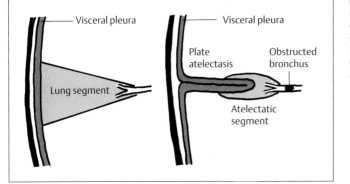

Fig. 13.**48**   The pleural hypothesis of plate atelectasis. Subsegmental lung contraction due to bronchial obstruction leads to indrawing and folding of the visceral pleura, which forms a band-like opacity on the chest radiograph (from Müller and Fraser 2001).

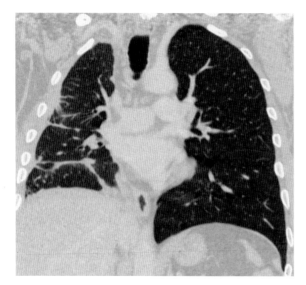

Kerley Lines

Kerley lines represent thickened interlobular septa. Kerley B lines are most common, are up to 1 cm in length, and are seen most frequently in the lateral costophrenic angles.

The less common Kerley A lines are thin lines up to 5 cm in length which radiate from the hilum into the lung especially into the upper zones. They are thinner than vascular shadows and are not branched. They represent thickened interlobular septa in the anterior portions of the upper lobe. A reticular pattern is occasionally referred to as "Kerley C lines."

Fig. 13.**49** Lung encasement with linear shadowing in a patient with malignant pleural mesothelioma.

8. Reticular Shadowing

■ Diagnostic Approach

Many pathologic processes involve the interstitial connective tissue of the lung. Interstitial thickening may be due to edema, inflammatory or neoplastic infiltration, or fibrosis. Interstitial fibrosis is characterized by increased collagen deposition and represents the end stage of a number of diseases.

The interstitium of the healthy lung generally forms a three-dimensional network that completely permeates the lung parenchyma. This includes the perivenous connective tissue, the connective tissue surrounding the bronchoarterial bundles, the interlobular connective tissue septa, the basement membrane of the alveoli, and the subpleural connective tissue. The perivascular connective tissue diminishes towards the periphery of the lung.

Interstitial lung disease in many cases is well advanced before changes are visible radiographically. Thus, it is not uncommon to find normal chest radiographs in patients who have significant clinical and spirometric evidence of restrictive ventilatory impairment. Thin collimation/high-resolution CT (HRCT) is much more sensitive than the chest radiograph to the presence of interstitial change.

The radiographic features that characterize interstitial lung disease include (Felson 1966, Table 13.**10**):

- The reticular pattern refers to a fine network of markings that may be diffusely or regionally distributed through the lungs. It is due to superimposition of thickened intralobular and interlobular septa. This pattern has occasionally been referred to as *Kerley C lines.*
- *Kerley B lines* are horizontal lines up to 1 mm in thickness and approximately 10 mm in length, which are seen most commonly in the lateral costophrenic angles. They represent thickened interlobular septa in the lung periphery. Anatomic studies have shown that interlobular septa are most numerous in the anterior and lateral regions of the lower zones and the anterior aspect of the upper zones.
- *Kerley A lines* are thin lines up to 5 cm in length that radiate from the hilum into the upper zones. They represent the thickened interlobular septa of the anterior portion of the upper lobe. They are seen much less frequently than Kerley B lines.
- The reticulonodular pattern refers to a reticular pattern combined with miliary nodulation. The miliary opacities are usually due to small nodules in the interstitium but sometimes they may represent a summation effect caused by intersecting line shadows.
- *Interlobar/subpleural thickening*: Infiltration or fibrosis of the subpleural connective tissue leads to accentuation of the interlobar fissures and accessory pleural lines.

Table 13.**10** Radiographic features of interstitial shadowing (from Felson)

- Kerley A, B, and C lines
- Miliary nodules
- Late radiographic signs, often appearing years after onset of clinical symptoms
- Honeycombing
- Thickened bronchovascular bundles

- The honeycomb pattern refers to a coarse reticular pattern that sometimes characterizes end-stage pulmonary fibrosis.

Only a small percentage of interstitial lung diseases can be diagnosed on the basis of clinical and radiographic findings.

Past radiographs, if available, will help determine the duration and progression of change. Determining if a process is acute or chronic may limit the differential diagnosis. Other associated radiographic findings including cardiomegaly, pulmonary vascular dilatation, and lymph node enlargement may suggest the diagnosis.

The history and clinical findings may also advance the diagnosis by disclosing factors such as toxic fume inhalation, dust exposure, a sudden or insidious disease onset, fever, cough, hemoptysis, and extrapulmonary symptoms and signs including joint and skin changes.

■ Differential Diagnosis (Table 13.11)

Interstitial Pulmonary Edema
(Cardiogenic and Noncardiogenic, Fig. 13.**50a, b**)
Vascular shadows have ill-defined borders, there is peribronchial cuffing, and reticular markings and Kerley B lines are most distinct in the dependent posterobasal lung. There may be associated cardiomegaly and features of pulmonary venous hypertension. Noncardiogenic edema is most commonly seen in patients on renal dialysis when it is a manifestation of fluid overload. Longstanding untreated/treatment-resistant pulmonary edema may eventually lead to some degree of interstitial fibrosis (see below).

Viral/Mycoplasma Interstitial Pneumonia
Reticular and linear shadowing is most marked in the perihilar lung (see also Chapter 3, p. 65).

Subacute Pulmonary Hemorrhage
Areas of resolving pulmonary hemorrhage may give a fine reticular pattern (see also Fig. 3.**77**).

Pulmonary Lymphangitis Carcinomatosa
Pulmonary lymphangitis carcinomatosa is manifest as interstitial thickening with in particular interlobular septal thickening which frequently is most marked in the perihilar regions and lower zones. An associated pleural effusion is frequent (see also Chapter 6, p. 174).

Idiopathic Interstitial Pneumonias
The chest radiograph may show a reticular pattern characteristically with a lower zone and subpleural distribution in both *usual interstitial pneumonia* (UIP) and *nonspecific interstitial pneumonia* (NSIP). End-stage UIP is characterized by honeycombing in this distribution (Figs. 13.**51a, b**, 13.**52**; see also Idiopathic Interstitial Pneumonias, Chapter 3, p. 95).

Table 13.**11**   Interstitial and reticular shadowing

- Interstitial edema
- Acute interstitial pneumonia
- Subacute parenchymal hemorrhage
- Pulmonary lymphangitis carcinomatosis
- Idiopathic interstitial pneumonias
- Sarcoidosis
- Chronic hypersensitivity pneumonitis
- Drug-induced pneumonitis
- Connective-tissue associated interstitial lung disease
- Asbestosis
- Hemosiderosis
- Chronic bronchitis (dirty lung)
- Bronchiectasis

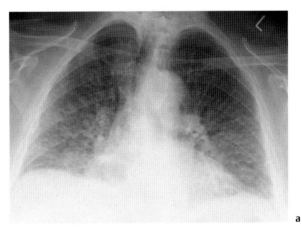

a

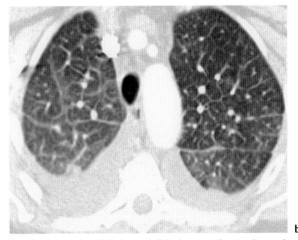

b

Fig. 13.**50a, b**   Interlobular septal thickening: Chest radiograph (**a**) shows marked bilateral septal thickening. CT (**b**) through the upper lung zones shows marked interlobular septal and centrilobular thickening.

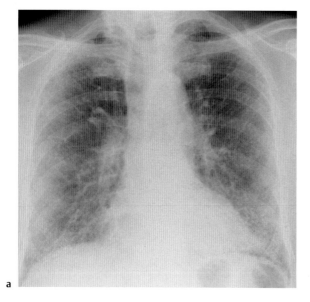

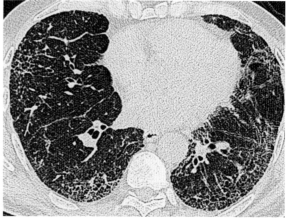

Fig. 13.**51 a, b** Interstitial-reticular pattern. Chest radiograph (**a**) shows bilateral interstitial thickening. CT (**b**) shows subpleural reticular change and some honeycombing.

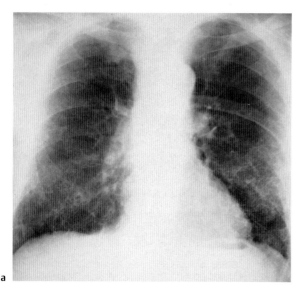

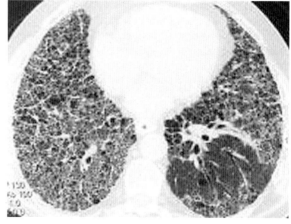

Fig. 13.**52 a, b** Pulmonary fibrosis with cicatricial emphysema and honeycombing.

Connective Tissue-Associated Interstitial Pneumonias
See Chapter 3, p. 100.

Sarcoidosis
Radiographs in stage II disease show miliary nodules and a reticular pattern that is most pronounced in the perihilar lung (Fig. 13.**53**). Associated bilateral hilar lymph node enlargement is frequently present.

Stage III disease is characterized by pulmonary fibrosis with a honeycomb pattern, which again tends to be most marked in the perihilar midzones (Fig. 13.**54**).

Chronic Hypersensitivity Pneumonitis/Extrinsic Allergic Alveolitis (EAA)
Reticular change develops with progression to pulmonary fibrosis in individuals chronically exposed to the allergen.

Asbestosis
Asbestos-induced interstitial fibrosis characteristically has a lower zone distribution. Reticular shadowing may be accompanied by asbestos-induced benign pleural disease, thus helping in differentiation from UIP.

Chronic Bronchitis

Chronic recurrent bronchitis may lead to peribronchial fibrosis with a radiographic interstitial pattern that is most marked in the lower zones. There may be radiographic features of associated emphysema.

Drug-Induced Interstitial Pneumonitis and Fibrosis

Drugs including bleomycin, methotrexate, and amiodarone may give an interstitial pneumonia in a basal and subpleural distribution. This may progress to interstitial fibrosis (see also Chapter 3, p. 108).

Radiation-Induced Pulmonary Fibrosis

Radiotherapy may induce a pneumonitis which over time progresses to an interstitial fibrosis. Reticular change is characteristically confined to the radiation portal with involvement of the medial lung postmediastinal radiotherapy and with involvement of the anterior 2 cms of the lung in breast radiotherapy.

Chronic Pulmonary Edema and Hemosiderosis

Chronic, recurring pulmonary edema induces connective tissue proliferation in the interstitium. Chest radiographs show a relatively coarse reticular pattern in the mid- and lower zones, usually accompanied by a cardiac silhouette consistent with mitral stenosis. Micronodular opacities are occasionally present in the mid- and lower zones and indicate hemosiderosis.

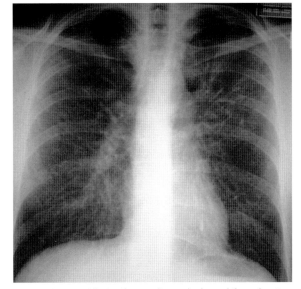

Fig. 13.**53**   Sarcoidosis: chest radiograph shows bilateral reticular change in sarcoidosis.

Fig. 13.**54 a–c**   Pulmonary fibrosis in end-stage sarcoidosis.

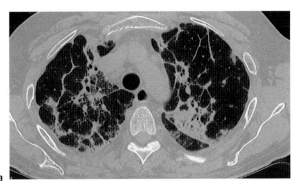

a

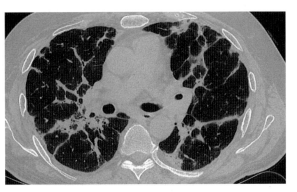
b

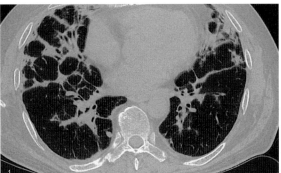
c

9. Cavitating Lung Lesions

■ Diagnostic Approach

Cavities are formed when pus from an inflammatory process or liquefied necrotic material from a neoplasm erodes into a bronchus and then is expectorated. If all of the fluid is not expectorated, radiographs will demonstrate an air–fluid level within the cavity (Table 13.**12**).

■ Differential Diagnosis

- Lung abscess and septic pulmonary emboli: Figures 13.**55**, 13.**56**.
- Pulmonary tuberculosis: Figures 13.**57**, 13.**58**.
- Echinococcal cyst: (Fig. 13.**59**) Echinococcosis (hydatid disease) is endemic in Mediterranean regions, Australia, and Africa. Chest radiographs show isolated, or rarely, multiple homogeneous round masses 1–10 cm in diameter in the central lung. The pericyst may erode into a bronchial lumen, causing a crescent of air to form around the endocyst (meniscus sign). With rupture of the endocyst, the collapsed chitin membrane may float on the fluid contents (water lily sign).

Table 13.**12**   Cavitating lung lesions

- Pyogenic lung abscess and septic pulmonary emboli
- Pulmonary tuberculosis
- Mycotic abscess (invasive pulmonary aspergillosis)
- Echinococcal cyst
- Amebic abscess
- Wegener granulomatosis
- Rheumatoid nodules
- Progressive massive fibrosis
- Bronchial carcinoma
- Pulmonary metastases from extrapulmonary squamous cell primary

- Angioinvasive pulmonary aspergillosis.
- Wegener granulomatosis.
- Bronchial carcinoma: Fig. 13.**60**.
- Pulmonary metastasis from extrapulmonary squamous cell primary.

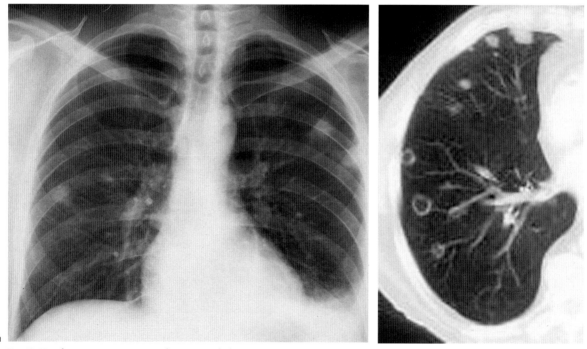

a   b

Fig. 13.**55 a, b**   Cavitation: septic pulmonary emboli.

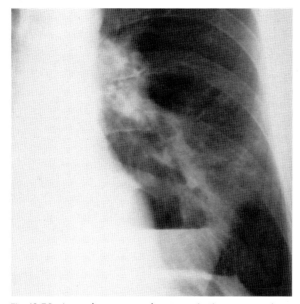

Fig. 13.**56**   Lung abscess secondary to aspiration pneumonia.

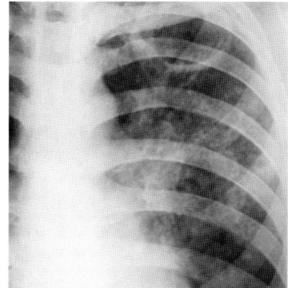

Fig. 13.**57**   Cavitation: tuberculosis. Cavitating lesion is seen at the left lung apex with adjacent poorly-defined nodular opacification.

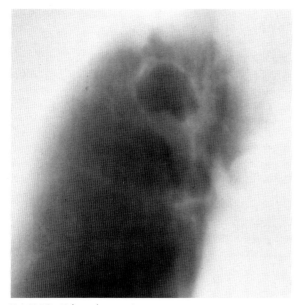

Fig. 13.**58**   Tuberculous cavity.

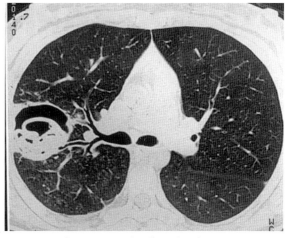

Fig. 13.**59**   Echinococcus with collapsed endocyst.

- Rheumatic nodules: Rheumatoid nodules are characteristically found in a subpleural distribution in the lower zones. Central necrosis and cavitation is occasionally seen.
- Silicosis and coal worker's pneumoconiosis: Silicosis and coal worker's pneumoconiosis (anthracosilicosis)

may lead to the formation of large, confluent fibrotic masses or plaques in the upper lobes. In this setting, cavitation usually signifies tuberculous reactivation but is occasionally due to idiopathic liquefactive necrosis of the lesion.

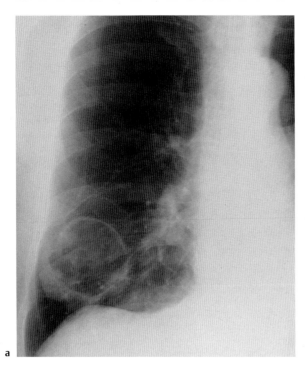

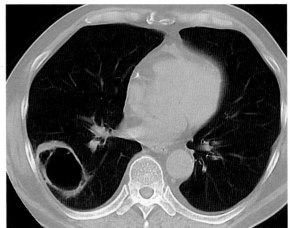

a

Fig. 13.**60 a, b**   Necrotizing large cell carcinoma.

10. Ring Shadows and Cystic Lung Disease (Table 13.**13**)

▓ Diagnostic Approach

Air-filled spaces ranging from a few millimeters to several centimeters in size may develop within the lung parenchyma in a number of disease processes (Fig. 13.**61**). These spaces appear as *ring shadows* when surrounded by aerated lung but they appear as radiolucencies when they lie within consolidated lung.

Table 13.**13**   "Cystic" lesions of the lung

- Emphysematous bullae
- Cystic bronchiectasis
- Honeycombing
- Lymphangiomyomatosis (LAM)
- Tuberous sclerosis
- Pulmonary Langerhans cell histiocytosis (PLCH)
- Lymphocytic interstitial pneumonia
- AIDS-related cystic lung change
- Pneumatocele
- Congenital lung cysts

▓ Differential Diagnosis

- Emphysematous bullae: These thin-walled air-containing lesions are found in all forms of emphysema. When subpleural in distribution, they may rupture into the pleural space to give a pneumothorax.
- Cystic bronchiectasis: Foci of cystic bronchiectasis may give ring shadows of variable wall thickness.
- Pulmonary Langerhans cell histiocytosis: Figure 13.**62**.
- Lymphocytic interstitial pneumonia.
- Lymphangiomyomatosis (Figs. 13.**63**, 13.**64**).
- Tuberous sclerosis.
- Traumatic lung cysts (Fig. 13.**65**): These lesions result from pulmonary lacerations and most commonly involve the subpleural parenchyma. They begin as hemorrhagic areas appearing as patchy opacities and progress to elliptical air-filled cavities.
- Pneumatoceles: A check-valve mechanism may give rise to giant cysts that occupy more than one-third of the lung and cause vascular and mediastinal displacement. Pneumatoceles most often develop in children and adolescents with staphylococcal pneumonia, but they also may form secondary to an infected lung cyst or abscess.
- Congenital lung cysts: Figure 13.**66**.
- AIDS-related cystic lung change.

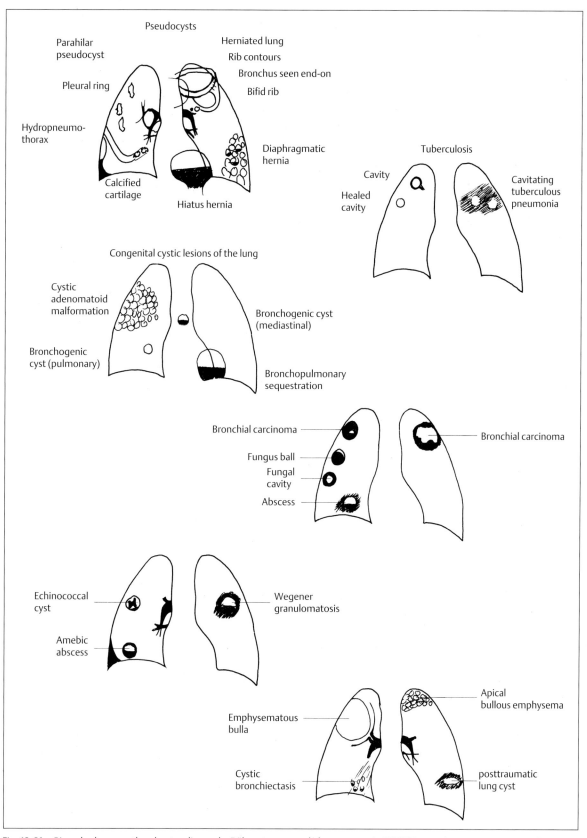

Fig. 13.**61**   Ring shadows on the chest radiograph. Dähnert proposed the mnemonic CAVITY = carcinoma, autoimmune (Wegener granulomatosis, rheumatoid disease, etc.), vascular (septic emboli), infection, trauma, young (= congenital).

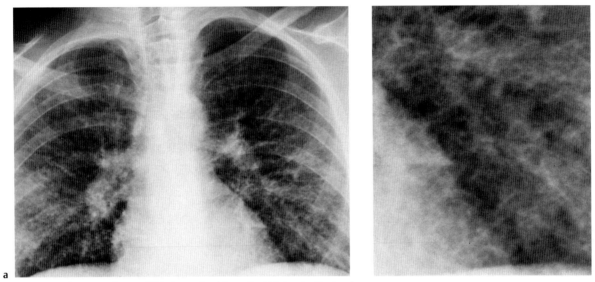

a   b

Fig. 13.**62 a, b**   Langerhans cell histiocytosis with marked bilateral reticular change.

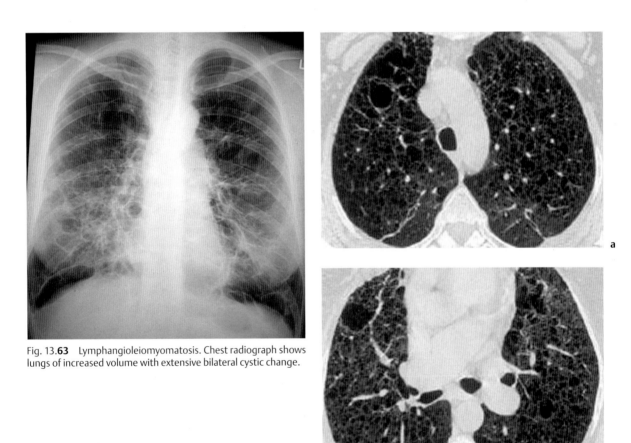

Fig. 13.**63**   Lymphangioleiomyomatosis. Chest radiograph shows lungs of increased volume with extensive bilateral cystic change.

a

b

Fig. 13.**64 a, b**   Lymphangioleiomyomatosis.

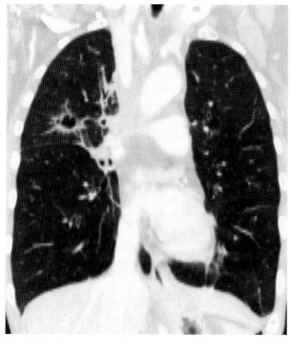

Fig. 13.**65**   Posttraumatic lung cyst.

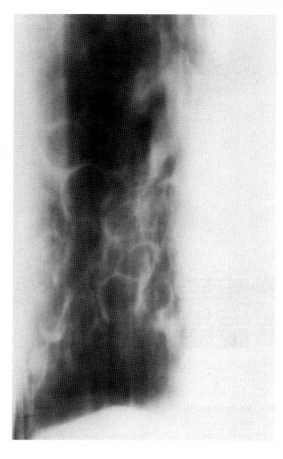

Fig. 13.**66**   Multiple congenital lung cysts.   ▷

11. Pulmonary Hypertransradiancy (Table 13.**14**)

■ Diagnostic Approach

Pulmonary vascular shadows chiefly determine the transradiancy of the lung and the density of its linear markings. Hypertransradiancy, whether generalized or regional may be due to:

1. A decrease in the caliber and number of intrapulmonary vessels
2. Pulmonary hyperinflation which leads to decreased density of vessels

The "darkness" of the lung on the chest radiograph has limited value in assessing pulmonary transradiancy since radiographic density is determined to a large extent by exposure factors and beam attenuation by the chest wall.

Table 13.**14**   Pulmonary hypertransradiancy

Extrapulmonary factors
- Overexposure
- Grid cutoff
- Thoracic asymmetry (scoliosis, mastectomy, congenital pectoral aplasia, unilateral soft tissue compression)
- Pneumothorax

Pulmonary factors
Emphysema
- In COPD and alpha-1 antitrypsin deficiency
- Localized emphysema (cicatricial emphysema, apical bullous emphysema, progressive pulmonary dystrophy)
- Compensatory emphysema (atelectasis, lobectomy)

Air Trapping
- Aspirated foreign body, endobronchial tumors, inflammatory strictures
- Bronchiolitis obliterans

Pulmonary vasoconstriction
- Acute and chronic thromboembolism
- Pulmonary artery hypoplasia

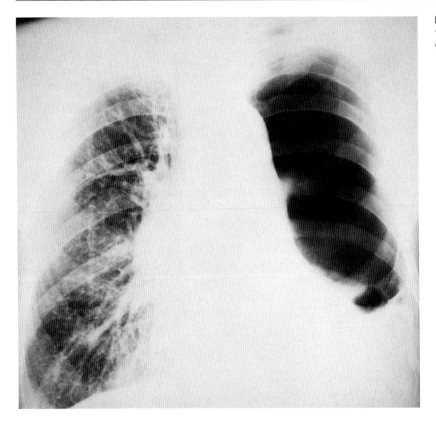

Fig. 13.**67**   Left pneumonectomy with air-filled left hemithorax in early postoperative period.

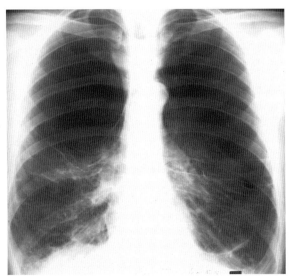

Fig. 13.**68**   "Vanishing" lung.

Vessel caliber and the number of vascular shadows per square centimeter may be more reliable indicators of pulmonary transradiancy.

Typical causes of thoracic/pulmonary hypertransradiancy are listed below.

- Extrapulmonary causes. These include exposure factors, overlying soft tissues, recent pneumectomy, and pneumothorax (Fig. 13.**67**).

- Pulmonary hyperinflation leads to hypertransradiancy.
- Pulmonary oligemia. Stenosis or occlusion of central pulmonary arteries leads to distal vasoconstriction.

Diffuse Bilateral Hypertransradiancy

- Overexposure: On an overexposed radiograph, both lungs appear abnormally hypertransradiant as do the soft tissues of the chest wall and mediastinum.
- Generalized emphysema: The chest radiograph shows signs of hyperexpansion including barrel chest, depressed diaphragmatic leaflets, expansion of the retrosternal space, and widening of the intercostal spaces (Fig. 13.**68**).
- Bronchiolitis obliterans—constrictive bronchiolitis.
- Pulmonary oligemia in pulmonary artery hypertension.

Unilateral Hypertransradiancy

Thoracic Asymmetry
Severe scoliosis, mastectomy (Fig. 13.**69**), or congenital absence of pectoral major may cause apparent variations in radiographic lung density.

Swyer–James Syndrome (Fig. 13.70)
An entire lung may appear hypertransradiant and significant air trapping is noted on expiratory views. The syn-

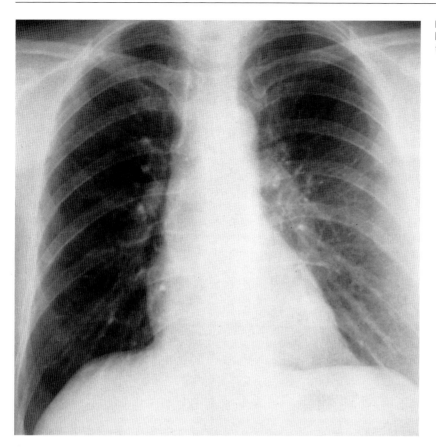

Fig. 13.**69** Hypertransradiant hemithorax following a right mastectomy.

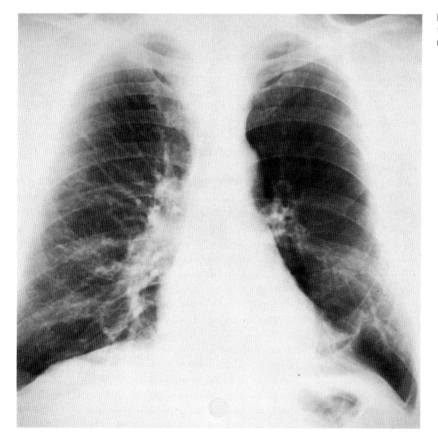

Fig. 13.**70** Swyer–James syndrome with markedly decreased vascular markings in the left hemithorax.

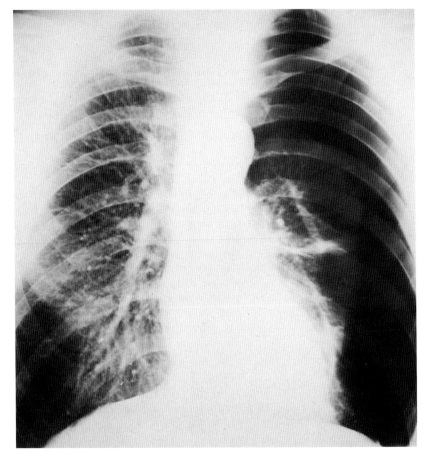

Fig. 13.**71**   Pneumothorax.

drome has been interpreted as a sequel to constrictive bronchiolitis in childhood. While initial radiographic descriptions of this entity suggested unilateral change, HRCT in most cases shows bilateral air trapping.

Pulmonary Artery Hypoplasia

This congenital anomaly is usually characterized by a unilateral hypertransradiant lung and a small hemithorax. Perfusion scintigraphy documents a marked perfusion deficit. The expiratory view does not show the air trapping which is seen in Swyer–James syndrome. CT angiography and conventional arteriography show decreased vascularity and occasional vascular occlusions. In the latter case, the lung parenchyma derives its blood supply from the bronchial arteries.

Regional Hypertransradiancy

Pneumothorax (Fig. 13.71)

Lateral to the thin line of the visceral pleura is a hyperlucent area devoid of pulmonary vascular markings. With a large pneumothorax or tension pneumothorax, the collapsed lung appears dense, the hemithorax is hypertransradiant, and there is contralateral mediastinal shift.

Localized Emphysema

Emphysematous lung change shows regional variation in many cases and in addition, associated bullous change may give regional hypertransradiancy. Special forms of "localized emphysema" include progressive pulmonary dystrophy and congenital lobar emphysema.

Compensatory Emphysema

Normal lung tissue expands to fill the void produced by atelectasis or lobectomy and may show decreased vascular markings and increased transradiancy.

Poststenotic Hypertransradiancy

Bronchial stenosis is associated with impairment of aeration as well as a reflex decrease in vascularity. The stenosis also may function as a check-valve leading to air trapping in the distal lung.

Pneumatocele

A large air-containing cyst may occupy the entire hemithorax. It can develop as a result of staphylococcal pneumonia, especially in children. The volume of the lesion changes within a few days. Tomography or CT can define the wall of the pneumatocele.

Thromboembolism
Most thromboemboli do not cause radiographic abnormalities, although circumscribed hypovascularity (the Westermark sign) may be present. The diagnosis is based on the clinical presentation (thrombosis in the lower extremities, acute chest pain), CT evidence of thromboemboli in major vessels, and perfusion scintigraphy, which shows wedge-shaped perfusion defects.

12. Hilar Enlargement

See Table 13.15.

▮ Diagnostic Approach

Detection of hilar abnormality is important as an enlarged hilum is frequently an indicator of significant pathology. However, variability in hilar shape is a normal phenomenon since the hilum is a summation shadow formed by both pulmonary arteries and veins.

A normal hilum is characterized by the following:
- The lateral border is concave.
- The diameter of the right interlobar artery is less than 16 mm.

Hilar enlargement may be due to:
- Pulmonary artery dilatation
- Pulmonary venous dilatation
- Hilar lymph node enlargement
- Bronchial carcinoma

Table 13.**15** Hilar Enlargement

Vascular
- Vascular ectasia
- Pulmonary venous hypertension
- Pulmonary artery hypertension
- Asymmetric pulmonary perfusion
- Pulmonary artery aneurysm

Lymph node enlargement
- Lymphoma
- Hilar lymph node metastases
- Tuberculous lymphadenitis
- Fungal infections (histoplasmosis, coccidioidomycosis, blastomycosis)
- Castleman disease
- Sarcoidosis
- Silicosis

Primary Neoplasia
- Central bronchial carcinoma
- Carcinoid

▮ Differential Diagnosis

Pulmonary Artery Ectasia in the Elderly
The age-related variant of an ectatic or elongated pulmonary artery may produce a unilateral hilar bulge or general enlargement of the hilum. Ectasia is particularly common in elderly patients due to age-related loss of vessel wall elasticity.

Pulmonary Artery Hypertension
There is dilatation of the main and central pulmonary arteries with bilateral symmetric hilar enlargement and with preservation of lateral hilar concavity (Fig. 13.**72**). There also may be radiographic features consistent with right heart dilatation (see Chapter 7, p. 184).

Pulmonary Venous Hypertension ± Congestive Heart Failure
The central pulmonary veins are dilated giving bilateral symmetric hilar enlargement. In addition, they may be poorly defined due to perivascular edema.

Asymmetrical Pulmonary Perfusion
Unilateral decreased pulmonary perfusion is associated with a compensatory increase in contralateral lung perfusion with associated unilateral hilar enlargement. This discrepancy may result from unilateral vascular occlusion in pulmonary thromboembolic disease or unilateral hypoventilation with reflex vasoconstriction such as occurs in carcinoma-associated bronchial stenosis.

Pulmonary Artery Aneurysm
Congenital aneurysms of the pulmonary artery are extremely rare. Turbulence caused by pulmonary artery stenosis may occasionally lead to poststenotic dilatation (Fig. 13.**73**).

Lymphoma (Fig. 13.**74 a, b**)
There may be uni-or bilateral hilar lymph node enlargement often in association with mediastinal lymph node enlargement.

Sarcoidosis (Fig. 13.75)
Hilar lymph node enlargement in sarcoidosis is usually bilateral and symmetric. In contrast to lymphoma and

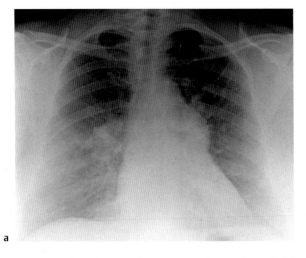

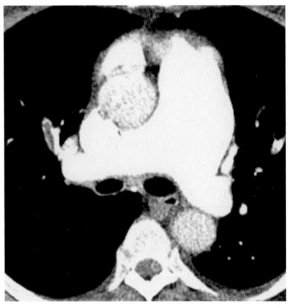

Fig. 13.**72 a, b** Pulmonary hypertension: Chest radiograph (**a**) shows dilated main pulmonary artery and bilateral hilar enlargement. CT (**b**) confirms that changes are due to central pulmonary artery dilatation.

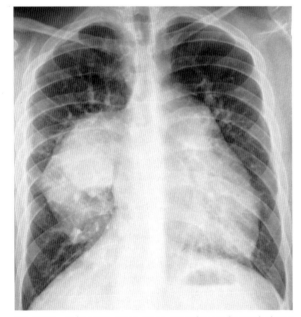

Fig. 13.**73** Pulmonary artery aneurysm: Chest radiograph shows central pulmonary artery dilatation with marked right hilar enlargement in patient with longstanding Eisenmenger's reaction. Right hilar enlargement was due to a pulmonary artery aneurysm.

carcinoma, aerated lung is occasionally present between the hilar nodes and mediastinum.

Central Bronchial Carcinoma
This may manifest as unilateral hilar enlargement (Fig. 13.**76**). "Spiculate" shadowing radiating from the hilum may be present and signifies lymphatic involvement.

Hilar Lymph Node Metastases
Asymmetric lymph node enlargement is usually present. The most common primary tumors are bronchial and breast carcinoma.

Bacterial and Viral Infection
Pulmonary infections may be associated with ipsilateral hilar lymph node enlargement although parenchymal opacification is usually the dominant radiographic finding.

Tuberculous Infection
Unilateral hilar lymph node enlargement may signify tuberculous lymphadenitis particularly in children and these enlarged nodes may compress the right middle lobe bronchus leading to atelectasis.

Mycotic Infection
Histoplasmosis, coccidiomycosis, and sporotrichosis may give uni- or bilateral hilar lymph node enlargement. The diagnosis is confirmed by identification of fungi in biopsy specimens and by elevated titers of precipitating antibody.

Silicosis
Symmetrical enlargement of bronchopulmonary and hilar lymph nodes is common in silicosis and is usually associated with nodular parenchymal disease. The lymph nodes may show an eggshell pattern of calcification (see Fig. 5.**15**).

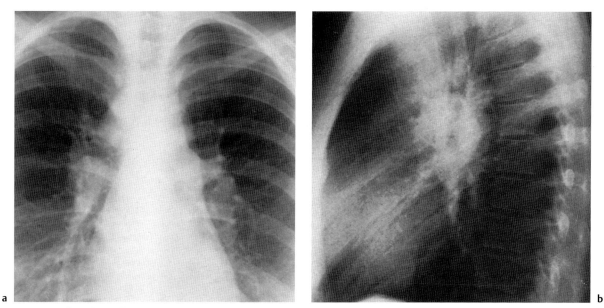

a   b

Fig. 13.**74 a, b**   Bilateral hilar and mediastinal lymph node enlargement in Hodgkin's lymphoma.

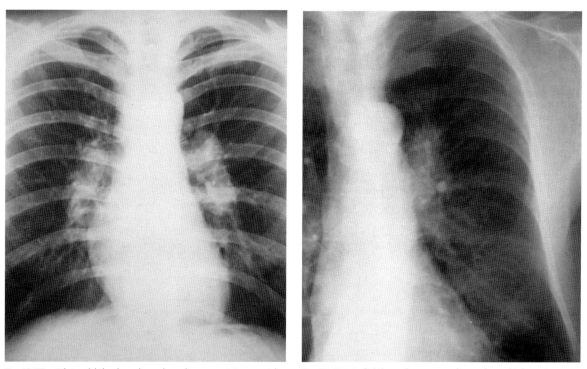

Fig. 13.**75**   Bilateral hilar lymph node enlargement in sarcoidosis.

Fig. 13.**76**   Left hilar enlargement due to bronchial carcinoma.

13. Intrathoracic Calcifications

Calcifications are a common finding on chest radiographs (Felson 1969). With its high atomic number, calcium is a stronger absorber of roentgen rays than a soft-tissue lesion of similar size. Most intrathoracic calcifications are recognized by their flocculent, granular, or punctate appearance (Figs. 13.**77**, 13.**79**).

Intrathoracic calcifications may be classified as dystrophic, which generally signify an inactive or degenerative process, and metastatic which are much less common and are found in disorders of calcium metabolism.

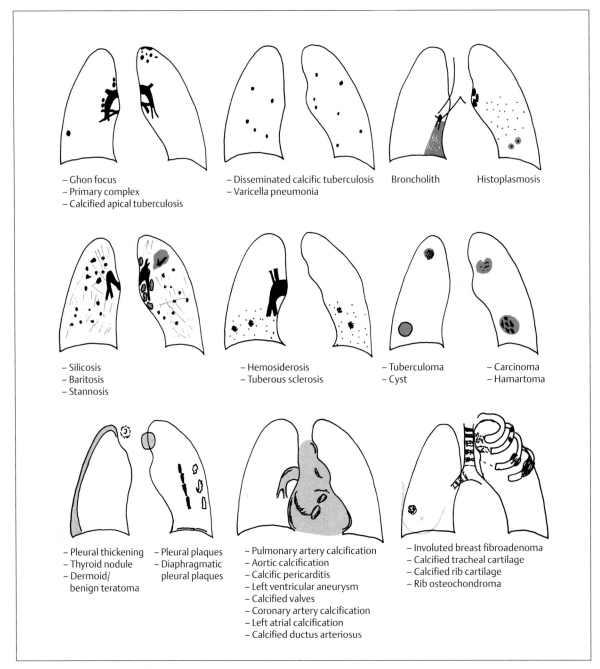

- Ghon focus
- Primary complex
- Calcified apical tuberculosis

- Disseminated calcific tuberculosis
- Varicella pneumonia

Broncholith   Histoplasmosis

- Silicosis
- Baritosis
- Stannosis

- Hemosiderosis
- Tuberous sclerosis

- Tuberculoma
- Cyst

- Carcinoma
- Hamartoma

- Pleural thickening
- Thyroid nodule
- Dermoid/
  benign teratoma

- Pleural plaques
- Diaphragmatic
  pleural plaques

- Pulmonary artery calcification
- Aortic calcification
- Calcific pericarditis
- Left ventricular aneurysm
- Calcified valves
- Coronary artery calcification
- Left atrial calcification
- Calcified ductus arteriosus

- Involuted breast fibroadenoma
- Calcified tracheal cartilage
- Calcified rib cartilage
- Rib osteochondroma

Fig. 13.**77**   Intrathoracic calcifications.

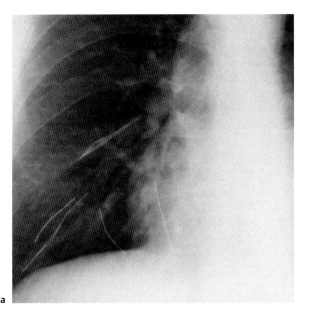

a

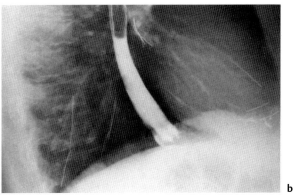

b

Fig. 13.**78 a, b** Intrapulmonary foreign body emboli. Patient with a history of psychiatric disease inserted paper clips into the antecubital vein. They embolized to the pulmonary arteries through the right heart but produced no symptoms.

Pulmonary Calcifications

▓ Differential Diagnosis

Pulmonary Tuberculosis
- Old Ghon Focus. This round opacity measuring 3–10 mm in diameter showing flocculent or homogeneous calcification is usually located peripherally in the midzone. It represents the calcified, healed primary focus of tuberculosis.
- Tuberculoma (Fig. 13.**79**). These nodules may reach a diameter of 4–5 cm and show patchy or homogeneous calcification.
- Calcified Apical Tuberculosis. Speckled and focal calcifications at both apices are usually associated with fibrocirrhotic tuberculosis and apical pleural thickening.
- Disseminated Calcific Tuberculosis (Fig. 13.**80**). This reflects healed miliary tuberculosis in which multiple calcific nodules are scattered throughout the lungs.

Histoplasmosis
This disease is common in the U.S. and rare in Europe. Radiographs in the healed stage show multiple calcific foci in the lung parenchyma, often in association with calcified hilar lymph nodes.

Past Varicella Pneumonia (Fig. 13.81)
Healed granulomas following varicella pneumonia appear as nodular calcifications distributed uniformly throughout both lungs.

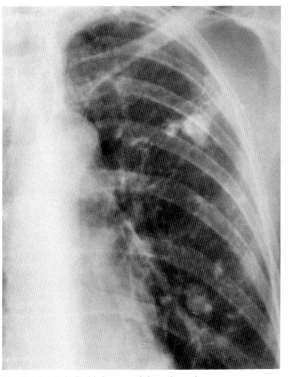

Fig. 13.**79**   Calcified left upper lobe tuberculoma.

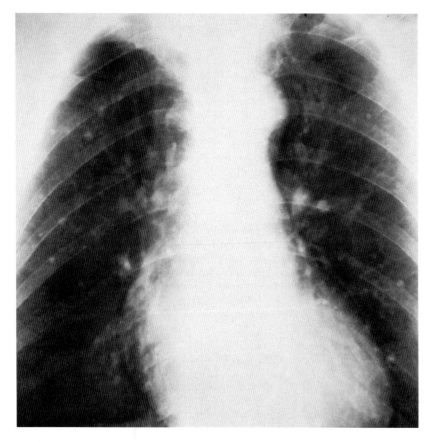

Fig. 13.**80**   Calcified granulomata in old tuberculosis.

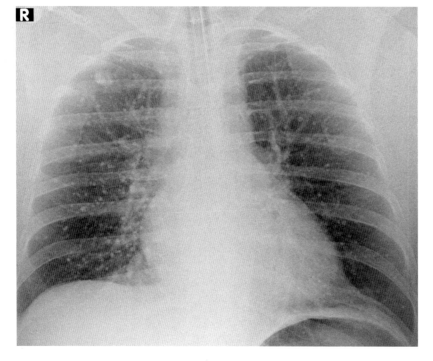

Fig. 13.**81**   Varicella pneumonia. Chest radiograph shows multiple bilateral calcified nodules consistent with past varicella pneumonia.

Healed Parasitic Infestation

Disseminated miliary to pea-sized calcifications are sometimes seen in persons who have lived in regions where cysticercosis, schistosomiasis, and paragonimiasis (Fig. 13.**82**) are endemic.

Hemosiderosis

Chronic pulmonary edema particularly when found in association with mitral stenosis may lead to development of small, calcified hemosiderin granulomas. Located mainly in the lower zones, they may reflect an inflammatory response to small parenchymal hemorrhages.

Pneumoconioses (see Fig. 13.**83**)

Intrapulmonary silicotic nodules may calcify, and often there is concomitant eggshell calcification of the hilar lymph nodes. Baritosis and stannosis may also be associated with multiple granular calcium deposits of very high density scattered throughout the lung parenchyma.

Metabolic Calcification

Metabolic calcification in the lung often can be detected histologically in patients with abnormal calcium metabolism (i. e., primary or secondary hyperparathyroidism, hypervitaminosis D, sarcoidosis). This calcification, however, tends to be so diffuse that it is seldom visible on radiographs except when it is precipitated in pneumonic exudates or sarcoid granulomas.

Scleroderma

The occurrence of Thibièrge–Weissenbach syndrome in the setting of scleroderma is a possible but infrequent cause of miliary pulmonary calcification.

Alveolar Microlithiasis

This is a familial disease of unknown etiology that probably has an autosomal recessive mode of inheritance (Prakash 1983). Amyloid bodies containing calcium phosphate are found in a large number of alveoli. Patients present clinically with exertional dyspnea and function tests show abnormal diffusion. The disease generally has a good prognosis. Chest radiographs show myriad micronodular opacities of calcific density located predominantly in the mid-to-lower zones (*sandstorm lung*). Radionuclide scintigraphy shows increased uptake of bone-avid radiotracer in the lung. CT demonstrates intra-acinar microliths accompanied by reactive interstitial fibrosis. Occasionally, the pleura may appear as a lucent stripe which contrasts sharply with the calcified lung (*black pleural stripe* sign as described by Felson 1973 b).

Idiopathic Pulmonary Ossification

This rare disorder also termed ossifying pneumonitis predominantly affects elderly men. Chest radiographs show reticular calcium deposits (Schmitt et al. 1978).

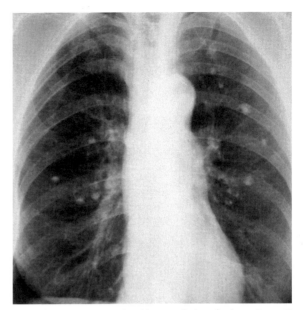

Fig. 13.**82** Paragonimiasis with some lesions having a "target" pattern of calcification.

Tracheobronchial Calcifications

■ Differential Diagnosis

Calcified Tracheobronchial Cartilage

The cartilage rings may be heavily calcified in elderly patients. Plain radiographs in these cases may define the tracheobronchial system peripherally to the level of the subsegmental bronchi.

Tracheopathia osteochondroplastica

This condition is characterized by the presence of very slow-growing, osteocartilaginous nodules in the submucosa of the trachea and proximal bronchi. The calcified nodules arise from the cartilage rings and usually do not cause significant respiratory impairment until after age 50.

Broncholiths

These are concretions up to 5 mm in diameter that are formed by inspissated and calcified bronchial secretions. They are commonly associated with bronchiectasis (Vix 1978). Calcified peribronchial lymph nodes (histoplasmosis, TB, fungi) may gain access to the bronchial lumen through inflammatory fistulae and give rise to broncholiths. A radiologic diagnosis is possible only if the calculi migrate, are expectorated (lithoptysis), or if CT can define clearly their endobronchial location (Conces et al. 1991).

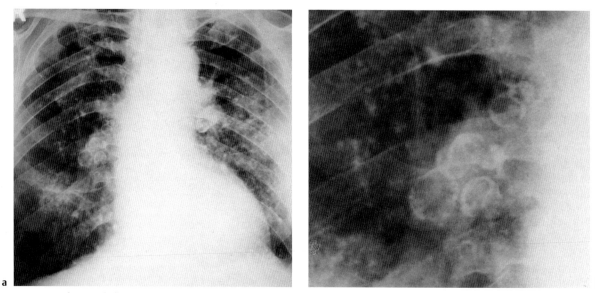

Fig. 13.**83 a, b**   Eggshell calcification of hilar lymph nodes and calcified pulmonary nodules in silicosis.

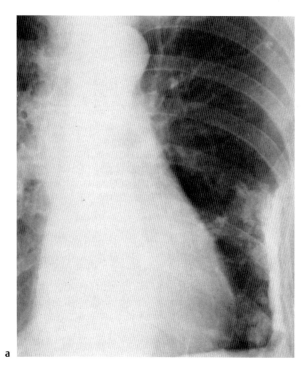

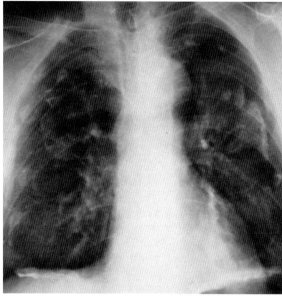

Fig. 13.**84 a, b**   Pleural calcification secondary to hemothorax (**a**) and asbestos-induced pleural disease (**b**).

Lymph Node Calcification

■ Differential Diagnosis

- Tuberculous lymph node calcification.
- Eggshell calcification in sarcoidosis and silicosis (Fig. 13.**83**).

Pleural Calcifications

■ Differential Diagnosis

- Calcified fibrothorax (Fig. 13.**84 a**). See also p. 224.
- Calcified asbestos-induced pleural plaques: Pleural plaques may undergo hyaline degeneration (Fig. 13.**84 b**) and subsequently may calcify.

14 Thoracic Intervention

Radiologic interventions are minimally invasive diagnostic and therapeutic procedures which may be performed under ultrasound, computed tomography (CT), or fluoroscopic guidance.

The following interventions will be discussed:

- Biopsy
- Drainage
- Foreign body retrieval/extraction
- Bronchial artery embolization
- Coil embolization of pulmonary arteriovenous malformations (PAVM)
- Embolization/occlusion of pulmonary artery false aneurysms

Biopsy

■ Clinical Features and Indications

Diagnostic fine needle aspiration (FNA) and core biopsy can provide cytologic, histologic, and microbiologic information on pulmonary, pleural, chest wall, and mediastinal lesions. FNA and core biopsy of pulmonary and mediastinal lesions are usually performed under CT guidance whereas more superficial lesions of the pleura and chest wall sometimes may be biopsied under ultrasound guidance.

■ Contraindications

- *Uncooperative patient* (may require general anesthesia).
- Lung biopsy in a patient with *severe respiratory impairment* (i. e., FEV1 of less than 1 liter). This group will tolerate a pneumothorax poorly due to lack of respiratory reserve.
- *Coagulopathy* (minimum requirements: platelet count $> 50\,000/\mu L$, Quick PT $> 50\%$, PTT > 50 s or INR $< 1.3–1.4$).
- *Suspected mesothelioma* is considered a contraindication in some centers. This is due to the risk of seeding tumor cells along the needle track. However, this risk may be minimized by subsequent therapeutic irradiation of the biopsy track.

■ Technique

The imaging procedure must define clearly the biopsy needle path, the target lesion, and surrounding critical structures.

When ultrasound guidance and a transcostal approach are used, the needle is introduced at the superior rib margin to protect the intercostal arteries.

For biopsy of pulmonary and mediastinal lesions, CT is employed to accurately localize the target lesion and the biopsy needle can be advanced under CT/CT-fluoroscopic guidance avoiding surrounding vessels and other critical structures (Fig. 14.1).

It is easiest for the patient to keep still when imaging is performed at functional residual capacity or in slight inspiration.

Histologic and cytologic specimens are acquired from solid lesions. Spring-loaded 18-gauge cutting needles (TruCut type) are most commonly used (Fig. 14.2).

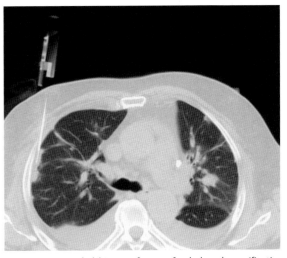

Fig. 14.1 CT-guided biopsy of area of subpleural opacification using 18G TruCut needle.

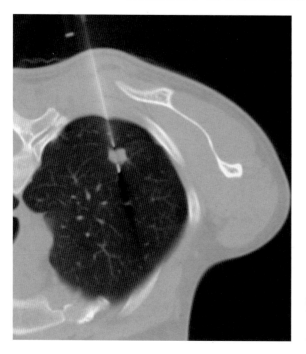

Fine needle diagnostic or therapeutic aspirates may be taken from fluid collections. The needle gauge depends on the viscosity of the fluid contents.

■ Complications

A small *pneumothorax* is commonly seen after percutaneous lung biopsy with a reported incidence of 25–30%. Most of these, however, resolve spontaneously and needle aspiration and/or percutaneous tube drainage are required in just a small number of cases.

Biopsy-related pulmonary hemorrhage and hemoptysis may also occur.

Fig. 14.**2**   CT-guided biopsy of left upper lobe lesion with patient in prone position and using 18G TruCut needle. The inner needle with specimen notch has been advanced into the lesion. The outer cutting sheath has not yet been deployed.

Drainage

■ Clinical Features and Indications

Percutaneous needle aspiration and catheter drainage is employed for treatment of pleural effusion, empyema, and pneumothorax. It is usually performed under local anesthesia.

Prerequisites include a clear anatomical drainage path and a discrete well-defined collection which has not become significantly loculated. Simple needle aspiration may be sufficient or a catheter may be inserted using a "direct" or Seldinger technique and this may be left in-situ for a few days until adequate drainage has occurred (Fig. 14.**3a, b**).

■ Contraindications

- *Coagulopathy* (see above)
- *Absence of a safe drainage pathway*

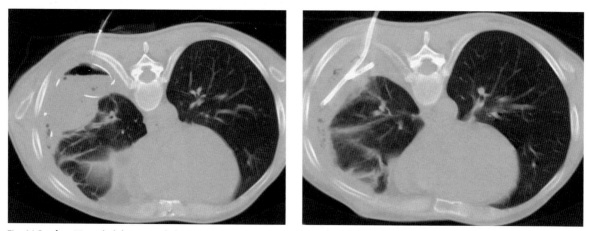

Fig. 14.**3a, b**   CT-guided drainage of pleural empyema using Seldinger technique. Fig. (**a**) shows guidewire which has been advanced through the introducer needle into the collection. Fig. (**b**) shows correct placement of 12F pigtail catheter.

■ Technique

Pleural effusions and empyemas in many cases may be visualized sufficiently well with ultrasound to allow ultrasound-guided drainage. CT-guided drainage may be performed if the collection cannot be visualized adequately with ultrasound due to its small size, anatomic position, or due to large patient body habitus. Collections containing significant amounts of gas may also be better visualized with computed tomography.

These procedures are usually performed under local anesthesia.

■ Complications

Potential complications include *hemorrhage* and *infection*.

Foreign Body Retrieval-Extraction

■ Clinical Indications

Foreign bodies in the major systemic veins, right heart, and pulmonary arteries may reflect fragments which have become detached from venous catheters. Other foreign bodies include fragments of puncture sets, guidewires, pacemaker leads, and embolization materials from treatment of arteriovenous shunts. These foreign bodies tend to become lodged in the right atrium, superior vena cava, and left pulmonary artery. For percutaneous retrieval to be feasible the foreign body must be *radiographically visible* and it must be possible *to "mechanically" grasp the object* under fluoroscopic visualization. The object should not have been present long enough to allow endothelialization and vascular adhesion to occur.

■ Contraindications

The potential for complications from the foreign body should be weighed against the risk of its retrieval.

■ Technique

The standard technique involves femoral venous access and use of a large-bore sheath. If the foreign body has been present for some time, diagnostic angiography should be performed to exclude secondary thrombus. Otherwise the retrieval may be preceded by lytic therapy. The preferred instrument is a gooseneck snare, which is maneuvered over one end of the foreign body under fluoroscopic guidance and tightened so that it forms a U-shaped loop when withdrawn. The retrieval catheter and snared foreign body are withdrawn into the sheath and extracted with it (Fig. 14.**4a, b**). The alterna-

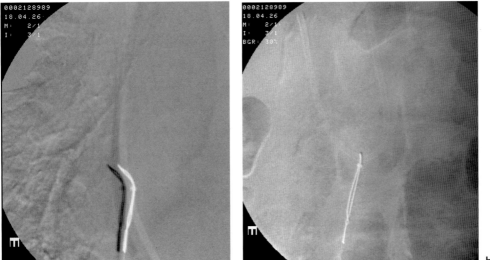

a   b

Fig. 14.**4a, b**
Catheter fragment retrieval. (**a**) Fragment of a ventriculoatrial CSF catheter which has been "snared" within the superior vena cava. (**b**) Catheter fragment has been pulled inferiorly into the inferior vena cava.

tive use of a forceps catheter carries a higher risk of vessel wall injury and does not grasp the object as securely as the snare.

■ Complications

Complications are rare but include *vascular injury* including damage to the femoral vein and *cardiac arrhythmias*.

■ Results

Success rates of approximately 90% are reported in the literature with some rate variation related to the clinical indication.

Bronchial Artery Embolization

■ Clinical Features and Indications

Hemoptysis is alarming for the patient and when severe, constitutes a life-threatening emergency. Primary management may include oxygen administration, bronchoscopic suction ± coagulation of the bleeding lesion and bronchial tamponade. Most severe hemoptyses result from chronic inflammatory processes in the setting of bronchiectasis, tuberculosis, aspergilloma, or pneumoconiosis. Neoplastic lesions and vascular anomalies in the form of systemic-pulmonary arterial shunts (SPAS) less commonly cause severe hemoptysis. If hemoptysis persists, interventional radiology in the form of bronchial artery embolization is indicated. The systemic nutrient bronchial arteries are by far the most common source of hemorrhage and hemostasis is achieved by identification and occlusion of the bleeding vessel.

The procedure is technically demanding and to date there have been no study-based reports offering definitive criteria for patient selection. We (S. Lange and colleagues) can recommend the following criteria based on our own experience of more than 150 procedures:

- Recurrent bleeding episodes over a period of at least several months (bleeds within a one-month period are considered one episode).
- A single life-threatening bleeding episode.
- No real prospect of effective treatment of the primary disease.
- Good correlation between the bronchoscopically identified bleeding site and the bleeding source indicated by angiography.

■ Contraindications and Potential Risks

The systemic blood supply is part of a comprehensive arterial network that supplies all thoracic organs. We are limited in our ability to fully define the cross-connections within this network due to flow dynamics and this can lead to *unintended embolization and ischemia of the trachea, esophagus, coronary arteries, or even the spinal cord with an associated risk of paraplegia*. Other issues include *systemic-pulmonary arterial shunts*, which very often originate from the bronchial arteries, regardless of the precipitating cause. If angiography detects this type of cross-connection or shunt, it will be necessary to either modify the embolization technique or terminate the procedure.

The pulmonary arteries to the region must be patent as the residual systemic bronchial supply postembolization may be insufficient to prevent pulmonary ischemia.

Intervention is contraindicated during *active bleeding* and should be performed only after the patient has been stabilized hemodynamically.

■ Technique

The procedure commences with an angiographic survey of the thoracic aorta and the supra-aortic branches. In a cooperative patient, this makes it possible to identify abnormal bronchial arteries and other systemic arteries supplying the lung; these are highly variable in their origin and number.

This is followed by selective visualization of the identified bleeding sites and a systematic search for typical sources of bleeding.

If it is likely that the bronchoscopically- and angiographically-identified bleeding sites correspond (a search is made for vascular pathology rather than acutely bleeding vessels), it is appropriate to proceed with vessel embolization.

If multiple bronchial arteries in both lungs are identified as potential causes of the hemoptysis, it may be preferable to occlude just one artery in a sitting due to the risk of bronchial ischemia.

The interventional phase of the procedure immediately follows the diagnostic phase (Fig. 14.5 a–c). With the selective catheter placed in the orifice of the bronchial artery, a smaller-caliber tube is passed through it into the bronchial artery and advanced toward the target site. This coaxial technique prevents embolization material from backing up into the aorta or accessing extrapulmonary organs through periaortic

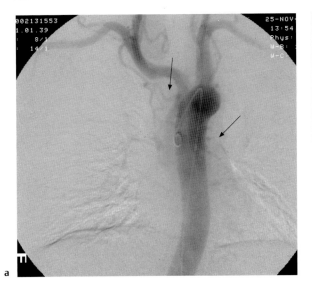

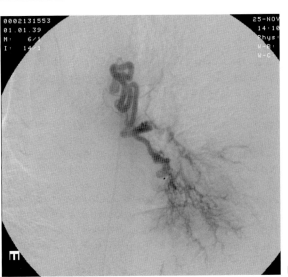

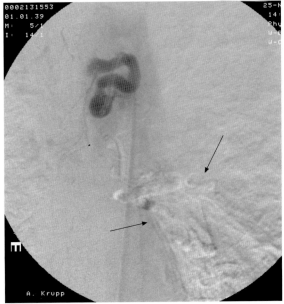

Fig. 14.5a–c 63-year-old male with known bronchiectasis and recurrent episodes of bleeding from left lower lobe. (**a**) Initial aortogram shows dilated bronchial arteries bilaterally (*arrows*). (**b**) Selective angiography shows elongation and dilatation of the left bronchial artery. Peripheral pulmonary vessels are opacified via systemic-pulmonary arterial shunts. (**c**) Angiogram post embolization shows stasis of contrast medium within the proximal bronchial artery. *Arrows* indicate the Ethibloc-occluded segments.

collaterals. When the catheter has been securely positioned and diagnostic angiograms show no significant systemic-pulmonary arterial shunts, the embolization material may be injected. Our favorite embolization agent is Ethibloc, a corn protein that solidifies in blood. Lipiodol is added to the agent to improve visualization and prolong the liquid phase so that the embolization material may be deposited along a significant arterial segment. Any misdirection of the material can be detected with reasonable certainty so that the injection can be stopped. Coils produce a very localized occlusion which is rapidly bypassed by direct or collateral revascularization and particles may be difficult to confine to the target site.

The procedure concludes with a diagnostic angiographic evaluation of the treated vessel.

■ Complications

In addition to *ischemic complications* as described above, there is an approximately 20% incidence of *retrosternal pain and fever* following embolization. This usually resolves within a few days.

■ Results

Sixty percent of our patients are free of recurrent hemoptysis for periods of up to 10 years, but our results vary considerably depending on the causative disease and the degree of angiographic change. We know of no comparative studies in treated and untreated patients.

Coil Embolization of Pulmonary Arteriovenous Malformations

■ Clinical Features and Indications

Solitary pulmonary arteriovenous malformations (AVM) occur sporadically but these lesions are most commonly seen in hereditary hemorrhagic telangiectasia (HHT, Osler disease) where they develop in approximately 20 % of patients. They tend to enlarge and become more complex over time and a simple AVM composed of one afferent artery and one efferent vein may progress to a complex lesion involving multiple afferent and efferent vessels. The efferent veins lying adjacent to the shunt dilate and this venous ectasia may mimic tumor "spiculations" on radiographs.

Pulmonary AVMs allow direct flow of deoxygenated blood from pulmonary arteries to the pulmonary venous system thus bypassing the capillary bed and effectively producing a right-to-left shunt. Large untreated malformations carry a long-term risk of biventricular decompensation.

Pulmonary AVMs also compromise the capillary filtration function of the lung allowing venous emboli to enter the systemic arterial circulation (*paradoxical emboli*) with complications including cerebral infarction. This risk of systemic emboli constitutes the main indication for treatment of AVMs.

Treatment of pulmonary AVMs with a diameter of ≥ 3 mm is recommended but smaller lesions that are easily accessible to angiography may also be treated. Surgical treatment of AVMs has been largely abandoned as these lesions generally can be occluded more selectively and at less risk with an interventional technique. The only exceptions to this rule are cases in which a lo-

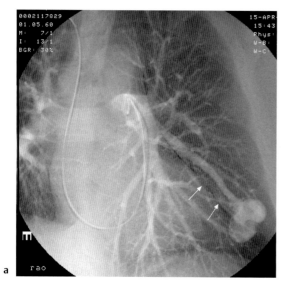

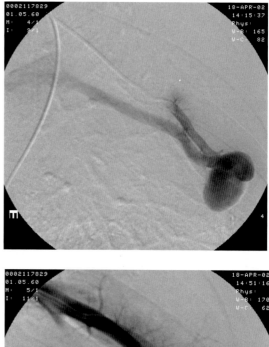

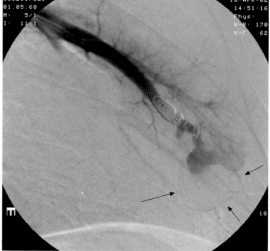

Fig. 14.**6a–c** Embolization of pulmonary arteriovenous malformation. (**a**) Selective left pulmonary angiogram shows pulmonary arteriovenous malformation (PAVM). *Arrows* indicate early opacification of draining vein. (**b**) PAVM selectively visualized in the LAO projection prior to embolization. There is rapid venous filling. (**c**) Pulmonary angiogram immediately post coil embolization shows some residual flow in the AVM which will cease when thrombosis occurs. *Arrows* indicate venous ectasia.

calized area of lung contains a high concentration of AVMs. Surgical resection in these cases may be preferable to numerous radiologic interventions.

■ Technique

Preprocedure helical CT studies ± diagnostic angiography define the morphology and distribution of the AVMs and allow planning of the intervention.

The femoral approach is preferred to the cubital route for pulmonary artery interventions as it provides a straighter route thus facilitating catheter control in the pulmonary arteries. This route also increases the distance between the operator and the image intensifier resulting in lower occupational radiation exposure.

Fiber coils are preferred for embolization of pulmonary AVMs. Detachable balloons offer the advantage of immediate and total AVM occlusion but they are much more difficult to deploy and are extremely difficult to use at peripheral sites. They are also difficult to retrieve if they enter the systemic circulation during the procedure.

For the embolization procedure, the feeding artery is selectively catheterized and the catheter is stabilized in position. An inner coaxial catheter is then placed at the narrowest point between the feeding artery and the venous ectasia. It is used to introduce the coils, which are applied in a close-packed arrangement to occlude at least a 1.5-cm segment of the artery. Definitive occlusion is not produced by the coils but by the thrombosis that the coils induce (Fig. 14.**6a–c**). Additional shunts are

treated using the same technique. In our experience, it takes approximately 60 min for coil embolization of each AVM. Patients with respiratory impairment may be treated on a number of successive occasions.

■ Complications

In a total of 80 procedures, we have seen two instances of *coil displacement*. Both cases were managed easily by retrieval from the systemic arteries. There is virtually no risk of late displacement owing to secondary thrombosis in the occluded segment. Rarely, the occlusion may incite an *inflammatory reaction in the adjacent pleura*. Occasionally, it may be necessary for technical reasons to include smaller, healthy pulmonary arteries in the occlusion and this may give a *circumscribed pulmonary infarction*. Both of these complications have a reported incidence of less than 10% and neither is associated with significant sequelae.

■ Results

This technique will provide definitive closure of the AVM if the coils are placed in a close-packed arrangement. We have had to reocclude several AVMs from earlier procedures due to residual patency. We have seen no instances of late displacement. Patients with HHT require ongoing follow-up for the early detection of new AVMs.

Coil Embolization of Pulmonary Artery False Aneurysms

■ Clinical Features and Indications

Traumatic false aneurysms have largely replaced mycotic aneurysms as the most common form of pulmonary artery false aneurysm. Traumatic false aneurysms are an iatrogenic complication which occur rarely (1:3000) as a complication of Swan–Gantz catheter use in assessment of pulmonary capillary wedge pressure. The pulmonary arterial wall may be damaged due to balloon overinflation or there may be vascular perforation by the catheter leading to secondary development of a false aneurysm.

The primary mortality rate of false aneurysm rupture is very high and in the range of 45–65%, with asphyxia and blood loss as the immediate causes of death. Among patients who survive this complication, 30–40% experience recurrent bleeding with subsequent mortality rates of 40–70%.

Clinical presentation of rupture is most commonly with hemoptysis. The chest radiograph characteristically

shows a well-circumscribed pulmonary nodule. Helical CT may show the vascular origin of the lesion and surrounding ground-glass opacification consistent with hemorrhage (Fig. 14.**7a–d**).

■ Technique

The procedure may be performed under general anesthesia in uncooperative patients.

A femoral approach is again favored and initial pulmonary angiography with subsequent selective catheterization defines the morphology of the aneurysm and parent artery. Because the false aneurysm and surrounding lung parenchyma offer very little mechanical resistance, the aim of the procedure is not to obliterate the aneurysmal sac but to occlude the parent artery just proximal to the site of injury. This procedure therefore is feasible only if this vascular segment is present. Once again a coaxial system is employed as in the treatment of

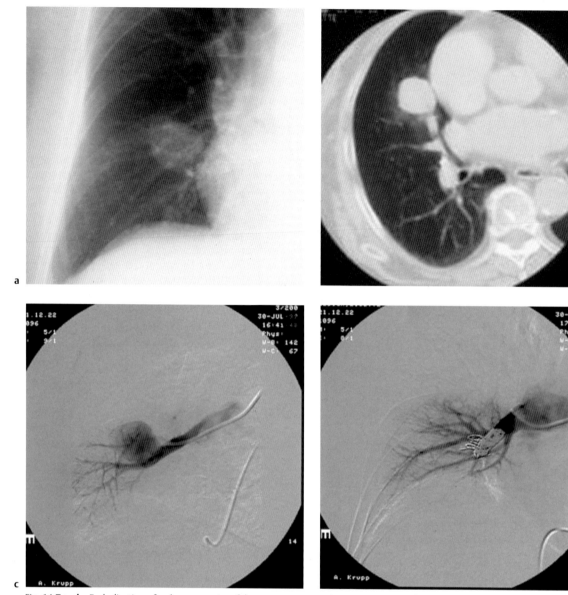

Fig. 14.**7 a–d** Embolization of pulmonary artery false aneurysm. (**a**) Chest radiograph shows new pulmonary nodule following recent placement of a Swan–Gantz catheter; appearance highly suggestive of development of false aneurysm. (**b**) Contrast-enhanced CT demonstrates right middle lobe lesion with afferent pulmonary artery and rim of surrounding parenchymal hemorrhage. (**c**) Selective angiography demonstrates the aneurysm arising from a middle lobe vessel. (**d**) Postprocedure angiogram shows satisfactory occlusion of the injured artery and exclusion of the "false aneurysm" from the pulmonary circulation.

pulmonary AVMs and this provides access for precise placement of close-packed fiber coils that exclude the affected pulmonary artery and false aneurysm from the circulation.

lead to significant occlusion. A significant pulmonary artery occlusion may cause ischemic pulmonary infarction similar to that associated with pulmonary embolism.

■ Complications

Coil displacement into the vessel distal to the site of false aneurysm formation is of no consequence. Isolated coils migrating into other pulmonary arteries usually do not

■ Results

There appears to be no risk of recurrence in cases where the procedure is technically feasible.

Reference List

Aberle DR, Gamsu G, Ray CS. High resolution CT of benign asbestos-related diseases: clinical and radiographic correlation. *AJR*. 1988;151:883–891.

Aberle DR, Balmes JR. Computed tomography of asbestos related pulmonary parenchymal and pleural diseases. *Clin Chest Med*. 1991;12:115–131.

Abrams DI. Asymptomatic lymphadenopathy and other early presentations of AIDS. *Front Radiat Ther Oncol*. 1985;19:59.

Achenbach S, Giesler T, Ropers D et al. Detection of coronary artery stenoses by contrast-enhanced, retrospectively electrocardiographically-gated, multislice spiral computed tomography. *Circulation*. 2001;103:2535–2538.

Agatston AS, Janowitz WR, Hildner FJ, Zusmer NR, Viamonte M, Detrano R. Quantification of coronary artery calcium using ultrafast computed tomography. *J Am Coll Cardiol*. 1990;15:827–832.

Ahn JM, Im JG, Seo JW et al. Endobronchial hamartoma: CT findings in three patients. *AJR*. 1994;163:49–50.

Akira M, Yamamoto S, Yokoyama K et al. Asbestosis: high-resolution CT–pathologic correlation. *Radiology*. 1990; 176:389–394.

Aksamit TR. Mycobacterium avium complex hot tub lung: Infection, inflammation or both? *Chest Meeting Abstracts*. 2003;124:213.

Alder SC, Silverman JF. Anomalous venous drainage of the left upper lobe. *Radiology*. 1973;108:563–565.

Alford BA, Keats TE. The Infant and Young Child. In: Grainger RG, Allison DJ, eds. *Diagnostic Radiology*. 2nd ed. Edinburgh: Churchill Livingstone; 1992:1:383–409.

Allen RP, Taylor R, Reiquam C. Congenital lobar emphysema with dilated septal lymphatics. *Radiology*. 1966;86:929.

Al-Saadi N, Nagel E, Gross M et al. Noninvasive detection of myocardial ischemia from perfusion reserve based on cardiovascular magnetic resonanace. *Circulation*. 2000; 101(12):1379–83.

Amundsen P. The diagnostic value of conventional radiological examination of the heart in adults. *Acta Radiol*. 1959:Suppl. 18:1–87

Aoki T, Nakata H, Watanabe H et al. Evolution of peripheral lung adenocarcinomas. *AJR*. 2000;174:763–768.

Arita T, Kuramitsu T, Kawamura M et al. Bronchogenic carcinoma: incidence of metastases to normal sized lymph nodes. *Thorax*. 1995;50:1267–1269.

Arita T, Matsumoto T, Kuramitsu T et al. Is it possible to differentiate malignant mediastinal nodes from benign nodes by size: reevaluation by CT, transesophageal echocardiography and nodal specimen. *Chest*. 1996;110: 1004–1008.

Armstrong P. The Mediastinum. In: Grainger RG, Allison DJ, eds. *Diagnostic Radiology*. 2nd ed. Edinburgh: Churchill Livingstone; 1992 a:1:185–211.

Armstrong P. The Normal Chest. In: Grainger RG, Allison DJ, eds. *Diagnostic Radiology*. 2nd ed. Edinburgh: Churchill Livingstone; 1992 b:1:127–147.

Armstrong P, Wilson AG, Dee P, Hansell DM, eds. Imaging of Diseases of the Chest. 2nd ed. St Louis: Mosby; 1995: 145–228.

Armstrong P. Mediastinal and Hilar Disorders. In: Armstrong P, Wilson AG, Dee P, Hansell DM, eds. *Imaging of Diseases of the Chest*. 3rd ed. London: Mosby; 2000: 789–892.

Aubry MC, Wright JL, Myers JL. The pathology of smoking-related diseases. *Clin Chest Med*. 2000;21:11–35.

Auerbach O, Garfinkel L. The changing pattern of lung carcinoma. *Cancer*. 1991;68:1973–1977.

Auger WR, Channick RN, Kerr KM, Fedullo PF. Evaluation of patients with suspected chronic thromboembolic pulmonary hypertension. *Semin Thorac Cardiovasc Surg*. 1999; 11:179–190.

Barakos JA, Brown JJ, Bresain RJ et al. High signal intensity lesions of the chest in MR imaging. J Comput Assist Tomogr. 1989;13:797–802

Basset F, Corrin B, Spencer H et al. Pulmonary histiocytosis X. *Am Rev Respir Disease*. 1978;118:811–820.

Battler A, Karliner JS, Higgins CB et al. The initial chest X-ray film in acute myocardial infarction prediction of early and late mortality and survival. *Circulation*. 1980;61: 1004–1009.

Baum GL. *Textbook of Pulmonary Diseases*. Boston: Little, Brown; 1974.

Bayer AS. Fungal pneumonias: coccidioidal syndroms. *Chest*. 1981;79:575–583.

Becker CR, Kleffel T, Crispin A. Coronary artery calcium measurement: agreement of multi-row detector and electron beam CT. *AJR*. 2001;176:1295–1298.

Bell J, McGivern D, Bullimore J et al. Diagnostic imaging of post-irradiation changes in the chest. *Clin Radiol*. 1988; 39:109–119.

Benito Hernandez N, Moreno Camacho A, Gatell Artigas JM. Infectious pulmonary complications in HIV-infected patients in the highly active antiretroviral therapy era in Spain. *Med Clin(Barc)*. 2005;125(14):548–555.

Bergin CJ, Wirth RL, Berry GJ et al. Pneumocystis carinii pneumonia: CT and HRCT observations. *J Comput Assist Tomogr*. 1990;14:756–759.

Bergin D, Ennis R, Keogh C et al. The 'dependent viscera' sign in CT diagnosis blunt traumatic diaphragmatic rupture. *AJR*. 2001;177:1137–1140.

Berkmen J. Radiologic aspects of intrathoracic sarcoidosis. *Semin Roentgenol*. 1985;20:356–375.

Berman L, Stringer DA, Ein S et al. Childhood diaphragmatic hernias presenting after the neonatal period. *Clin Radiol*. 1988;39:237–244.

Berrocal T, Madrid C, Novo S, Gutierrez J, Arjonilla A, Gomez-Leon N. Congenital anomalies of the tracheobronchial tree, lung and mediastinum: Embryology, radiology and pathology. *Radiographics*. 2003;24:e17.

Bessen LJ, Hymes KB, Greene JB. Human Immunodeficiency Virus: Epidemiology, Biology and Spectrum of Clinical Syndromes. In: Federle MD, Megilow AJ, Naidich DP, eds. *Radiology of AIDS*. New York: Raven; 1988:1–20.

Bjoraker JA, Jay H, Mark K et al. Prognostic significance of histopathologic subsets in idiopathic pulmonary fibrosis. *Am J Respir Crit Care Med.* 1998;157:199–203.

Blunt DM, Padley SPG. Radiographic manifestations of AIDS-related lymphoma in the thorax. *Clin Radiol.* 1995;50: 607–612.

Boer JS, Henry WL, Epstein SE. Echocardiographic findings in patients with systemic infiltrative diseases of the heart. *Am J Cardiol.* 1977;39:184.

Bohlig H. *Lunge und Pleura.* 2 nd ed. Stuttgart: Thieme; 1975.

Boiselle PM, Crans CA, Kaplan MA. The changing face of pneumocystis carinii pneumonia in AIDS patients *AJR.* 1999;172:1301–1309.

Boring CC, Brynes RK, Chan WC et al. Increase in high grade lymphoma in young men. *Lancet.* 1985;1:857–859.

Boxt LM, Rich S, Fried R et al. Automated morphologic evaluation of pulmonary arteries in primary pulmonary hypertension. Invest Radiol. 1986;21:906–909.

Bragg DG. The diagnosis and staging of primary lung cancer. *Radiol Clin North Am.* 1994;32(1):1–14.

Bragg DG, Chor PJ, Murray KA et al. Lymphoproliferative disorders of the lung: histopathology, clinical manifestations and imaging features. *AJR.* 1994;163:273–281.

Brauner MW, Grenier P, Mouelhi MM, Mompoint D, Lenoir S. Pulmonary histiocytosis X: evaluation with high-resolution CT. *Radiology.* 1989;172:255–258.

Bruckner BA, DiBardino DJ, Cumbie TC et al. Critical evaluation of chest computed tomography scans for blunt descending thoracic aortic injury. *Ann Thorac Surg.* 2006; 81(4):1339–1346.

Buff SJ, McLelland R, Gallis HA et al. Candida albicans pneumonia: radiographic appearance. *AJR.* 1982;138:645–648.

Burke AP, Farb A, Virmani R. The pathology of primary pulmonary hypertension. *Mod Pathol.* 1991;4:269–282.

Bury T, Dowlati A, Paulus P et al. Evaluation of the solitary pulmonary nodule by positron emission tomography imaging. *Eur Respir J.* 1996;9:410–414.

Cadranel J, Wislez M, Antoine M. Primary pulmonary lymphoma. *Eur Respir J.* 2002;20:750–762.

Callister TQ, Cooil B, Raya SP, Lippolis NJ, Russo DJ, Raggi P. Coronary artery disease; improved reproducibility of calcium scoring with an electron-beam CT volumetric method. *Radiology.* 1998;208:807–814.

Cappelluti E, Fraire AE, Schaefer OP. A case of 'hot tub lung' due to mycobacterium avium complex in an immunocompetent host. *Arch Intern Med.* 2003;163(7):845–848.

Carabello BA, Crawford FA. Valvular heart disease. *N Engl J Med.* 1997;307:1362–1367.

Carrington CB, Gaensler EA, Couto RE et al. Natural history and treated course of usual and desquamative interstitial pneumonia. *N Engl J Med.* 1978;298:801–809.

Case Records of the Massachusetts General Hospital. # 30–1988, N Engl J Med. 1988;319:227–237.

Centers for Disease Control. Revision of case definitions of acquired immunodeficiency syndrome for national reporting United States. *MMWR.* 1985;34:373–375.

Cervantes-Perez P, Toro-Perez AH, Rodriguez-Jurado P. Pulmonary involvement in rheumatoid arthritis. *J Am Med Ass.* 1980;243:1715.

Chechani V, Kamholz SL. Pulmonary manifestations of disseminated cryptococcosis in patients with AIDS. *Chest.* 1990;98:1060–1066.

Cheely R, McCartney WH, Perry JR et al. The role of noninvasive tests versus pulmonary angiography in the diagnosis of pulmonary embolism. *Am J Med.* 1981;70:17–22.

Chong S, Lee KS, Chung MJ, Han J, Kwon OJ, Kim TS. Neuroendocrine tumors of the lung: Clinical, pathologic and imaging findings. *Radiographics.* 2006;26:41–57.

Chong S, Lee KS, Chung MJ, Han J, Kwon OJ, Kim TS. Pneumoconiosis: Comparison of imaging and pathologic findings. *Radiographics.* 2006;26:59–77.

Chuck SL, Sande MA. Infections with *Cryptococcus neoformans* in the acquired immunodeficiency syndrome. *N Engl J Med.* 1989;321:794–799.

Coady MA, Rizzo JA, Elefteriades JA. Pathologic variants of thoracic aortic dissections: penetrating atherosclerotic ulcers and intramural hematomas. *Cardiol Clin North Am.* 1999;17:637–657.

Colby TV. *Pulmonary Angiitis and Granulomatosis.* Proceedings of the Fleischner Society: 26 th Annual Conference on Chest Disease. Vancouver: 1996.

Conces DJ Jr, Tarver RD, Vix VA. Broncholithiasis. CT features in 15 patients. *AJR.* 1991;157:249–253.

Connell JV Jr, Muhm JR. Radiographic manifestations of pulmonary histoplasmosis, a 10-year review. *Radiology.* 1976; 121:281–285.

Cooper JAD, Matthay RA. Drug-induced pulmonary disease. *Disease-a-month.* 1987;33:61–120.

Coussement A, Butori PJ. Le poumon normal ses variantes et se pièges. Nice: Coussement; 1978.

Cowie RL. The epidemiology of tuberculosis in gold miners with silicosis. *Am J Respir Crit Care Med.* 1994;150: 1460–1462.

Crawford ES. The diagnosis and management of aortic dissection. *JAMA.* 1990;264:2537–2541.

Davis SD, Henscke CI, Yankelevitz DF et al. MR imaging of pleural effusions. *J Comput Assist Tomogr.* 1990;14: 192–198.

Dawson WB, Müller NL. High-resolution computed tomography in pulmonary sarcoidosis. *Semin Ultrasound, CT and MR.* 1990;11:423–429.

Dee P. AIDS and Other Forms of Immunocompromise. In: Armstrong P, Wilson AG, Dee P, Hansell DM, eds. *Imaging of Diseases of the Chest.* 2 nd ed. St Louis: Mosby; 1995 a:229–271.

Dee P. Chest Trauma. In: Armstrong P, Wilson AG, Dee P, Hansell DM, eds. *Imaging of Diseases of the Chest.* 2 nd ed. St Louis: Mosby; 1995 b:869–893.

Dee P. Congenital Disorders of the Lungs and Airways. In: Armstrong P, Wilson AG, Dee P, Hansell DM, eds. *Imaging of Diseases of the Chest.* St Louis: Mosby; 1995 c: 609–640.

Dee P. Drug and Radiation-Induced Lung Disease. In: Armstrong P, Wilson AG, Dee P, Hansell DM, eds. *Imaging of Diseases of the Chest.* 2 nd ed. St Louis: Mosby; 1995 d: 461–484.

DeLorenzo LJ,Huang CT, Maguire GP et al. Roentgenographic patterns of Pneumocystis carinii pneumonia in 104 patients with AIDS. *Chest.* 1987;91:323–327.

DeRemee RA, Weiland LH, McDonald TJ. Respiratory vasculitis. Mayo Clin Proc. 1980;55:492

Desai SR, Wells AU, Rubens MB, Evans TW, Hansell DM. Acute respiratory distress syndrome: CT abnormalities at long-term follow-up. *Radiology.* 1999;210:29–35.

DesJarlais DC, Stoneburner R, Thomas P et al. Decline in proportion of Kaposi's sarcoma among cases of AIDS in multiple risk groups in New York City. Lancet. 1987;2: 1024–1025.

Detrano R, Tang W, Kang X et al. Accurate coronary calcium phosphate mass measurements from electron beam computed tomograms. *Am J Card Imaging.* 1995;9:167–173.

Dewan NA, Shehan CJ, Reeb SD, Gobar LS, Scott WJ, Ryschon K. Likelihood of malignancy in a solitary pulmonary nodule: comparison of Bayesian analysis and results of FDG-PET scan. *Chest.* 1997;112:416–422.

DiLorenzo M, Collin PP, Vaillancourt R et al. Bronchogenic cysts. *J Pediatr Surg.* 1989;24:988–991.

Didier D. Assessment of valve disease qualitative and quantitative. *Magn Reson Imaging Clin N Am.* 2003;11:115–134.

Diethelm L, Dery R, Lipton MJ et al. Atrial level shunts: sensitivity and specificity of MR in diagnosis. *Radiology.* 1987;162:181–186.

Doerr W. Spezielle pathologische Anatomie. Vol XVI, *Pathologie der Lunge.* Berlin: Springer; 1983.

Dunning J, McNeil K. Pulmonary thromboendarterectomy for chronic thromboembolic pulmonary hypertension. *Thorax.* 1999;54:755–756.

Dwamena BA, Sonnad SS, Angobaldo JO, Wahl RL. Metastases from non-small cell lung cancer. mediastinal staging in the 1990s—meta-analytic comparison of PET and CT. *Radiology.* 1999;213:530–536.

Earnest F, Muhm JR, Sheedy PF. Roentgenographic findings in thoracic aortic dissection. *Mayo Clin Prac.* 1979;54:43–50.

Earnest F, Swenson SJ, Zink FE. Respecting patient autonomy: screening at CT and informed consent. *Radiology.* 2003;226:633–644.

Egan TJ, Neiman HL, Herman RJ et al. Computed tomography in the diagnosis of aortic aneurysm dissection or traumatic injury. *Radiology.* 1980;136:141–146.

Ellis SJ, Cleverley JR, Muller NL. Drug-induced lung disease: HRCT findings. *AJR.* 2000;175:1019–1024.

Engler R et al. The clinical assessment and follow up of functional capacity in patients with chronic congestive cardiomyopathy. *Am J Cardiol.* 1982;49:1832–1837.

Erasmus JJ, Connolly JE, McAdams HP, Roggli VL. Solitary pulmonary nodules 1. Morphologic evaluation for differentiation of benign and malignant lesions. *Radiographics.* 2000;20:43–58.

Falaschi F, Batolla L, Mascalchi M et al. Usefulness of MR signal intensity in distinguishing benign from malignant pleural disease. *AJR.* 1996;166:963–968.

Fauci AS, Haynes BF, Katz P et al. Wegener's granulomatosis: prospective clinical and therapeutic experience with 85 patients for 21 years. *Ann Intern Med.* 1983;98:76–85.

Faulkner SL, Vernon R, Brown PP et al. Hemoptysis and pulmonary aspergilloma: operative versus non-operative treatment. *Ann Thorac Surg.* 1978;25:389–392.

Faustini A, Hall AJ, Percucci CA. Risk factors for multidrug resistant tuberculosis in Europe: asystemic review. *Thorax.* 2006;61(2):158–163.

Felson B. Röntgendiagnostik der alveolären und interstitiellen Lungenerkrankungen. In: Fuchs WA, Voegele E, eds. *Aktuelle Probleme der Röntgendiagnostik.* Vol II. *Röntgendiagnostik der Lunge.* Bern: Huber; 1973a.

Felson B. *Chest Roentgenology.* Philadelphia: Saunders; 1973b.

Felson B. Disseminated interstitial diseases of the lung. *Ann Radiol.* 9 1966;9:325–345.

Felson B. Thoracic calcifications. *Chest.* 1969;56:330–343.

Fenlon HM, Doran M, Sant SM, Breatnach E. High-resolution chest CT in systemic lupus erythematosus. *AJR.* 1996;166:301–307.

Fenoglio JJ, McAlister HA Jr, DeCastro CM et al. Congenital bicuspid valve after age 20. *Am J Cardiol.* 1977;39:164–169.

Fishman AP, Pietra GG. Primary pulmonary hypertension. *Ann Rev Med.* 1980;31:421–431.

Flower CDR. Chest Trauma. In: Grainger RG, Allison DJ, eds. *Diagnostic Radiology.* 2nd ed. Edinburgh: Churchill Livingstone; 1992:1:349–355.

Flower CDR. *Pulmonary Eosinophilia.* Proceedings of the Seminar in Pulmonary Radiology. London: Royal Brompton National Heart and Lung Institute; January 1995.

Fontana RS. Early diagnosis of lung cancer. *Am Rev Resp Dis.* 1977;116:399–402.

Fraser RG, Paré JAP. *Synopsis of Diseases of the Chest.* Philadelphia: Saunders; 1983.

Frazier AA, Rosado de Christenson ML, Stocker JT, Templeton PA. Intralobar sequestration: radiologic-pathologic correlation. *Radiographics.* 1997;17:725–745.

Frazier AA, Galvin JR, Franks TJ, Rosado-de-Christenson ML. Pulmonary Vasculature: Hypertension and infarction. *Radiographics.* 2000;20:491–524.

Freundlich IM, Israel HL. Pulmonary aspergillosis. *Clin Radiol.* 1973;24:248–253.

Friedman AC, Fiel SB, Radecki PD et al. Computed tomography of benign pleural and pulmonary parenchymal abnormalities related to asbestos exposure. *Semin Ultrasound, CT and MR.* 1990;11:393–408.

Friedman PJ, Liebow AA, Sokoloff J. Eosinophilic granuloma of lung: clinical aspects of primary pulmonary histiocytosis in the adult. *Medicine.* 1981;60:385–396.

Fry WA, Phillips JL, Menck HR. Ten year survey of lung cancer treatment and survival in hospitals in the United States: a national cancer data base report. *Cancer.* 1999;86:1867–1876.

Fuchs WA, Voegeli E. *Röntgendiagnostik der Lunge.* Bern: Huber; 1973.

Furin JJ, Johnson JL. Recent advances in the diagnosis and management of tuberculosis. *Curr Opin Pulm Med.* 2005;11(3):189–194.

Gaensler EA, Carrington CB. Peripheral opacities in chronic eosinophilic pneumonia: the photographic negative of pulmonary edema. *AJR.* 1977;128:1–13.

Gaerte SC, Meyer CA, Winer-Muram HT, Tarver RD, Conces DJ. Fat-containing lesions of the chest. *Radiographics.* 2002;22:61–78.

Geary L, Kashlan MB, Hunker FD, Fraser RG. Diffuse lung disease in a compromised host. *Invest Radiol.* 1980;15:85–91

Geddes DM, Corrin B, Brewerton DA et al. Progressive airway obliteration in adults in association with rheumatoid disease. *Q J Med.* 1977;46:427–444.

Gefter WB, Epstein DM, Miller WT. Allergic bronchopulmonary aspergillosis: less common patterns. *Radiology.* 1981;140:307–312.

Gelman R, Mirvis SE, Gens D. Diaphragmatic rupture due to blunt trauma: sensitivity of plain chest radiographs. *AJR.* 1991;156:51–57.

German Central Committee on Tuberculosis Control. Information Report. 1994.

Ghersin E, Litmanovich D, Dragu R et al. 16-MDCT coronary angiography versus invasive coronary angiography in acute chest pain syndrome: a blinded prospective study. *AJR.* 2006;186:177–184.

Glazer HS, Kaiser LR, Anderson DJ et al. Indeterminate mediastinal invasion in bronchogenic carcinoma: CT evaluation. *Radiology.* 1989;173:37–42.

Gleeson FV, Traill ZC, Hansell DM. Evidence on expiratory CT scans of small-airway obstruction in sarcoidosis. *AJR.* 1996;166:1052–1054.

Glimp RA, Bayer AS. Fungal pneumonias. 3. Allergic bronchopulmonary aspergillosis. *Chest.* 1981;80:85–94.

Goedert JJ, Biggar RJ, Melbye M et al. Effect of T4 count and cofactors on the incidence of AIDS in homosexual men infected with human immunodeficiency virus. *JAMA.* 1987;257:331–334.

Goodman LR, Curtin JJ, Mewissen MW et al. Detection of pulmonary embolism in patients with unresolved clinical and scintigraphic diagnosis: helical CT versus angiography. *AJR.* 1995;164:1369–1374.

Goodman LR, Gulsun M, Washington L, Nagy PG, Piacsek KL. Inherent variability of CT lung nodule measurements in vivio using semiautomated volumetric measurements. *AJR.* 2006;186:989–994.

Goodman PC. Pneumocystis carinii pneumonia. *J Thorac Imaging.* 1991;6:16–21.

Gottlieb MS, Schanker H, Fan P et al. Pneumocystis pneumonia-Los Angeles. *MMWR.* 1981 a;30:250–252.

Gottlieb MS, Schroff R, Schanker H et al. Pneumocystis carinii pneumonia and mucosal candidiasis in previously healthy homosexual men: evidence of a new acquired cellular immunodeficiency. *N Engl J Med.* 1981 b;305:1425–1431.

Grainger RG, Donner RM. Central Cyanosis. In: Grainger RG, Allison DJ, eds. *Diagnostic Radiology.* 2nd ed. Edinburgh: Churchill Livingstone; 1992:1:565–592.

Grainger RG, Donner RM. Left to Right Shunts. In: Grainger RG, Allison DJ, eds. *Diagnostic Radiology.* Edinburgh: Churchill Livingstone; 1992:1:545–563.

Grainger RG. Other Congenital Heart Anomalies. In: Grainger RG, Allison DJ, eds. *Diagnostic Radiology.* 2nd ed. Edinburgh: Churchill Livingstone; 1992:1:593–613.

Greene R, McLoud TC, Stark P. Pneumothorax. *Semin Roentgenol.* 1977;12:313–325.

Greene R. Adult respiratory distress syndrome: acute alveolar damage. *Radiology.* 1987;163:57–66.

Grenier P, Mourey-Gerosa I, Benali K et al. Abnormalities of the airways and lung parenchyma in asthmatics: CT observations in 50 patients and inter- and intraobserver variability. *Eur Radiol.* 1996;6:199–206.

Gross GW, Dougherty CH. Pleural hemorrhage in neonates on extracorporeal membrane oxygenation and after repair of congenital diaphragmatic hernia: imaging findings. *AJR.* 1995;164:951–955.

Gross SC, Barr I, Eyler WR et al. Computed tomography in dissection of the thoracic aorta. *Radiology.* 1980;136:135–139.

Guest JL, Anderson JN. Major airway injury in closed chest trauma. *Chest.* 1977;72:63–66.

Gullotta W, Wenzl H. Posttraumatische Lungenhämatome und Pneumatozelen. *Fortschr Röntgenstr.* 1974;121:35.

Gupta NC, Maloof J, Gunel E. Probability of malignancy in solitary pulmonary nodules using fluorine-18FDG and PET. *J Nucl Med.* 1996;37:943–948.

Gürtler KF, Erbe W, Kreysel HW, Bücheler E. Röntgenologische Verlaufsbeobachtungen am Thorax bei progressiver Sklerodermie. *Fortschr Röntgenstr.* 1979;126:97.

Hampton AO, Castleman B. Correlation of postmortem chest teleroentgenograms with autopsy findings. With special reference to pulmonary embolism and infarction. *AJR.* 1940;43:305.

Han J, Lee KS, Yi CA et al. Thymic epithelial tumors classified according to a newly established WHO scheme: CT and MR findings. *Korean J Radiol.* 2003;4:46–53.

Hanak V, Ryu J, Hartman T. Radiologic pattern of pulmonary disease associated with mycobacterium intracellulare-avium in hot tub users (hot tub lung). *Chest Meeting Abstracts.* 2005;128:347.

Hanke R, Kretschmar R. Die Rundatelektase. *Fortschr Röntgenstr.* 1983;138:151.

Hansell DM, Peters AM. Pulmonary Vascular Diseases and Pulmonary Edema. In: Armstrong P, Wilson AG, Dee P, Hansell DM, eds. Imaging of Diseases of the Chest. 2nd ed. St Louis: Mosby; 1995:369–425.

Harris JA, Bis KG, Glover JL et al. Penetrating atherosclerotic ulcers of the aorta. *J Vasc Surg.* 1994;19:83–89.

Harris NL. Extranodal lymphoid infiltrates and mucosa-associated lymphoid tissue (MALT): a unifying concept. *Am J Surg Pathol.* 1991;15:879–884.

Hartman TE, Primack SL, Müller NL et al. Diagnosis of thoracic complications in AIDS: accuracy of CT. *AJR.* 1994;162:547–553.

Hartman TE, Swensen SJ, Hansell DM et al. Nonspecific interstitial pneumonia: Variable appearance at high-resolution chest CT. *Radiology.* 2000;217:701–705.

Hatipoglu ON, Osma E, Manisali M et al. High resolution computed tomographic findings in pulmonary tuberculosis. *Thorax.* 1996;51:397–402.

Heelan RT, Rusch VW, Begg CB et al. Staging of malignant pleural mesothelioma: Comparison of CT and MR imaging. *AJR.* 1999;172:1039–1047.

Heidenreich PA, Steffens J, Fujita N et al. Evaluation of mitral stenosis with velocity-encoded cine-magnetic resonance imaging. *Am J Cardiol.* 1995;5:365–369.

Heilmann HP, Doppelfeld E. Ergebnisse der Strahlenbehandlung des Bronchialkarzinoms. *Dtsch Med Wschr.* 1976;101:1557.

Heinrich M, Uder M, Tscholl D, Grgic A, Kramann B, Schafers HJ. CT scan findings in chronic thromboembolic pulmonary hypertension: predictors of hemodynamic improvement after pulmonary thromboendarterectomy. *Chest.* 2005;127:1606–1613.

Heitzman ER. *The Lung.* St. Louis: Mosby; 1993.

Hendren W, McKee DM. Lobar emphysema of infancy. *J Pediatr Surg.* 1966;1:24–39.

Henschke CI, McCauley DI, Yankelevitz DF et al. Early lung cancer action project: overall design and findings from baseline screening. *Lancet.* 1999;354:99–105.

Henschke CI, Yankelevitz DF, Mirtcheva R et al. CT screening for lung cancer: frequency and significance of part solid and non-solid nodules. *AJR.* 2002;178:1053–1057.

Henschke CI, Yankelevitz DF, Naidich DP et al. CT screening for lung cancer: suspiciousness of nodules according to size on baseline scans. *Radiology.* 2004;231:164–168.

Herbert A, Walters MT, Cawley ID et al. Lymphocytic interstitial pneumonia identified as lymphoma of mucosa-associated lymphoid tissue. *J Pathol.* 1985;146:129–138.

Hering KG. Die Weiterentwicklung der Internationalen Staublungenklassifikation – von der ILO 1980 zur ILO 2000 und zur ILO 2000/Version Bundesrepublik Deutschland. *Pneumologie.* 2003;57:1–9.

Herold CJ, Kramer J, Serti K et al. Invasive pulmonary aspergillosis: evaluation with MR imaging. *Radiology.* 1989;173:717–721.

Heyneman LE, Ward S, Lynch DA, Remy-Jardin M, Johkoh T, Muller NL. Respiratory bronchiolitis, respiratory bronchiolitis-associated interstitial lung disease, and desquamative interstitial pneumonia: Different entities or part of the spectrum of the same disease process. *AJR.* 1999;173:1617–1622.

Higgins CB. *Essentials of Cardiac Radiology and Imaging.* New York: Lippincott; 1992.

Hillerdal G, Neu E, Osterman K et al. Sarcoidosis: epidemiology and prognosis, a 15 year European study. *Am Rev Respir Disease.* 1984;130:29–32.

Hillman BJ, Schnall MD. American College of Radiology Imaging Network: future clinical trials. *Radiology*. 2003; 227:631–632.

Hlavac M, Cook J, Ojala R, Town I, Beckert L. Latex-enhanced immunoassay d-dimer and blood gases can exclude pulmonary embolism in low-risk patients presenting to an acute care setting. *Chest*. 2005;128(4):2183–2189.

Hofner W, Küster W, Seidl G, Kummer F. Röntgenologische Aspekte beim Emphysem. *Fortschr Röntgenstr*. 1977;127: 520.

Hogg K, Dawson D, Mackway-Jones K. Outpatient diagnosis of pulmonary embolism. The MIOPED (Manchester Investigation of Pulmonary Embolism Diagnosis) study. *Emerg Med J*. 2006;23(2):123–127.

Hollingsworth HN, Mark EJ. Case records of the Massachusetts General Hospital. *New Engl J Med*. 2001;345(16): 1193–1200.

Honda O, Johkoh T, Ichikado K et al. Differential diagnosis of lymphocytic interstitial pneumonia and malignant lymphoma on high-resolution CT. *AJR*. 1999;173:71–74.

Hood RM, Sloan HE. Injuries of the trachea and major bronchi. *J Thorac Cardiovasc Surg*. 1959;38:458–480.

Hossein JH, Strauss W, Segall GM. SPECT and PET in the evaluation of coronary artery disease. *Radiographics*. 1999; 19:915–926.

Howling SJ, Hansell DM, Wells AU, Nicholson AG, Flint JDA, Muller NL. Follicular bronchiolitis: thin section CT and histologic findings. *Radiology*. 1999;212:637–642.

Hruban RH, Meziane MA, Zerhouni EA et al. Radiologic-pathologic correlation of the CT halo sign in invasive pulmonary aspergillosis. *J Comput Assist Tomogr*. 1987;11: 534–536.

Huzly A. Bronchus und Tuberkulose aus aktueller Sicht. *Internist (Berlin)*. 1973 b;4:88.

Ichikado K, Suga M, Muranaka H et al. Prediction of prognosis for acute respiratory distress syndrome with thin-section CT: validation in 44 cases. *Radiology*. 2005;238: 321–329.

Ikezoe J, Murayama S, Godwin JD, Done SL, Verschakelen JA. Bronchopulmonary sequestration: CT assessment. *Radiology*. 1990;176:375–379

ILO. *ILO guidelines for the use of the ILO classification of radiographs of Pneumokonioses*. Geneva: International Labour Office 2002 (Occupational Safety and Health Series No 22); 2000.

Im JG, Itoh H, Shim YS et al. Pulmonary tuberculosis: CT findings—early active disease and sequential change with antituberculous therapy. *Radiology*. 1993;186:653–660.

Im JG, Kyung SL. CT in adults with tuberculosis of the chest: characteristic findings and role in management. *AJR*. 1995;164:1361–1367.

Iochum S, Ludig T, Walter F, Sebbag H, Grosdidier G, Blum AG. Imaging of diaphragmatic injury: A diagnostic challenge? *Radiographics*. 2002;22:103–116.

Janower ML, Blennerhassett JB. Lymphangitic spread of metastatic cancer to the lung. A radiologic-pathologic classification. *Radiology*. 1971;101:267–273.

Jederlinic PJ, Sicilian L, Gaensler EA. Chronic eosinophilic pneumonia: a report of 19 cases and a review of the literature. *Medicine*. 1988;67:154–162.

Jeong YJ, Lee KS, Kim J et al. Does CT of thymic epithelial tumors enable us to differentiate histologic subtypes and predict prognosis? *AJR*. 2004;183:283–289.

Jewkes J, Kay PH, Paneth M et al. Pulmonary aspergilloma: analysis of prognosis in relation to hemoptysis and survey of treatment. *Thorax*. 1983;38:572–578.

Johkoh T, Muller NL, Taniguchi H, Kondoh Y, Akira M, Ichikado K et al. Acute interstitial pneumonia: thin section CT findings in 36 patients. *Radiology*. 199;211:859.

Kanemoto N, Furuya H, Etoh T, Sasamoto H, Matsuyama S. Chest roentgenograms in primary pulmonary hypertension. *Chest*. 1979;76:45–49.

Kaplan MH, Susin M, Puhwa SG et al. Neoplastic complications of HTLV-III infection: lymphomas and solid tumors. *Am J Med*. 1987;82:389–396.

Kapoor V, McCook BM, Torok FS. An introduction to PET-CT imaging. *Radiographics*. 2004;24:523–543.

Katz AS, Niesenbaum L, Mass B. Pleural effusion as the initial manifestation of disseminated cryptococcosis in acquired immunodeficiency syndrome: diagnosis by pleural biopsy. *Chest*. 1989;96:440–441.

Katzenstein AL, Fiorelli RF. Nonspecific interstitial pneumonia/fibrosis: histologic features and clinical significance. *Am J Surg Pathol*. 1994;18:136–147.

Katzenstein AL. Katzenstein and Askin's surgical pathology of non-neoplastic lung disease. 3 rd ed. Philadelphia, Pa: Saunders; 1997.

Kauffmann GW, Reinbold WD, Hagedorn M. Röntgenmorphologische Befunde bei Sklerodermie. *Fortschr Röntgenstr*. 1983 a; 138:607.

Kauffmann GW, Vogel W, Rühle KH, Friedburg HH, Papacharalampous X. Verlaufsbeobachtungen bei überlebter Schocklunge. (ARDS). *Fortschr Röntgenstr*. 1983 b;138:292.

Kazama T, Faria SC, Varavithya V, Phongkitkarun S, Ito H, Macapinlac HA. FDG PET in the evaluation of treatment for lymphoma: clinical usefulness and pitfalls. *Radiographics*. 2005;25:191–207.

Kehdy F, Richardson JD. The utility of 3-D CT scan in the diagnosis and evaluation of sternal fractures. *J Trauma*. 2006; 60(3):635–636.

Kennedy CD. Lobar emphysema. Long term imaging follow up. *Radiology*. 1991;180:189.

Killeen KL, Mirvis SE, Shanmuganathan K. Helical CT of diaphragmatic rupture caused by blunt trauma. *AJR*. 1999; 173:1611–1616.

Kilner PJ, Firmin DN, Rees RSO et al. Valve and great vessel stenosis: assessment with MR jet velocity mapping. *Radiology*. 1991;178:229–235.

Kim RJ, Wu E, Rafael A et al. The use of contrast-enhanced magnetic resonance imaging to identify reversible myocardial dysfunction. *N Engl J Med*. 2000;343(20):1445–1453.

Klose P, Thelen M, Erbel R. *Bildgebende Verfahren in der Diagnostik von Herzerkrankungen*. Stuttgart; Thieme: 1991.

Ko SM, Seo JB, Hong MK et al. Myocardial enhancement pattern in patients with acute myocardial infarction on two-phase contrast-enhanced ECG-gated multidetector-row computed tomography. *Clinical Radiology*. 2006;61: 417–422.

Kuhlman JE. Pneumocystis carinii pneumonia: spectrum of parenchymal CT findings. *Radiology*. 1990;175:711.

Kuhlman JE. The role of chest computed tomography in the diagnosis of drug-related reactions. *J Thorac Imaging*. 1991;6:52–61.

Kuhlman JE. Diseases of the Chest in AIDS. In: *Proceedings of the Fleischner Society: 26th Annual Conference on Chest Disease*. Vancouver: 1996: 57–71.

Kuhlman JE. Pneumocystic infection: the radiologist's perspective. *Radiology*. 1996;198:623–635.

Kuhlman JE, Fishman EK, Burch PA. Invasive pulmonary aspergillosis in acute leukemia: the contribution of CT to early diagnosis and aggressive management. *Chest*. 1987; 92:95–99.

Kuhlman JE, Fishman EK, Burch PA et al. Pictorial essay. CT of invasive pulmonary aspergillosis. *AJR*. 1988;150: 1015–1020.

Kuhlman JE, Fishman EK, Hruban RH et al. Diseases of the chest in AIDS: CT diagnosis. *Radiographics*. 1989;9: 827–857.

Kuhlman JE, Knowles MC, Fishman EK et al. Premature bullous pulmonary damage in AIDS: CT diagnosis. *Radiology*. 1989;173:23–26.

Kumpe DA, Oh KS, Wyman SM. A characteristic pulmonary finding in unilateral complete bronchial transection. *AJR*. 1970;110:704.

Lange S, Minck C. Die Lymphangiosis carcinomatosa der Lungen bei metastasierten Mammakarzinomen. *Fortschr Röntgenstr*. 1983;140:411.

Lanham JG, Elkon KB, Pusey CD et al. Systemic vasculitis with asthma and eosinophilia: a clinical approach to the Churg-Strauss syndrome. *Medicine*. 1984;63:65–81.

Laubenberger T. *Leitfaden der medizinischen Röntgentechnik*. Köln: Deutscher Ärzteverlag; 1980.

Ledbetter S, Stuk JL, Kaufman JA. Helical (spiral) CT in the evaluation of emergent thoracic aortic syndromes: traumatic aortic rupture, aortic aneurysm, aortic dissection, intramural hematoma, and penetrating atherosclerotic ulcer. *Radiol Clin North Am*. 1999;37:575–589.

Lee JS, Tuder R, Lynch DA. Lymphomatoid granulomatosis: Radiologic features and pathologic correlations. *AJR*. 2000;175:1335–1339.

Lee VW. Pulmonary kaposi sarcoma in patients with AIDS. *Radiology*. 1991;180:409.

Lesur O. Computed tomography in the etiologic assessment of idiopathic spontaneous pneumothorax. *Chest*. 1990; 98:341.

Leung AN, Müller NL, Miller RR. CT in differential diagnosis of diffuse pleural disease. *AJR*. 1990;154:487–492.

Levin B. The continuous diaphragm sign: a newly recognized sign of pneumomediastinum. *Clin Radiol*. 1973;24: 337–338.

Libshitz HI, Atkinson EW, Israel HI. Pleural thickening as a manifestation of Aspergillus superinfection. *AJR*. 1974; 120:883–886.

Liebow AA, Carrington CB. The Interstitial Pneumonias. In: Simon M, Potchen EJ, Le May M, eds. *Frontiers of Pulmonary Radiology*. New York: Grune and Stratton; 1969: 102–141.

Lien HH, Brodahl U, Telhaug R et al. Pulmonary changes at computed tomography in patients with testicular carcinoma treated with cis-platinum, vinblastine and bleomycin. *Acta Radiol (Diagn)*. 1985;26:507–510.

Light RW. *Pleural Diseases*. Philadelphia; Lea & Febiger: 1983.

Logan PM, Primack SL, Miller RR et al. Invasive aspergillosis of the airways: radiographic, CT and pathologic findings. *Radiology*. 1994;193:383–388.

Lowe VJ, Fletcher JW, Gobar L et al. Prospective investigation of positron emission tomography in lung nodules. *J Clin Oncol*. 1998;16:1075–1084.

Ludomirsky A, Huhta JC, Vick W III et al. Colour Doppler detection of multiple ventricular septal defects. *Circulation*. 1986;74:1317–1322.

Lui YQ. Radiology of aortoarteritis. *Radiol Clin North Am*. 1985;23:671–688.

Lundell CJ, Quinn M, Rinck E. Traumatic laceration of the ascending aorta: angiographic assessment. *AJR*. 1985;145: 715–719.

Lynch DA. Computed tomography in pulmonary sarcoidosis. *J Comput Assist Tomogr*. 1989;13:405.

Lynch DA. Imaging of asthma and allergic bronchopulmonary mycosis. *RCNA*. 1998;36(1):129–142.

Lynch DA. Nonspecific interstitial pneumonia: evolving concepts. *Radiology*. 2001;221:583–584.

Lynch DA, Newell JD, Tschomper BA et al. Uncomplicated asthma in adults: Comparison of CT appearance of the lungs in asthmatic and healthy subjects. *Radiology*. 1993; 188:829.

MacMahon H, Austin JHM, Gamsu G et al. Guidelines for management of small pulmonary nodules detected on CT scans: A statement from the Fleischner Society. *Radiology*. 2005;237:395–400.

Maguire R, Fauci AS, Doppman JL, Wolff SM. Unusual radiographic features of Wegener's granulomatosis. *AJR*. 1978; 130:233.

Mahadeva R, Walsh G, Flower CDR, Shneerson JM. Clinical and radiological characteristics of lung disease in inflammatory bowel disease. *Eur Respir J*. 2000;15:41–48.

Malo JL, Pepys J, Simon G. Studies in chronic allergic bronchopulmonary aspergillosis: 2. radiological findings. *Thorax*. 1977;32:262–268.

Malone PS, Brain AJ, Kiely EM et al. Childhood diaphragmatic defects that present late. *Archives of Diseases in Childhood*. 1989;64:1542–1544.

Manning WJ, Atkinson DJ, Parker JA et al. Assessment of intracardiac shunts with Gadolinium-enhanced ultrafast MR imaging. *Radiology*. 1992;184:357–361.

Maraj R, Rerkpattanapipat P, Jacobs LE et al. Meta-analysis of 143 reported cases of aortic intramural hematoma. *Am J Cardiol*. 2000;86:664–668.

Marchiori E, Ferreira A, Muller NL. Silicoproteinosis: high resolution CT and histologic findings. *J Thorac Imaging*. 2001;16:127–129.

Marom EM, McAdams PH, Erasmus JJ et al. Staging non-small cell lung cancer with whole-body PET. *Radiology*. 1999;212:803–809.

Marti-Bonmati L. CT findings in Swyer-James Syndrome. *Radiology*. 1989;172:477.

Martini N, Heelan R, Westcott J et al. Comparative merits of conventional, computed tomographic, and magnetic imaging in assessing mediastinal involvement in surgically confirmed lung carcinoma. *J Thorac Cardiov Sur*. 1985; 90:639–648.

Maskell GF, Lockwood CM, Flower CDR. Computed tomography of the lung in Wegener's granulomatosis. *Clin Radiol*. 1993;48:377–380.

Mathys H. *Klinische Pneumologie*. Berlin: Springer; 2001.

Matsumoto S, Miyake H, Oga M, Takaki H, Mori H. Diagnosis of lung cancer in a patient with pneumoconosis and progressive massive fibrosis using MRI. *Eur Radiol*. 1998;8: 615–617.

Mayo JR, Müller NL, Road J et al. Chronic eosinophilic pneumonia: CT findings in six cases. *AJR*. 1989;153:727–730.

McAdams HP, Erasmus J, Winter JA. Radiologic manifestations of pulmonary tuberculosis. *Radiol Clin North Am*. 1995;33(4):655–678.

McDonald TJ, Neel HB, DeRemee RA. Wegener's granulomatosis of the subglottis and the upper portion of the trachea. *Ann Otol Rhinol Laryngol*. 1982;91:588–592.

McGahan JP, Graves DS, Palmer PES, Stadalnik RC, Dublin AB. Classic and contemporary imaging of coccidioidomycosis. *AJR*. 1981:136;393.

McGonigal MD, Schwab CW, Kauder DR et al. Supplemented emergent chest computed tomography in the management of blunt torso trauma. *J Trauma*. 1990;30:1431–1435.

McGuinness G, Scholes JV, Jagirdar JS et al. Unusual lympho-proliferative disorders in nine adults with HIV or AIDS. CT and pathologic findings. *Radiology*. 1995;197:59–65.

McLoud TC, Flower CDR. Imaging the pleura: sonography, CT and MR imaging. *AJR*. 1991;156:1145–1153.

Meduri GU, Stover DE, Lee M et al. Pulmonary Kaposi's sarcoma in the acquired immunodeficiency syndrome: clinical, radiographic and pathologic manifestations. *Am J Med*. 1986;81:11–18.

Mendelson DS. Imaging of the thymus. *Chest Surg Clin N Am*. 2001;11:269–293.

Meng XY. Peforated amebic liver abscess: clinical analysis of 110 cases. *South Med J*. 1994;87:985.

Mergo PJ, Williams WF, Gonzalez-Rothi R et al. Three-dimensional volumetric assessment of abnormally low attenuation of the lung from routine helical CT. *AJR*. 1998; 170:1355–1360.

Meschan I. *An Atlas of Anatomy Basic to Radiology*. Philadelphia: Saunders; 1975.

Meschan I. Analyse der Röntgenbilder. Klinische Radiologie. Vol II. *Atemwege, Herz. Enke*. Stuttgart: Enke; 1981.

Midthun DE, Swenson SJ, Jett JR. Approach to the solitary pulmonary nodule. *Mayo Clin Proc*. 1993;68:378–385.

Miles KA, Griffiths MR, Fuentes MA. Standardized perfusion value: Universal CT contrast enhancement scale that correlates with FDG PET in lung nodules. *Radiology*. 2001; 220:548.

Miller RR. Limitations of computed tomography in the assessment of emphysema. *Am Rev Resp Dis*. 1989; 139:980.

Mills SR, Jackson DC, Ovder RA, Heaston DK, Moore AV. The incidence, etiologies, and avoidance of complications of pulmonary angiography in a large series. *Radiology*. 1980; 36:295–299.

Mino M, Noma S, Taguchi Y, Tomii K, Kohri Y, Oida K. Pulmonary involvement in polymyositis and dermatomyositis: sequential evaluation with CT. *AJR*. 1997;169:83–87.

Mirvis SE, Shanmuganathan K. MR imaging of thoracic trauma. *Magn Reson Imaging Clin N Am*. 2000;8:91–104.

Mitchell L, Jenkins JPR, Watson Y et al. Diagnosis and assessment of mitral and aortic valve disease by cine-flow magnetic resonance imaging. *Magn Reson Med*. 1989;12: 181–197.

Moore ADA, Godwin JD, Dietrich PA et al. Swyer-James syndrome: CT findings in eight patients. *AJR*. 1992;158: 1211–1215.

Morgan PW, Goodman LR, Aprahamian C et al. Evaluation of traumatic aortic injury: does dynamic contrast-enhanced CT play a role? *Radiology*. 1992;182:661–666.

Moskowitz H, Platt RT, Schachar R, Mellins H. Roentgen visualization of minute pleural effusion. *Radiology*. 1973; 109:33–35.

Mountain CF. A new international staging system for lung cancer. *Chest*. 1986;89:225–233.

Mountain CF. Revisions in the international system for staging lung cancer. *Chest*. 1997;111:1710–1717.

Müller KH. Lungentumoren. In: Doerr W, ed. *Spezielle pathologische Anatomie*. Vol XVI. , Berlin: Springer; 1983.

Müller NL, Fraser RG, Paré JAP. *Diagnosis of Diseases of the Chest*. 2nd ed. Philadelphia: Saunders; 2001.

Müller NL, Miller RA. Diffuse pulmonary hemorrhage. *Radiol Clin North Am*. 1991;29:5:965–971.

Müller NL, Miller RR. Acute Diffuse Lung Disease. In: Putman CE, ed. *Diagnostic Imaging of the Lung. Lung Biology in Health and Disease*. Vol 46. New York: Marcel Dekker; 1990:337–441.

Murata K, Itoh H, Todo G et al. Centrilobular lesions of the lung: demonstration by high resolution CT and pathologic correlation. *Radiology*. 1986;161:641–645.

Murray JF. Pulmonary tuberculosis: update 1996. In: *Proceedings of the Fleischner Society; 26th Annual Conference on Chest Disease*. Vancouver: 1996:47–51.

Murray JF, Nadel JA. *Textbook of Respiratory Medicine*. Philadelphia: Saunders; 2000.

Murray JG, Caoili E, Gruden JF et al. Acute rupture of the diaphragm due to blunt trauma: diagnostic sensitivity and specificity of CT. *AJR*. 1996;166:1035–1039.

Musset D, Grenier P, Carette MF et al. Primary lung cancer staging: prospective comparative study of MR imaging with CT. *Radiology*. 1986;160:607–611.

Nagai S, Kitaichi M, Itoh H, Nishimura K, Izumi T, Colby TV. Idiopathic nonspecific interstitial pneumonia/fibrosis: comparison with idiopathic pulmonary fibrosis and BOOP. *Eur Respir J*. 1998;12:1010–1019.

Nagel E, Al-Saadi N, Paetsch I. Magnetic resonance myocardial perfusion reserve for the detection of coronary artery disease in an unselected patient population. Presented at the meeting of the American Heart Association, Atlanta, Georgia; 1999.

Naidich DP, McCauley DI, Leitman BS et al. CT of Pulmonary Tuberculosis. In: Siegelman SS, ed. *Computed Tomography of the Chest*. New York: Churchill Livingstone; 1984: 175–217.

Naidich DP, McGuinness G. Pulmonary manifestations of AIDS: CT and radiographic correlations. *Radiol Clin North Am*. 1991;29:999–1017.

Naidich DP, Rumanak WM, Ettenger NA et al. Congenital anomalies of the lungs in adults: MR diagnosis. *AJR*. 1988; 151:13–19.

Naidich DP, Webb WR, Muller NL, Krinsky GA, Zerhouni EA, Siegelmann SS. Computed tomography and magnetic resonance of the thorax. Philadelphia, Pa: Lippincott-Raven; 1999.

Naidich DP, Zerhouni EA, Siegelman SS. The Pleura and Chest Wall. In: *Computed Tomography of the Thorax*. New York: Raven Press; 1984:243–268.

Naidich DP, Zerhouni EA, Siegelmann SS. *Computed Tomography and Magnetic Resonance of the Thorax*. New York: Raven; 1991.

Ng CS, Wells AU, Padley SPG. A CT sign of chronic pulmonary arterial hypertension: the ratio of main pulmonary artery to aortic diameter. *J Thorac Imaging*. 1999;14:270–278.

Nieman K, Cademartiri F, Lemos PA et al. Reliable non-invasive coronary angiography with fast submillimeter multislice spiral computed tomography. *Circulation*. 2002;106: 2051–2054.

Nikolaou K, Schoenberg SO, Attenberger U et al. Pulmonary arterial hypertension: diagnosis with fast perfusion MR imaging and high-spatial-resolution MR angiography—preliminary experience. *Radiology*. 2005;236:694–703.

Nishimura K, Kitaichi M, Izumi T et al. Usual interstitial pneumonia: histologic correlation with high resolution CT. *Radiology*. 1992;182:337–342.

Nishino M, Ashiku SK, Kocher ON et al. The thymus: A comprehensive review. *Radiographics*. 2006;26(2):335–348.

Noguchi M, Morikawa A, Kawasaki M et al. Small adenocarcinoma of the lung. *Cancer*. 1995;75:2844–2852.

Nolan RL, McAdams HP, Sporn TA, Roggli VL, Tapson VF, Goodman PC. Pulmonary cholesterol granulomas in patients with pulmonary artery hypertension: chest radiographic and CT findings. *AJR*. 1999;172:1317–1319.

Ognibene FP, Steis RG, Macher AM et al. Kaposi's sarcoma causing pulmonary infiltrates and respiratory failure in the acquired immunodeficiency syndrome. *Ann Intern Med.* 1985;102:471–475.

Oh YW, Kim JH, Lee NJ et al. High resolution CT appearance of miliary tuberculosis. *J Comput Assist Tomogr.* 1994; 18(6):862–866.

Oldham SAA, Castillo M, Jacobson FL et al. HIV associated lymphocytic interstitial pneumonia: radiologic manifestations and pathologic correlation. *Radiology.* 1989;170: 83–87.

Orens JB, Martinez FJ, Lynch JP. Pleuropulmonary manifestations of systemic lupus erythematosus. *Rheum Dis Clin North Am.* 1994;20:159–193.

Orr DP, Myerowitz RL, Dubois PJ. Patho-radiologic correlation of invasive pulmonary aspergillosis in the compromised host. *Cancer.* 1978;41:2028–2039.

Ortiz E, Robinson PJ, Deanfield JE et al. Localisation of ventricular septal defects by simultaneous display of superimposed colour Doppler and cross sectional echocardiographic images. *Br Heart J.* 1985;54:53–60.

Otto H. Bedeutung, Morphologie und Entstehungsprinzipien des chronischen destruktiven Lungenemphysems. Atemwegs- u. Lungenkrankh. 1976;2:95.

Otto H., Reinhard H. Die Beteiligung der Lunge an der Sklerodermie. *Prax Pneumol.* 1970;34:753.

Padley SPG, Adler B, Hansell DM et al. High-resolution computed tomography of drug-induced lung disease. *Clin Radiol.* 1992;46:232–236.

Pagani JJ, Libshitz HI. Opportunistic fungal pneumonias in cancer patients. *AJR.* 1981;137:1033–1039.

Paganin F, Trussard V, Seneterre E et al. Chest radiography and high resolution computed tomography of the lungs in asthma. *Am Rev Respir Dis.* 1992;146:1084.

Palmer WE, Rivitz SM, Chew FS. Bilateral bronchogenic cysts. *AJR.* 1991;157:950.

Parker MS, Matheson TL, Rao AV et al. Making the transition. The role of helical CT in the evaluation of potentially acute thoracic aortic injuries. *AJR.* 2001;176:1267–1272.

Pastores SM, Naidich DP, Aranda CP et al. Intrathoracic adenopathy associated with pulmonary tuberculosis in patients with human immunodeficiency virus infection. *Chest.* 1993;103:1433–1437.

Patel S, Kazerooni EA. Helical CT for the evaluation of acute pulmonary embolism. *AJR.* 2005;185:135–149.

Patz EF Jr, Shaffer K, Piwnica-Worms DR et al. Malignant pleural mesothelioma: value of CT and MR imaging in predicting resectability. *AJR.* 1992;159:961–966.

Patz EF, Rusch VW, Heelan R. The proposed new international TNM staging system for malignant pleural mesothelioma: application to imaging. *AJR.* 1996;166: 323–327.

Patz EF, Connolly J, Herndon J. Prognostic value of thoracic FDG PET imaging after treatment for non-small cell lung cancer. *AJR.* 2000;174:769–774.

Pearson MC, Rigby MB. Congenital Heart Disease-Specific Conditions. In: Sutton D, ed. *A Textbook of Radiology and Imaging.* 4th ed. Edinburgh: Churchill Livingstone; 1987: 1:643–686.

Pilate I, Marcelis S, Timmerman H et al. Pulmonary asbestosis: CT study of subpleural curvilinear shadow (letter). *Radiology.* 1987;164:584.

PIOPED: a collaborative study by the PIOPED investigators. Value of the ventilation/perfusion scan in acute pulmonary embolism: results of the prospective investigation of pulmonary embolism diagnosis. *JAMA.* 1990;263: 2753–2759.

Pirolo JS, Hutchins GM, Moore GW. Infarct expansion: pathologic analysis of 204 patients with a single myocardial infarct. *J Am Coll Cardiol.* 1986;7(2):349–54.

Poustchi-Amin M, Gutierrez FR, Brown JJ et al. Performing cardiac MR imaging: An overview. *RCNA.* 2003;2(1):1–19.

Pretre R, von Segesser LK. Aortic dissection. *Lancet.* 1997; 349:1461–1464.

Quint LE, Park CH, Iannettoni MD. Solitary pulmonary nodules in patients with extrapulmonary neoplasms. *Radiology.* 2000;217:257–261.

Ranniger K, Valvassori GE. Angiographic diagnosis of intralobar pulmonary sequestration. *AJR.* 1964;92:540.

Raphael MJ, Gibson DG. Cardiomyopathies, Cardiac Tumours, Trauma. In: Grainger RG, Allison DJ, eds. *Diagnostic Radiology.* 2nd ed. Edinburgh: Churchill Livingstone; 1992:1:695–712.

Raptopoulos V, Sherman RG, Phillips DA et al. Traumatic aortic tear: screening with chest CT. *Radiology.* 1992; 182:667–673.

Rau WS. Die röntgenologische Feinstruktur der Lunge. *Fortschr Röntgenstr.* 1980;133:571.

Rawlin RN, Raval B, Finley R. Primary chylopericardium: combined lymphangiographic and CT diagnosis (case report). *J Comput Assist Tomogr.* 1980;4:869–870.

Reed JC, Sobonya RE. Morphologic analysis of foregut cysts in the thorax. *AJR.* 1974;120:851–860.

Reeder MM, Felson B. *Gamuts in Radiology.* Berlin: Springer; 2003.

Reid L. Reduction in bronchial subdivision in bronchiectasis. *Thorax.* 1950;5:233.

Reinhardt MJ, Herkel C, Altehoefer C, Finke J, Moser E. Computed tomography and 18F-FDG positron emission tomography for therapy control of Hodgkin's and non-Hodgkin's lymphoma patients: when do we really need FDG-PET? *Annals of Oncology.* 2005;16(9):1524–1529.

Reis-Filho JS, Carrilho C, Valenti C et al. Is TTF1 a good immunohistochemical marker to distinguish primary from metastatic lung adenocarcinomas? *Pathol Res Pract.* 2000; 196(12):835–840.

Remy-Jardin MJ, Remy J, Wattinne L et al. Central pulmonary thromboembolism: diagnosis with spiral volumetric CT with the single-breath-hold technique—comparison with pulmonary angiography. *Radiology.* 1992;185:381–387.

Remy-Jardin M, Remy J, Cortret B, Mauri F, Delcambre B. Lung changes in RA: CT findings. *Radiology.* 1994;193: 375–382.

Remy-Jardin M, Remy J. Spiral CT angiography of the pulmonary circulation. *Radiology.* 1999;212:615–636.

Remy-Jardin M, Duhamel A, Deken V, Bouaziz N, Dumont P, Remy J. Systemic collateral supply in patients with chronic thromboembolic and primary pulmonary hypertension: Assessment with multi-detector row helical CT angiography. *Radiology.* 2005;235:274–281.

Rendina EA, Bognolo DA, Mineo TC et al. Computed tomography for the evaluation of intrathoracic invasion by lung cancer. *J Thorac Cardiovasc Surg.* 1987;94:57–63.

Reston A, Maitre S, Humbert M et al. Pulmonary arterial hypertension: thin-section CT predictors of epoprostenol therapy failure. *Radiology.* 2002;222:782–788.

Reston A, Maitre S, Humbert M et al. Pulmonary hypertension: CT of the chest in pulmonary veno-occlusive disease. *AJR.* 2004;183:65–70.

Reynolds JH, Hansell DM. The interstitial pneumonias: understanding the acronyms. *Clinical Radiology.* 2000;55: 249–260.

Roberts CM, Citron KM, Strickland B. Intrathoracic aspergilloma: role of CT in diagnosis and treatment. *Radiology.* 1987;165:123–128.

Roberts WC. The congenitally bicuspid aortic valve. A study of 85 autopsy cases. *Am J Cardiol.* 1970;26:72–83.

Roberts WC. Aortic dissection: anatomy, consequences, and causes. *Am Heart J.* 1981;101:195–214.

Ropers D, Baum U, Pohle K et al. Detection of coronary artery stenoses with thin-slice multi-detector row spiral computed tomography and multiplanar reconstruction. *Circulation.* 2003;107:664–666.

Rosado de Christenson ML, Frazier AA, Stocker JT. Extralobar sequestration: radiologic-pathologic correlation. *Radiographics.* 1993;13:425–441.

Rosenberg ER. Ultrasound in the assessment of pleural densities. *Chest.* 1983;84:283–285.

Rübe W. *Der Lungenrundherd.* Stuttgart: Thieme; 1967.

Rübe W. Rundherde der Lunge. In: Teschendorf W, Anacker H, Thurn P, eds. *Röntgenologische Differentialdiagnostik.* Stuttgart: Thieme; 1975.

Rubinowitz JG, Ulreich S, Soriano C. The usual unusual manifestations of sarcoidosis and the "hilar haze": a new diagnostic aid. *AJR.* 1974;120:821–831.

Rusch VW, ed. The International Mesothelioma Interest Group. A proposed new international TNM staging system for malignant pleural mesothelioma. *Chest.* 1995;108:1122–1128.

Safrin S. New developments in the management of pneumocystis carinii disease. *AIDS Clin Rev.* 1993;95–112.

Safrin S. Pneumocystis carinii pneumonia in patients with the acquired immunodeficiency syndrome. *Semin Respir Infect.* 1993;8:96–103.

Saiduffin A, Arthur RJ. Congenital diaphragmatic hernia: a review of pre- and postoperative chest radiology. *Clin Radiol.* 1993;47:104–110.

Sakai F, Sone S, Kiyono K et al. MR imaging of thymoma: radiologic-pathologic correlation. *AJR.* 1992;158:751–756.

Sasaki M, Kuwabara Y, Ichiya Y et al. Differential diagnosis of thymic tumors using a combination of 11C-Methionine PET and FDG-PET. *J Nucl Med.* 1999;40:1595–1601.

Scadding JG. The late stages of pulmonary sarcoidosis. *Postgrad Med J.* 1970;46:530.

Scadding JG, Mitchell DN. *Sarcoidosis.* 2nd ed. London: Chapman and Hall Medical; 1985:101–180.

Schaefer NG, Hany TF, Taverna C et al. Non-Hodgkin lymphoma and Hodgkin Disease: Coregistered FDG PET and CT at Staging and Restaging—Do we need contrast-enhanced CT? *Radiology.* 2004;232:823–829.

Schermuly W. Differenzierung der Grundprozesse: Granulomatose und Fibrose bei der Sarkoidose. *Radiologe.* 1977;17:26.

Schettler G. *Innere Medizin.* Stuttgart: Thieme; 1990.

Schinz HR. *Radiologische Diagnostik in Klinik und Praxis.* Vol 2. Stuttgart: Thieme; 1983.

Schinz HR, Baensch WE, Frommhold W, Glauner R, Uehlinger E, Wellauer J. *Lehrbuch der Röntgendiagnostik.* Vol IV/1. Stuttgart: Thieme; 1983.

Schmidt M. Idiopathische fibröse Mediastinitis. Fortschr Rontgenstr. 1973;119:723

Schmitt WG, Menges V, Kühn H. Disseminierte verästelte Lungenverknöcherung, kombiniert mit heterotoper Knochenneubildung im Bereich der Muskulatur. *Fortschr Röntgenstr.* 1978;128:300.

Schoenhagen P, Halliburton SS, Stillman AE et al. Noninvasive imaging of coronary arteries: Current and future role of multi-detector row CT. *Radiology.* 2004;232:7–17.

Schoenhagen P, Ziada K, Kapadia SR et al: Extent and direction of arterial remodelling in stable versus unstable coronary syndromes. *Circulation.* 2000;101:598–603.

Schwickert H, Schweden F, Schild H et al. Darstellung der chronisch rezidivierenden Lungenembolie mit der Spiral-CT. *Rofo. Fortschritte auf dem Gebiete der Rontgenstrahlen und der neuen bildgebenden Verfahren.* 1993;158(4):308–313.

Scott WW. Focal pulmonary lesions in patients with AIDS. *Radiology.* 1991;180:419.

Scully RE, Galdabini JJ, McNeely BU. Case records of the Massachusetts General Hospital: case 18–1981. *N Engl J Med.* 1981;304:1090–1096.

Searles G, McKendry RJR. Methotrexate pneumonitis in rheumatoid arthritis: potential risk factors. Four case reports and a review of the literature. *J Rheumatol.* 1987;14:1164–1171.

Secci A, Wong N, Tang W, Wang S, Doherty T, Detrano R. Electron beam computed tomographic coronary calcium as a predictor of coronary events. *Circulation.* 1997;96:1122–1129.

Shanmuganathan K, Mirvis SE. Imaging diagnosis of nonaortic thoracic injury. *Radiol Clin North Am.* 1999;37:533–551.

Shanmuganathan K, Killeen K, Mirvis SE et al. Imaging of diaphragmatic injuries. *J Thorac Imaging.* 2000;15:104–111.

Sherrick AD, Swenson SJ, Hartman TE. Mosaic pattern of lung attenuation on CT scans: frequency among patients with pulmonary artery hypertension of different causes. *AJR.* 1997;169:79–82.

Shigematsu N, Emori K, Matsuba K et al. Clinicopathologic characteristics of pulmonary acinar sarcoidosis. *Chest.* 1978;73:186–188.

Shim SS, Kim Y, Lim SM. Improvement of image quality with b-blocker premedication on ECG-gated 16-MDCT coronary angiography. *AJR.* 2005a;184:649–654.

Shim SS, Lee KS, Kim B et al. Non-small cell lung cancer: prospective comparison of integrated FDG PET/CT and CT alone for preoperative staging. *Radiology.* 2005b;236:1011–1019.

Shimosato Y, Mukai K. Tumors of the Thymus and Related Lesions. In: Shimosato Y, Mukai K, eds. *Atlas of Tumor Pathology: Tumors of the Mediastinum.* Fasc 21, ser 3. Washington, DC: Armed Forces Institute of Pathology; 1997: 158–168.

Shinnick JP, Cudkowicz O, Blanco G et al. A problem in pulmonary hypertension. Part 1: The clinical course. *Chest.* 1974a: 65;65–69.

Shinnick JP, Cudkowicz L, Saldana M, Brodsky I. A problem in pulmonary hypertension. Part 2: The final course and autopsy findings. *Chest.* 1974b;65:192.

Sider L, Weiss AJ, Smith MD et al. Varied appearance of AIDS-related lymphoma in the chest. *Radiology.* 1989;171:629–632.

Sider L, Gabriel H, Curry DR et al. Pattern recognition of the pulmonary manifestations of AIDS on CT scans. *Radiographics.* 1993;13:771–784.

Siegelman SS, Khouri NF, Scott WW Jr et al. Pulmonary hamartoma: CT findings. *Radiology.* 1986;160:313–317.

Simon G, Pride N. Relation between abnormalities in the chest radiograph and changes in pulmonary function in bronchitis and emphysema. *Thorax.* 1973;28:15.

Small JH, Flower CDR, Traill ZC, Gleeson FV. Air-trapping in extrinsic allergic alveolitis on computed tomography. *Clin Radiol.* 1996;51:684–688.

Soler P, Bergeron A, Kambouchner M et al. Is high-resolution computed tomography a reliable tool to predict the histopathological activity of pulmonary Langerhan's cell histiocytosis? *Am J Respir Crit Care Med.* 2000;162:264–270.

Solomon A. Radiological features of asbestos-related visceral pleural changes. *Am J Int Med.* 1991;19:339–355.

Stanley RJ. Inherent dangers in radiologic screening. *AJR.* 2001;177:989–992.

Stark D, Bradley G. *Magnetic Resonance Imaging.* St. Louis: Mosby 1999.

Stein MG, Gamsu G, Webb WR et al. Computed tomography of diffuse tracheal stenosis in Wegener's granulomatosis. *J Comput Assist Tomogr.* 1986;10:868–870.

Stenhouse G, Fyfe N, King G, Chapman A, Kerr KM. Thyroid transcription factor 1 in pulmonary adenocarcinoma. *J Clin Pathol.* 2004;57(4):383–387.

St-Georges R, Deslauriers J, Duranceau A. Clinical spectrum of bronchogenic cysts of the mediastinum and lung in the adult. *Ann Thorac Surg.* 1991;52:6–13.

Stitik FP. Staging of lung cancer. *Radiographic Clinics of North America.* 1990;28:619–630.

Stocker JT. Sequestrations of the lung. *Semin Diagn Pathol.* 1986;3:106–121.

Sturm JT, Hankins DG, Young G. Thoracic aortography following blunt chest trauma. *Am J Emerg Med.* 1990;8: 92–96.

Suen HC, Mathisen DJ, Grills HC et al. Surgical management and radiological characteristics of bronchogenic cysts. *Ann Thorac Surg.* 1993;55:476–481.

Sueyoshi E, Matsuoka Y, Imada T et al. New development of an ulcerlike projection in aortic intramural hematoma: CT evaluation. *Radiology.* 2002;224:536–541.

Suzuki M, Takashima T, Itoh H et al. Computed tomography of mediastinal teratomas. *J Comput Assist Tomogr.* 1983;7: 74–76.

Swenson SJ, Viggiano RW, Midthun DE et al. Lung nodule assessment at CT: Multicenter study. *Radiology.* 2000;214: 73–80.

Swenson SJ. CT screening for lung cancer. *AJR.* 2002;179: 833–836.

Swenson SJ, Jett JR, Hartman T et al. Screening for lung cancer with CT: Mayo Clinic experience. *Radiology.* 2003; 226(3):756–761.

Swenson SJ, Jett JR, Hartman TE et al. CT screening for lung cancer: five-year prospective experience. *Radiology.* 2005; 235:259–265.

Tammilehto L, Kivisaari L, Salminen US et al: Evaluation of the clinical TNM staging system for malignant pleural mesothelioma: an assessment in 88 patients. Lung Cancer 1995; 12: 25–34.

Tan RT, Kuzo R, Goodman LR, Siegel R, Haasler GB, Presberg KW and the Medical College of Wisconsin Lung Transplant Group. Utility of CT scan evaluation for predicting pulmonary hypertension in patients with parenchymal lung disease. *Chest.* 1998;113:1250–1256.

Tanaka N, Kim JS, Newell JD et al. Rheumatoid arthritis—related lung diseases: CT Findings. *Radiology.* 2004;232: 81–91.

Taskinen SO, Salo JA, Halttumen PEA et al. Tracheobronchial rupture due to blunt chest trauma: a follow-up study. *Ann Thorac Surg.* 1989;48:846–849.

Tazi A, Soler P, Hance AJ. Adult pulmonary Langerhan's cell histiocytosis. *Thorax.* 2000;55:404–416.

Teates CD. Radiographic changes in the irradiated lung. *Radiology.* 1980;134:795.

Teschendorf W, Anacker H, Thurn P. *Röntgenologische Differentialdiagnostik.* 5 th ed. Vol I. Stuttgart: Thieme; 1975.

Thorsen MK, Scott JE, Mewissen MW, Youker JE. CT and MR imaging of partial anomalous pulmonary venous return to the azygos vein. *J Comput Assist Tomogr.* 1990;14: 1007–1009.

Thurlbeck MB, Müller NL. Noninfectious angiitis and granulomatosis: where we stand. *J Respir Dis.* 1989;10:19–34.

Thurlbeck WM, Muller NL. Emphysema: Definition, imaging and quantification. *AJR.* 1994;163:1017.

Tocino IM, Miller MH, Frederick PR et al. CT Detection of occult pneumothorax in head trauma. *AJR.* 1984;143: 987–990.

Tshcholakoff D, Sechtem U, de Goer G et al. Evaluation of pleural and pericardial effusions by magnetic resonance imaging. *Eur J Radiol.* 1978;7:169–174.

Tukiainen P, Taskinen E, Holsti P, Korhola O, Valle M. Prognosis of cryptogenic fibrosing alveolitis. *Thorax.* 1983;38: 349–355.

UICC. *TNM-Atlas.* Berlin: Springer; 1990.

Uthgenannt H. Streifenschatten. In: Teschendorf W, Anacker H, Thurn P, eds. *Röntgenologische Differentialdiagnostik.* 5 th ed. Vol I/1. Stuttgart: Thieme; 1975.

Vincent RG, Pickien JW, Lane WW et al. The changing histopathology of lung cancer: a review of 1682 cases. *Cancer.* 1977;39:1647–1653.

Virmani R, Roberts WC. Pulmonary Arteries in Congenital Heart Disease: A Structure-function Analysis. In: Roberts WC, ed. *Adult Congenital Heart Disease.* 1 st ed. Philadelphia, Pa: Davis; 1987:77–130.

Vix VA. Radiographic manifestations of broncholithiasis. *Radiology.* 1978;128:295–299.

Von Overbeck J. Update on HIV infection. *J Insur Med.* 2005;37(3):201–213.

Wagner A, Mahrholdt H, Sechtem U et al. MR imaging of myocardial perfusion and viability. *Magn Reson Imaging Clin N Am.* 2003;11:49–66.

Waldman AD. Subacute pulmonary granulomatous schistosomiasis. *Br J Radiol.* 2001;74:1052.

Waldschmidt ML, Laws HL. Injuries of the diaphragm. *J Trauma.* 1980;20:587–591.

Wall SD, Federle MP, Jeffrey RB et al. CT diagnosis of unsuspected pneumothorax after blunt abdominal trauma. *AJR.* 1983;141:919–921.

Webb WR. High resolution CT of the lung parenchyma. *Radiol Clin North Am.* 1989;27:1085–1097.

Webb WR, Gatsonis C, Zerhouni EA et al. CT and MR imaging in staging non-small cell bronchogenic carcinoma: report of the Radiologic Diagnostic Oncology Group. *Radiology.* 1991;178:705–713.

Webb WR, Muller NL, Naidich DP, eds. *High-Resolution CT of the Lung.* New York: Raven Press; 1992.

Webb WR, Muller NL, Naidich DP. Diseases characterized primarily by cysts and emphysema. In: Webb WR, Muller NL, Naidich DP, eds. *High Resolution CT of the Lung.* 3 rd ed. Philadelphia, Pa: Lippincott, Williams & Wilkins; 2001: 421–463.

Wegener OH. *Ganzkörpercomputertomographie.* Berlin: Blackwell; 1992.

Weiss W, Boucot KE, Cooper DA. The Philadelphia pulmonary neoplasm research project. Survival factors in bronchogenic carcinoma. *J Am Med Ass.* 1973;216:2119–2123.

Wells AU, Cullinan P, Hansell DM et al. Fibrosing alveolitis associated with systemic sclerosis has a better prognosis than lone cryptogenic fibrosing alveolitis. *Am J Respir Crit Care Med.* 1994;149:1538–1590.

Willens HJ, Kessler KM. Transesophageal echocardiography in the diagnosis of diseases of the thoracic aorta. 1. Aortic dissection, aortic intramural hematoma, and penetrating atherosclerotic ulcer of the aorta. *Chest.* 1999;116:1772–1779.

Wilson AG, Flower CDR. The Chest Wall, Pleura and Diaphragm. In: Grainger RG, Allison DJ, eds. *Diagnostic Radiology.* 2nd ed. Edinburgh: Churchill Livingstone; 1992:1: 163–184.

Wilson AG. Diseases of the Airways. In: Armstrong P, Wilson AG, Dee P, Hansell DM, eds. *Imaging of Diseases of the Chest.* 2nd ed. St Louis: Mosby; 1995 a:817–868.

Wilson AG. Immunologic Diseases of the Lungs. In: Armstrong P, Wilson AG, Dee P, Hansell DM, eds. *Imaging of Diseases of the Chest.* 2nd ed. St Louis: Mosby; 1995 b: 485–567.

Wilson AG. Pulmonary Diseases of Unknown Origin and Miscellaneous Lung Diseases. In: Armstrong P, Wilson AG, Dee P, Hansell DM, eds. *Imaging of Diseases of the Chest.* 2nd ed. St Louis: Mosby; 1995 c:568–608.

Wiot JF. The radiologic manifestations of blunt chest trauma. *J Am Med Ass.* 1975;231:500.

Wislez M, Cadranel J, Antoine M et al. Lymphoma of pulmonary mucosa-associated lymphoid tissue: CT scan findings and pathological correlations. *Eur Respir J.* 1999;14: 423–429.

Wood BP. Cystic fibrosis. *Radiology.* 1997;204:1.

World Health Organization. Report of an Expert Committee. Definition and diagnosis of pulmonary disease with special reference to chronic bronchitis and emphysema in chronic cor pulmonale. WHO Technical Report Ser. 1961; 213:14–19.

Worthy SA, Kang EY, Hartman TE et al. Diaphragmatic rupture: CT findings in 11 patients. *Radiology.* 1995;194: 885–888.

Wynder EL, Mushinsky M, Spivak JC. Tobacco and alcohol consumption in relation to the development of multiple primary cancers. *Cancer.* 1977;40:1872–1878.

Yamagishi M, Terashima M, Awano K et al. Morphology of vulnerable coronary plaque: insights from follow-up of patients examined by intravascular ultrasound before an acute coronary syndrome. *J Am Coll Cardiol.* 2000;35: 106–111.

Yankelevitz DF, Henschke CI. Does 2 year stability imply that pulmonary nodules are benign? *AJR.* 1997;168:325–328.

Yankelevitz DF, Henschke CI. Small pulmonary nodules: Volumetrically determined growth rates based on CT evaluation. *Radiology.* 2000;217:251–256.

Yoshida S, Akiba H, Tamakawa M et al. Thoracic involvement of type A aortic dissection and intramural hematoma: Diagnostic accuracy—comparison of emergency helical CT and surgical findings. *Radiology.* 2003;228:430–435.

Young RC, Bennett JE, Vogel CL et al. Aspergillosis: the spectrum of disease in 98 patients. *Medicine.* 1970;49:147–173.

Ziegler JL, Becstead JA, Volberling PA et al. Non Hodgkin's lymphoma in 90 homosexual men: relation to generalized lymphadenopathy and the acquired immunodeficiency syndrome. *N Engl J Med.* 1984;311:565–570.

Zimmer EA, Zimmer-Brossy M. Lehrbuch der röntgendiagnostischen Einstelltechnik. Berlin: Springer; 1992.

Ziskind MM, Weill H, Pagzant AR. The recognition and significance of acinus-filling processes of the lung. *Am Rev Respir Dis.* 1963;87:551–559.

Zylak CJ, Eyler WR, Spizarny DL, Stone CH. Developmental lung anomalies in the adult: Radiologic-pathologic correlation. *Radiographics.* 2002;22:25–43.

Index

Page numbers in **bold type** refer to illustrations.

Thieme Chest X-Ray Titles

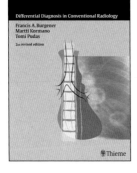

The Chest X-Ray
2nd edition
Differential Diagnosis in Conventional Radiology

Francis A. Burgener
Martti Kormano
Tomi Pudas

© 2006. 216 pp., 498 illus.,
hardcover

The Americas:
ISBN 978-1-58890-446-1
US$ 99.95

Rest of World:
ISBN 978-3-13-107612-0
€ 79.95

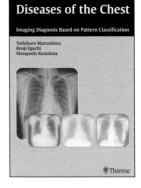

Diseases of the Chest
Imaging Diagnosis Based on Pattern Classification

Toshiharu Matsushima

© 2007. 184 pp., 591 illus.,
hardcover

The Americas:
ISBN 978-1-58890-562-8
US$ 109.95

Rest of World:
ISBN 978-3-13-143571-2
€ 89.95

The conventional chest x-ray remains the first line in the diagnostic imaging of thoracic disease. In the new edition of this classic, you will get the essential help you need to make preliminary diagnoses of a vast range of pulmonary, cardiovascular, and other thoracic conditions. The differential diagnostic information is provided in extensive tables, organized by classes of findings, and illustrated by hundreds of brilliant radiographs and, where helpful, schematic diagrams.

Professionals value the systematic structure of the information in the Burgener series, which aids in making diagnoses confidently and cost-effectively.

Contents Overview
– Cardiac Enlargement
– Mediastinal or Hilar Enlargement
– Pleural Effusion
– Intrathoracic Calcifications
– Alveolar Infiltrates and Atelectasis
– Interstitial Infiltrates
– Pulmunory Edema and Symmetrical Bilateral Infiltrates
– Pulmunory Nodules and Mass Lesions
– Pulmunory Cavitary and Cystic Lesions
– Hyperlucent Lung

The chest x-ray is the most commonly performed diagnostic x-ray examination. Highly illustrated and with only a minimum of necessary text, this new book takes a highly efficient pattern-based approach to evaluating the chest x-ray. Classes of findings, such as "increased radiolucency" or "alveolar shadow: atelectasis," are used to orient the reader toward the underlying medical problem. Tables help to organize the basic findings so as to be able to arrive at a differential diagnosis.

While the emphasis is on the chest x-ray, a supporting role is played by helpful CT images, schematics and drawings, and photographs of pathologic specimens, where these may be helpful to understand the chest x-ray appearance of the disease.

Chest x-rays are often performed routinely, prior to employment, prior to surgery or during immigration. The examining physician must be in a position to evaluate large numbers of chest x-rays confidently and speedily. This book succeeds admirably in helping the examiner to this end.

Easy ways to order:
Visit our homepage www.thieme.com

Prices subject to change.

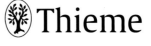

The Americas	Fax +1-212-947-1112	Thieme Publishers 333 Seventh Avenue New York, NY 10001, USA	E-mail customerservice @thieme.com	Call toll-free within the USA 1-800-782-3488
South Asia	Fax +91-11-23263522	Thieme Publishers Ansari Road, Daryaganj New Delhi-110002, India	E-mail thieme_vitasta@eth.net	
Rest of World	Fax +49-7 11-89 31-410	Thieme Publishers P.O. Box 30 11 20 70451 Stuttgart, Germany	E-mail custserv@thieme.de	

Thieme Chest X-Ray Titles

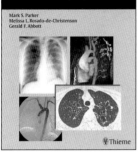

Teaching Atlas of Chest Imaging

Mark S. Parker

Melissa L. Rosado-de-Christenson

Gerald F. Abbott

© 2006. 800 pp., 1064 illus., hardcover

The Americas:
ISBN 978-1-58890-230-6
US$ 149.95

Rest of World:
ISBN 978-3-13-139021-9
€ 129.95

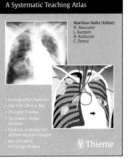

The Chest X-Ray
A Systematic Teaching Atlas

Matthias Hofer

© 2007. 224 pp., 825 illus., softcover

The Americas:
ISBN 978-1-58890-554-3
US$ 44.95

Rest of World:
ISBN 978-3-13-144211-6
€ 39.95

This lavishly illustrated book is your comprehensive, hands-on guide to evaluating chest images. It is ideal for reading cover-to-cover, or as a reference of radiological presentations for common thoracic disorders. With this book, you will learn to interpret chest images and recognize the imaging findings, generate an appropriate differential diagnosis, and understand the underlying disease process.

The atlas begins with a review of normal thoracic radiography, CT, and MR anatomy, and goes on to present cases on a wide range of congenital, traumatic, and acquired thoracic conditions. Each case is supported by a discussion of etiology, pathology, imaging findings, treatment, and prognosis in a concise, bullet format to give you a complete clinical overview of each disorder. More than 1,050 high-quality images demonstrate normal and pathologic findings, and complementary scans demonstrate additional imaging manifestations of disease entities.

Residents, fellows, and general radiologists called upon to interpret chest images will find this easy-to-use book invaluable as a learning tool and reference. It is also a must for thoracic radiologists, pulmonary physicians, and thoracic surgeons who must read chest images—especially of challenging cases.

For whom is this book designed?

For all students and physicians in training who want to learn more about the systematic interpretation of conventional chest radiographs, and for anyone who wants to learn how to insert chest tubes and central venous catheters.

What does this book offer?

- Detailed diagrams on topographical anatomy, with numerical labels for self-review.
- Coverage includes even relatively complex findings in trauma victims and ICU patients.
- Detailed, step-by-step instructions on the placement of CVCs and chest tubes.
- Simple aids and tricks, such as the "silhouette sign," that are helpful in image interpretation.
- Images to illustrate all common abnormalities (systematically arranged according to morphological patterns).

Easy ways to order:
Visit our homepage www.thieme.com

Prices subject to change.

Thieme

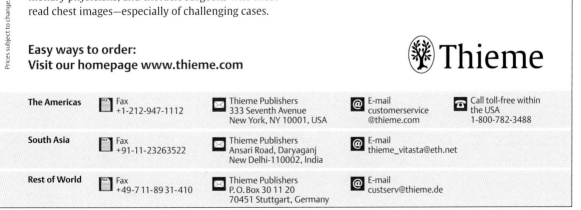